T0226413

Melanoma

Editor

F. STEPHEN HODI

HEMATOLOGY/ONCOLOGY
CLINICS OF NORTH AMERICA

www.hemonc.theclinics.com

Consulting Editors
GEORGE P. CANELLOS
H. FRANKLIN BUNN

June 2014 • Volume 28 • Number 3

ELSEVIER

1600 John F. Kennedy Boulevard • Suite 1800 • Philadelphia, Pennsylvania, 19103-2899

http://www.theclinics.com

HEMATOLOGY/ONCOLOGY CLINICS OF NORTH AMERICA Volume 28, Number 3
June 2014 ISSN 0889-8588, ISBN 13: 978-0-323-32014-6

Editor: Jessica McCool
Developmental Editor: Donald Mumford

Hematology/Oncology Clinics (ISSN 0889-8588) is published bimonthly by Elsevier Inc., 360 Park Avenue South, New York, NY 10010-1710. Months of issue are February, April, June, August, October, and December. Business and Editorial Offices: 1600 John F. Kennedy Blvd., Ste. 1800, Philadelphia, PA 19103—2899. Customer Service Office: 3251 Riverport Lane, Maryland Heights, MO 63043. Periodicals postage paid at New York, NY and at additional mailing offices. Subscription prices are $385.00 per year (domestic individuals), $633.00 per year (domestic institutions), $190.00 per year (domestic students/residents), $440.00 per year (Canadian individuals), $783.00 per year (Canadian institutions) $520.00 per year (international individuals), $783.00 per year (international institutions), and $255.00 per year (international and Canadian students/residents). International air speed delivery is included in all Clinics subscription prices. All prices are subject to change without notice. POSTMASTER: Send address changes to Hematology/Oncology Clinics of North America, Elsevier Health Sciences Division, Subscription Customer Service, 3251 Riverport Lane, Maryland Heights, MO 63043. Customer Service (orders, claims, online, change of address): Elsevier Health Sciences Division, Subscription Customer Service, 3251 Riverport Lane, Maryland Heights, MO 63043. Tel: 1-800-654-2452 (U.S. and Canada); 314-447-8871 (outside U.S. and Canada). Fax: 314-447-8029. E-mail: journalscustomerservice-usa@elsevier.com (for print support); journalsonlinesupport-usa@elsevier.com (for online support).

Reprints. For copies of 100 or more, of articles in this publication, please contact the Commercial Reprints Department, Elsevier Inc., 360 Park Avenue South, New York, New York 10010-1710; Tel.: 212-633-3874, Fax: 212-633-3820, E-mail: reprints@elsevier.com.

Hematology/Oncology Clinics of North America is covered in MEDLINE/PubMed (Index Medicus), EMBASE/Excerpta Medica, and BIOSIS.

Contributors

CONSULTING EDITORS

GEORGE P. CANELLOS, MD
William Rosenberg Professor of Medicine; Department of Medical Oncology, Dana-Farber Cancer Institute, Boston, Massachusetts

H. FRANKLIN BUNN, MD
Professor of Medicine; Division of Hematology, Brigham and Women's Hospital, Harvard Medical School, Boston, Massachusetts

EDITOR

F. STEPHEN HODI, MD
Leader, Melanoma Disease Center, Director, Center for Immuno-Oncology, Dana-Farber Cancer Institute, Harvard Medical School, Boston, Massachusetts

AUTHORS

MICHELLE T. ASHWORTH, MD
Clinical Fellow, Hematology/Oncology, University of California, San Francisco, San Francisco, California

ELIZABETH I. BUCHBINDER, MD
Instructor of Medicine, Division of Hematology/Oncology, Beth Israel Deaconess Medical Center, Boston, Massachusetts

RICHARD D. CARVAJAL, MD
Director, Developmental Therapeutics; Elizabeth and Felix Rohatyn Chair for Junior Faculty, Department of Medicine, Memorial Sloan-Kettering Cancer Center, New York, New York

GUO CHEN, PhD
Postdoctoral Fellow, Department of Melanoma Medical Oncology, The University of Texas MD Anderson Cancer Center, Houston, Texas

ADIL I. DAUD, MD
Director, Melanoma Clinical Research, University of California, San Francisco Helen Diller Family Comprehensive Cancer Center, San Francisco, California

MICHAEL A. DAVIES, MD, PhD
Associate Professor, Department of Melanoma Medical Oncology, The University of Texas MD Anderson Cancer Center, Houston, Texas

GLENN DRANOFF, MD
Department of Medical Oncology; Cancer Vaccine Center, Dana-Farber Cancer Institute; Department of Medicine, Brigham and Women's Hospital, Harvard Medical School, Boston, Massachusetts

DAVID E. FISHER, MD, PhD
Chairman, Department of Dermatology; Director, Melanoma Program, Massachusetts General Hospital Cancer Center; Professor of Dermatology, Harvard Medical School, Boston, Massachusetts

EDWARD F. FRITSCH, PhD
Department of Medical Oncology, Dana-Farber Cancer Institute, Boston; Broad Institute of Harvard and MIT, Cambridge, Massachusetts

GEOFFREY T. GIBNEY, MD
Assistant Member, Department of Cutaneous Oncology, Moffitt Cancer Center; Assistant Professor, Department of Oncologic Sciences, University of South Florida Morsani College of Medicine, Tampa, Florida

VIKRAM C. GORANTLA, MD
Division of Hematology/Oncology, Department of Medicine, School of Medicine, University of Pittsburgh, Pittsburgh, Pennsylvania

DAMIEN KEE, MBBS, DMedSc, FRACP
Division of Cancer Medicine and Research, Peter MacCallum Cancer Centre, East Melbourne; Department of Pathology, University of Melbourne, Parkville, Victoria, Australia

DANNY N. KHALIL, MD, PhD
Department of Medicine, Memorial Sloan-Kettering Cancer Center, New York, New York

JOHN M. KIRKWOOD, MD
Division of Hematology/Oncology, Department of Medicine, School of Medicine, University of Pittsburgh; Usher Professor of Medicine; Dermatology and Translational Science, Melanoma and Skin Cancer Program, University of Pittsburgh Cancer Institute, Pittsburgh, Pennsylvania

KIM MARGOLIN, MD
Professor, Medical Oncology, Seattle Cancer Care Alliance, University of Washington, Seattle, Washington

GRANT MCARTHUR, MBBS, PhD, FRACP
Professor, Division of Cancer Medicine and Research, Peter MacCallum Cancer Centre, East Melbourne; Department of Pathology, University of Melbourne, Parkville; Department of Medicine, St Vincent Hospital, University of Melbourne, Fitzroy, Victoria, Australia

DAVID F. MCDERMOTT, MD
Director, Biologic Therapy and Cutaneous Oncology Program; Associate Professor of Medicine, Division of Hematology/Oncology, Beth Israel Deaconess Medical Center, Boston, Massachusetts

JARUSHKA NAIDOO, MB, BCh, BAO
Medical Oncology Fellow, Department of Medicine, Memorial Sloan-Kettering Cancer Center, New York, New York

PATRICK A. OTT, MD, PhD
Department of Medical Oncology; Melanoma Disease Center; Center for Immuno-Oncology, Dana-Farber Cancer Institute; Assistant Professor, Department of Medicine, Brigham and Women's Hospital, Harvard Medical School, Boston, Massachusetts

DAVID B. PAGE, MD
Medical Oncology Fellow, Department of Medicine, Memorial Sloan-Kettering Cancer Center, New York, New York

VERNON K. SONDAK, MD
Chief, Department of Cutaneous Oncology, Moffitt Cancer Center; Professor, Departments of Oncologic Sciences and Surgery, University of South Florida Morsani College of Medicine, Tampa, Florida

RYAN J. SULLIVAN, MD
Center for Melanoma, Massachusetts General Hospital Cancer Center; Instructor of Medicine, Harvard Medical School, Boston, Massachusetts

AHMAD A. TARHINI, MD, PhD
Department of Medicine, Division of Hematology-Oncology, University of Pittsburgh Cancer Institute, Pittsburgh, Pennsylvania

PRASHANTH M. THALANAYAR, MD
Department of Internal Medicine, University of Pittsburgh Medical Center, Pittsburgh, Pennsylvania

JEDD D. WOLCHOK, MD, PhD
Lloyd J. Old Chair of Clinical Investigation; Service Chief, Melanoma and Immunotherapy Service; Associate Professor, Department of Medicine, Memorial Sloan-Kettering Cancer Center, Ludwig Center for Cancer Immunotherapy, New York, New York

CATHERINE J. WU, MD
Department of Medical Oncology; Cancer Vaccine Center, Dana-Farber Cancer Institute; Department of Medicine, Brigham and Women's Hospital, Harvard Medical School, Boston, Massachusetts

Contents

Preface   **xiii**

F. Stephen Hodi

State of Melanoma: An Historic Overview of a Field in Transition   **415**

Vikram C. Gorantla and John M. Kirkwood

The last 30 years has seen a revolution in melanoma. Fundamental elements of the surgical, adjuvant medical, and systemic therapy for the disease have been significantly altered toward improved management and better outcomes. The intent of this article is to reflect on past efforts and research in melanoma and the current landscape of treatment of melanoma. The authors also hope to capture the excitement currently rippling through the field and the hope for a cure. The intent of treatment of advanced melanoma, which was once considered incurable, has changed from palliative to potentially curative.

Understanding the Biology of Melanoma and Therapeutic Implications   **437**

Ryan J. Sullivan and David E. Fisher

From 1976 to 2010, only 2 medications were approved for treating metastatic melanoma. Between 2011 and 2013, 4 agents were approved and other therapies have shown great promise in clinical trials. Fundamental discoveries, such as the identification of oncogenic mutations in most melanomas, the elucidation of the molecular signaling resulting from these mutations, and the revelation that several cell surface molecules serve as regulators of immune activation, have been instrumental in this progress. This article summarizes the molecular pathogenesis of melanoma, describes the current efforts to target oncogene-driven signaling, and presents the rationale for combining immune and molecular targeting.

Surgical Management of Melanoma   **455**

Vernon K. Sondak and Geoffrey T. Gibney

Surgery remains the mainstay of treatment of every patient in whom complete excision of all disease is feasible. For clinically localized melanoma (clinical stages 0–II), wide excision and, when appropriate, sentinel lymph node biopsy are well established. The management of stage III melanoma is more contentious. Resection remains the first choice of therapy for patients with oligometastatic melanoma in accessible locations, but careful consideration of preoperative use of highly active drugs is appropriate. Decisions regarding surgical management of stage IV melanoma should routinely be made in the context of a multidisciplinary team approach.

Melanoma Adjuvant Therapy   **471**

Ahmad A. Tarhini and Prashanth M. Thalanayar

Adjuvant therapy targets melanoma micrometastases in patients with surgically resected disease that carry a high risk of death from melanoma recurrence. In this setting, adjuvant therapy provides the greatest opportunity for cure before progression into advanced inoperable stages. In randomized clinical trials, interferon-alfa has been shown to have a significant impact on relapse-free survival and, at high dosage, on overall survival compared with observation (E1684) and the GMK vaccine (E1694). This article reviews melanoma adjuvant therapy along with the ongoing and planned clinical trials.

Targeted Therapies for Cutaneous Melanoma   491

Damien Kee and Grant McArthur

Melanoma is resistant to cytotoxic therapy, and treatment options for advanced disease have been limited historically. However, improved understanding of melanoma driver mutations, particularly those involving the mitogen-activated protein kinase pathway, has led to the development of targeted therapies that are effective in this previously treatment-refractory disease. In cutaneous melanomas with *BRAF* V600 mutations the selective RAF inhibitors, vemurafenib and dabrafenib, and the MEK inhibitor, trametinib, have demonstrated survival benefits. Early signals of efficacy have also been demonstrated with MEK inhibitors in melanomas with *NRAS* mutations, and KIT inhibitors offer promise in melanomas driven through activation of their target receptor.

Treatments for Noncutaneous Melanoma   507

Danny N. Khalil and Richard D. Carvajal

Historically the approach to treating noncutaneous melanoma was largely guided by the experience with cutaneous melanoma, particularly in the metastatic setting. However, as genetic tools have allowed clinicians to better characterize these malignancies, their unique biology has become apparent. The ability to accurately distinguish the subtypes of melanoma and the genetic alterations that drive them is beginning to yield the tools that are shifting this disease from one that has proved to be intractable in the advanced setting to one that can be effectively treated.

Targeted Therapy Resistance Mechanisms and Therapeutic Implications in Melanoma   523

Guo Chen and Michael A. Davies

Although selective mutant BRAF inhibitors have revolutionized the treatment of metastatic melanoma, the magnitude and duration of their clinical benefit are significantly undermined by de novo and acquired resistance. Functional studies, molecular characterization of clinical samples, and clinical trials are providing insights into the landscape of resistance mechanisms in this disease. These findings have implications for the development of rational therapeutic approaches, and have identified several challenges that remain to be overcome if outcomes are to be improved in patients with metastatic melanoma.

Introduction to the Role of the Immune System in Melanoma   537

Kim Margolin

The concept of immunosurveillance of cancer has been widely accepted for many years, but only recently have the precise mechanisms of tumor-host immune interactions been revealed. Inflammatory and immune reactions play a role in melanomagenesis and may contribute to the eradication of tumor as well as potentiate its growth and proliferation. Studies of the role of tumor-immune system interactions are providing insights into the pathogenesis and opportunities for highly effective therapeutic strategies. Some patients, even with advanced disease, are now cured with immunotherapy, and increasing numbers of such cures are likely in the future.

Vaccines and Melanoma 559

Patrick A. Ott, Edward F. Fritsch, Catherine J. Wu, and Glenn Dranoff

The potential for therapeutic efficacy of a melanoma vaccine has been evident preclinically for many years. In melanoma patients, vaccines have resulted in the induction of immune responses, although clinical benefit has not been clearly documented. The recent achievements with immune-checkpoint blockade have shown that immunotherapy can be a powerful tool in cancer therapy. With increased understanding of tumor immunity, the limitations of previous cancer vaccination approaches have become evident. Rapid progress in technologies that enable better vaccine design raise the expectation that these limitations can be overcome, thus leading to a clinically effective melanoma vaccine in the near future.

Interferon, Interleukin-2, and Other Cytokines 571

Elizabeth I. Buchbinder and David F. McDermott

Cytokines are a diverse group of signaling molecules with immunomodulatory activity. This article reviews the application of cytokine therapy in melanoma with a focus on interferon-α and interleukin-2. In addition, it addresses the clinical considerations of these therapies including patient selection, reduction in toxicity, and combination regimens.

Immune Checkpoint Blockade 585

Jarushka Naidoo, David B. Page, and Jedd D. Wolchok

Since the development and approval of Ipilimumab, the first immune checkpoint inhibitor licensed for the treatment of metastatic melanoma, clinicians have gained a better understanding of the mode of action, management of toxicities, and assessment of response to this class of drugs. Several antibodies are now in development, aimed at blocking novel immune checkpoint molecules, such as PD-1 and it's corresponding ligand PD-L1. This article summarizes the mechanism of action, preclinical development, and subsequent clinical studies of immune checkpoint antibodies in melanoma.

Combinatorial Approach to Treatment of Melanoma 601

Michelle T. Ashworth and Adil I. Daud

There are multiple effective and well-tolerated systemic therapy treatments for the treatment of advanced melanoma, as well as new immunotherapy and targeted therapy agents in clinical trials. Traditional cytotoxic chemotherapy and targeted BRAF inhibitors can increase antigen presentation and can rebalance the intratumoral immune milieu. The combination of pulsed cytotoxic therapy and immunotherapy is a logical next step in designing treatment regimens. Combination radiotherapy and immuno-therapy also has experimental and clinical support. The standard of care for patients with advanced melanoma remains participation in clinical trials in order to enhance understanding of the effectiveness and toxicities of combination regimens.

Index   **613**

HEMATOLOGY/ONCOLOGY CLINICS OF NORTH AMERICA

FORTHCOMING ISSUES

August 2014
Iron Disorders
Matthew M. Heeney and
Alan R. Cohen, *Editors*

October 2014
Multiple Myeloma
Kenneth C. Anderson, *Editor*

December 2014
Colorectal Cancer
Leonard B. Saltz, *Editor*

RECENT ISSUES

April 2014
**Emerging Therapies Targeting the
Pathophysiology of Sickle Cell Disease**
Elliot P. Vichinsky, *Editor*

February 2014
Hodgkin Lymphoma
Volker Diehl and
Peter Borchmann, *Editors*

December 2013
Prostate Cancer
Christopher J. Sweeney, *Editor*

ISSUE OF RELATED INTEREST

Surgical Oncology Clinics of North America, October 2013 (Vol. 22, Issue 4)
Translational Cancer Research for Surgeons
William G. Cance, *Editor*
Available at: http://www.surgonc.theclinics.com/

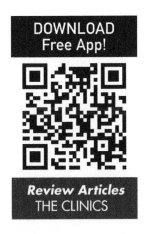

DOWNLOAD
Free App!

Review Articles
THE CLINICS

NOW AVAILABLE FOR YOUR iPhone and iPad

Preface

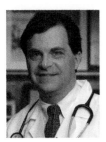

F. Stephen Hodi, MD
Editor

It is truly amazing to witness within the time of one's career the paradigm shift in the treatment of melanoma. Melanoma has transformed from a disease of limited options to one of continued hope, a reflection of turning scientific discoveries into therapeutic realities for patients. This has required enormous improvements in the basic knowledge of cancer biology, as well as rigorous clinical science in a fortuitous time. From manipulation of immune regulation of the host to selectively targeting melanoma driver mutations, translational medicine has converted a disease with the worst reputation into one whose connotations suggest a chronic disease or even the mention of cure.

In the current issue of *Hematology/Oncology Clinics of North America*, we have compiled leaders in melanoma biology and therapeutics to reveal the current state of the art. Drs Kirkwood and Gorantia provide an overview of melanoma therapeutics with highlights from the past to current understanding and practice. Dr Fisher analyzes the biology of melanoma development with a focus on therapeutic implications. Dr Sondak details the surgical management of melanoma. Dr McArthur examines targeted therapies for cutaneous melanoma including the paradigm shift in our molecular understanding, clinical approach, and patient care. Drs Carvajal and Khalil explore the recent advances in our understanding and treatment of noncutaneous (ocular and mucosal) melanoma. Dr Davies examines the resistant mechanisms to melanoma treatments, emphasizing the critical importance in understanding the complexities of cell biology to overcome these obstacles. Dr Margolin discusses the role of the immune system in melanoma biology with an emphasis on therapeutic implications. Drs Dranoff and Ott review vaccine development for the treatment of melanoma and recent developments in vaccine engineering with novel clinical applications. Drs McDermott and Buchbinder describe the roles for interleukin-2, interferon, and cytokines in the treatment of melanoma. Drs Naidoo, Wolchok, and Page detail the advances in immune checkpoint blockade and paradigm shift in clinical assessments, toxicities, and long-term patient benefits. Dr Tarhini discusses adjuvant treatments and the potential, greater than ever, to design trials with the intention for cure. Drs Adaud and Ashworth examine combinatorial approaches to melanoma therapy, a critical area of investigation currently and in the future, with the hope of providing synergistic benefits to patients but having the inherent hurdles of how best to do so.

Hematol Oncol Clin N Am 28 (2014) xiii–xiv
http://dx.doi.org/10.1016/j.hoc.2014.04.001
0889-8588/14/$ – see front matter © 2014 Published by Elsevier Inc.

We hope that this issue proves useful to students and investigators in continuing to advance our understanding and treatment of melanoma and serve as a model for cancer therapeutics.

F. Stephen Hodi, MD
Center for Immuno-Oncology
Dana-Farber Cancer Institute
Harvard Medical School
450 Brookline Avenue
Boston, MA 02215, USA

E-mail address:
Stephen_Hodi@dfci.harvard.edu

State of Melanoma
An Historic Overview of a Field in Transition

Vikram C. Gorantla, MD[a], John M. Kirkwood, MD[a,b],*

KEYWORDS

- Melanoma • Prognosis • Biology • Immunotherapy • Targeted therapies
- Neoadjuvant • Adjuvant • Combination therapy

KEY POINTS

- The last 30 years has seen a revolution in melanoma.
- Fundamental elements of the surgical, adjuvant medical, and systemic therapy for the disease have been significantly altered toward improved management and better outcomes.
- The intent of treatment of advanced melanoma, which was once considered incurable, has changed from palliative to potentially curative.

If I have seen a little further, it is by standing on the shoulders of giants.
—Isaac Newton

INTRODUCTION

In 2014, an estimated 76,100 patients will develop new primary melanoma in the United States, and 9710 will die of this disease.[1] In the United States, melanoma accounts for less than 5% of all skin cancers but is the leading cause of skin cancer mortality.[2] The annual rate of increase of melanoma incidence is currently estimated at 3% compared with 6% in the 1970s to 1980s, but the overall mortality has been relatively stable since 1990.[3] Worldwide the incidence of melanoma continues to increase; despite advances in local and systemic therapy, mortality continues to increase, with 80% of skin cancer-related deaths attributable to melanoma.[4] Progress in the basic molecular biology and immunology of melanoma over the past 50 years has translated into improved outcomes for patients with localized disease as well as for

[a] Division of Hematology/Oncology, Department of Medicine, School of Medicine, University of Pittsburgh, 5150 Centre Avenue, Pittsburgh, PA 15232, USA; [b] Melanoma and Skin Cancer Program, University of Pittsburgh Cancer Institute, 5115 Centre Avenue, Suite 1.32, Pittsburgh, PA 15232, USA
* Corresponding author. University of Pittsburgh Cancer Institute, 5115 Centre Avenue, Suite 1.32, Pittsburgh, PA 15232.
E-mail address: kirkwoodjm@upmc.edu

Hematol Oncol Clin N Am 28 (2014) 415–435
http://dx.doi.org/10.1016/j.hoc.2014.02.010
0889-8588/14/$ – see front matter © 2014 Elsevier Inc. All rights reserved.

those with systemic disease. The distribution of the burden of disease may be seen as inversely related to the opportunities to improve outcome. Advanced disease represents a smaller fraction of cases compared to earlier *operable* disease, associated with higher morbidity/mortality affording us greater opportunities for improved outcomes.[5] Outcomes for patients with deeper primary lesions show a different picture. Those patients with deeper localized American Joint Committee on Cancer (AJCC) stage IIB/IIC disease have an increased risk of relapse and death, whereas patients with microscopic regional stage IIIA disease detectable with sentinel lymph node (SLN) mapping and biopsy have an intermediate risk. Recurrent nodal disease and bulky nodal IIIB-C disease have a relapse and mortality risk that approaches 70% or more at 5 years.[5] Treatment and outcomes for advanced melanoma have improved over the past 20 years because of rapid advances in tumor cell biology, immunology, surgical techniques, radiosurgery, and imaging that are likely to further transform the field in the decade to come. This review reflects on the progress made in the past century and familiarizes the reader with the current state and management of melanoma.

HISTORICAL PERSPECTIVES

Described in antiquity as a *fatal black tumor*, the term derived from Greek (*melas* "dark" and *oma* "tumor") was coined by Dr Robert Carswell in 1838. References to this *fatal black tumor* can be found in the writings of the Greek physician Hippocrates in the fifth century BC, whereas those of Rufus of Ephesus emanate from the first century AD.[6] Hunter is credited with the first resection of melanoma in 1787. Renè Laennec described melanoma as a disease entity and coined the term *melanose* to describe the tumor in 1804.[7] Dr William Norris noted the heterogeneous appearance of the tumor and its propensity to metastasize in 1820[8] and first noted the heritable nature of melanoma and familial atypical multiple melanoma. In further publications, he observed that most of his patients had fair skin with light colored hair and the futility of surgery and medical therapy in the setting of distant metastases.[9] Thomas Fawdington[10] described one of the first cases of uveal melanoma and despaired at the lack of knowledge of therapies for this "insidious" process in 1820. In 1844, British surgeon Samuel Cooper[11] recognized the benefit of the early removal of tumors and the untreatable nature of advanced disease.

PATHOGENESIS

Melanocytes in the epidermis of the skin produce the pigment melanin, which occurs in several forms that variably protect the skin from UV radiation. Most melanoma is sporadic. Environmental insults followed by proto-oncogene activation coupled with the suppression of tumor suppressor genes and defects in the DNA repair mechanism further exacerbated by the inability of the immune system to contain these insults result in melanoma. William Norris presciently observed the hereditary nature of melanoma and light hair and complexion associated with melanoma in 1857. He proposed that nevi and environmental exposures predispose to melanoma, observations that were validated in the discovery of the Familial Atypical Multiple Mole and Melanoma (FAMM) syndrome[12,13] and the sporadic dysplastic nevus syndrome.[14] The connection between UV radiation exposure and increased risk of melanoma in the Australian Caucasian population was described by Henry Lancaster in 1956 whose later work demonstrated the importance of skin characteristics in the cause of melanoma.[15] These observations gave impetus to efforts to understand the genetics of melanoma. The discovery of the melanocortin receptor 1 (MC1R) on skin/hair phenotype[16] and its highly polymorphic nature helped make the association between pale skin/fair hair with poor tanning response (English/Celtic ancestry) and melanoma. Approximately 40% of familial melanomas were attributed to a heritable germline mutation in the cyclin-dependent kinase (CDK) gene CDKN2A.[17] Defects in CDK4, xeroderma pigmentosum, and MC1R genes have been implicated in familial melanomas.[18–21] The discovery of the role of the Ras oncogene family in the 1980s and their effects on downstream signaling were the first steps toward the identification of driver mutations in melanoma.[22] NRAS was first identified in a melanoma cell line in 1984.[23] The identification of the mitogen-activated protein kinase (MAPK)/ERK and PI3K/Akt pathways of melanoma tumorigenesis followed. The mutations termed *rapidly accelerated fibrosarcoma* (RAF) were initially identified in Ewing sarcoma. Systematic genetic typing identified the V600E variant to be frequent in cutaneous melanoma in 2002.[24] This mutation and its constitutive activation of the MAPK pathway have become the target of multiple pharmaceutical trials of small molecule inhibitors resulting in several new therapies approved by the Food and Drug Administration (FDA). The evaluation of other histologic subtypes led to the discovery of cKIT in acral and mucosal melanomas.[25] Uveal melanomas exhibit driver mutations in GNAQ, GNA11, and BAP1 with a low incidence of BRAF.[26] The differing pattern of driver mutations in different histologic subtypes of melanoma and the numeric burden of mutations in different melanoma cell lines from single tumors and in tumor samples ex vivo[27,28] reflect the genetic heterogeneity of melanoma and are likely to have profound implications for the molecular and immunologic therapy for melanoma.

RISK FACTORS

Melanoma is a disease that afflicts Caucasian Americans 20 times more commonly than African Americans. The lifetime risk of melanoma is approximately 2.0% (1 in 50) for Caucasians, 0.1% (1 in 1000) for African Americans, and 0.5% (1 in 200) for Hispanics. The risk of melanoma increases with age. The average age at incidence is 61 years; but it is not uncommon among those younger than 30 years, especially young women. Men have a higher lifetime risk than women. Previous history of melanoma is associated with an approximately 7% chance of developing a second primary melanoma. Exposure to UV radiation is the predominant environmental risk factor leading to melanoma. Cumulative solar exposure and sunburn events (UV-B) are both suspected as causative. UV-A exposure from tanning beds has been implicated in the risk and incidence of melanoma, particularly among women younger than 35 years.[29] This finding has led to the labeling of sun beds/lamps as human carcinogens by multiple health organizations, including the National Institutes of Health (NIH). Most melanomas arise as new lesions in the skin, although a significant fraction (25%–40%) seems to arise from preexisting nevi. The latter type, clinically described as atypical[30] and pathologically identified as dysplastic nevi[31] along with congenital nevi, has long been considered a risk marker and nonobligate precursor warranting surveillance. Giant congenital nevi (>20 cm) carry an increased risk of melanoma and are excised when possible.[32] Family history of melanoma increases an individual's risk of melanoma up to 8 fold.[33–36] Population studies have shown an increased incidence of skin cancers, including melanoma, in patients with chronic lymphocytic leukemia.[37] BRCA2 mutation carriers are noted to have a 2.58 times greater risk than noncarriers of developing melanoma.[38]

DIAGNOSIS

Patients may present with an unusual, new, or changing skin lesion to their primary care physician or dermatologist. Melanoma can present as amelanotic flesh-colored or nodular lesions. The ABCDEs of melanoma guide the decision to biopsy. The American Academy of Dermatology recommends an excisional biopsy with narrow margins as the preferred biopsy technique over shave and incisional biopsy.[39] A deeper saucerization biopsy is acceptable, and incisional biopsy is appropriate for lesions suspicious for melanoma that are not suitable for excisional biopsy. If a punch biopsy is performed, it should be deep enough to encompass the base of the lesion.[40] The stains traditionally used to identify melanoma include a combination of S100B (in some centers, this has been replaced with a pooled mixture of antibodies to Melan-A/MART1), HMB-45, and tyrosinase. Newer targets for IHC assessment include SOX10 and Mitf. Growth phase (radial vs vertical), morphotype (nodular or superficial spreading) mitotic rate, ulceration, and presence of tumor regression and tumor infiltration by lymphocytes are conventionally reported for their prognostic implications. Melanoma can be categorized morphologically and anatomically into the uveal, cutaneous, mucosal, and acral types, which have differing molecular patterns of driver oncogenes. Invasive cutaneous melanomas have historically been subdivided based on growth patterns into superficial spreading (most common), nodular (next most common), and acral lentiginous mucosal and lentigo maligna morphotypes, which have differing biologic behavior, prognosis, and molecular driver gene patterns.

STAGING

The foundation for the current staging system was laid by the pioneering work of Wallace Clark and Alexander Breslow. In 1966, Clark proposed a system that derived from the assessment of the tissue level of invasion subsequently termed *Clark level* to assist in the pathologic assessment of the prognosis of melanoma. Invasion of the layers of skin reflect prognosis (Clark levels I–V representing the junction, upper papillary, full papillary, reticular, and subcutaneous zones of the skin) with decreasing survival rates associated with increased level of invasion. In 1970, Breslow observed that prognosis was affected by tumor thickness and worsened with increasing thickness measured from the granular layer of the epidermis. These systems were incorporated into clinical trial structure building the framework for surgical and medical management and serving as a common language for physicians to communicate and compare patients in clinical experiences. The AJCC Melanoma Staging Committee has periodically reassessed the staging of melanoma for prognostic assessment and last revised the staging system in 2009 (seventh edition), which was put it into practice after a period of commentary in 2010.[5] The committee based its actions on a multivariate analysis of approximately 38,000 patients (7972 with stage IV disease) from North America, Europe, and Australia to revise/clarify the TNM classifications and overall stage grouping criteria. It incorporated key prognostic features, including Breslow thickness, ulceration, mitotic rate for thin melanomas (replaced Clark level), involvement of lymph nodes (LN) including manifestations of lymphatic spread (satellite lesions, in-transit disease), and the presence of distant metastatic disease (lung vs other). The system also integrated prognostic data for survival and risk of relapse within each stage. The staging system reflects excellent long-term survival for AJCC stage I and II melanoma, approaching 90% and 80%, respectively, at 20 years, whereas stages IIB and greater have an increased risk of relapse and death, with stage IIIB-C approaching 70% or greater relapse/mortality at 5 years.[5]

PROGNOSIS

The prognosis at diagnosis is largely defined by the stage of disease. Staging incorporates clinical and pathologic features and determines diagnostic and therapeutic pathways for a given individual. The extent of disease including the presence or absence of LN involvement and any distant metastases are the most important prognostic factors. The staging system also incorporates other important prognostic microstaging factors of the primary, such as Breslow thickness, presence or absence of ulceration, and mitotic rate of the primary tumor. Older patients have a worse prognosis regardless of the stage of disease compared with younger patients.[41] Among the morphotypes of melanoma, nodular melanoma by virtue of its predominant vertical growth phase and more frequent presence of ulceration carries a worse prognosis. Acral lentiginous melanomas are more difficult to detect (inconspicuous location) and are generally first detected at more advanced stages. Lentigo maligna melanomas are generally often of longer gestation and may be detected and operated at lesser depths of invasion. Anatomically, extremity melanomas have better outcomes than truncal or head/neck melanomas. Women tend to do better than men. Ulceration serves as a marker for aggressive tumor biology and propensity to metastasize. In thin melanomas, a mitotic rate of 1 or more serves as an indication of higher risk and, therefore, warrants SLN evaluation. NRAS and BRAF mutations are also associated with differing patterns of disease aggressiveness. NRAS is associated with thicker primaries and higher mitotic rates.[42] These markers seem to correlate with aggressive tumor biology reflecting a propensity for distant invasion.

SURGICAL TREATMENT
Primary Tumor

In 1857, William Norris first recognized the importance of local disease control and advocated for a wide excision of the primary tumor with surrounding unaffected tissue to prevent local recurrence.[9] This recommendation formed the basis of the subsequent policy for wide local excision (WLE), which is still the standard of practice today. Its scientific basis can be found in the concept that melanoma forms discontinuous nests of tumor cells in the dermal lymphatics adjacent to the primary tumor. William Handley proposed the removal of 2 in (5 cm) of surrounding tissue down to the level of muscle fascia for local control,[43] and margins of 5 cm were accepted until the 1990s. This hypothesis was tested in multiple large trials, which looked at the impact of larger margins on overall survival (OS), local recurrence, and disease-free survival (DFS).[44–47] No benefit was associated with a 3-, 4-, or 5-cm margin in terms of local recurrence, DFS, or OS. Thomas and colleagues[48] reported the inadequacy of 1-cm compared with 3-cm WLE margins. A 1-cm WLE margin arm demonstrated an increased risk of locoregional recurrence, although the OS was similar. Data from these and other trials were summarized in a meta-analysis by Haigh and colleagues[49] showing 1 cm margins adequate for primary melanomas of 1 mm Breslow thickness but 2-cm margins preferable for 1 to 2 mm thickness and 2-cm margins recommended for greater than 2 mm. Margins should always be negative at the time of the final pathology evaluation. Mohs micrographic surgery (MMS) is inadequately evaluated. Generally, it has been done by dermatologists who have not had facility with sentinel node biopsy, so has left patients often with margins that are hard to assess in terms of their en bloc pathologic status and lacking in the regional sentinel node assessment that has, since 2000, been recommended by the AJCC and other melanoma expert groups. The Mohs approach for cutaneous melanoma in general has been discouraged given the concern that this surgical technique ignores the biology of melanoma and the prognostic significance of discontinuous lymphatic spread and is done without the capacity to verify adequate margins in that the successive layers of skin taken in this procedure are not subjected to peer-reviewed pathologic assessment in the manner that formal wide-excision specimens conventionally may be. The fact that Mohs surgery is performed in a relatively limited number of isolated silos suggests that the lack of prospective clinical trials comparing MMS with WLE to provide more rigorous evidence-based analysis of this open question is a problem that will not soon be rectified.

Lymphadenectomy

Early on, physicians realized the aggressive nature of melanoma and its propensity for lymphatic and hematogenous metastasis and the futility of aggressive locoregional surgery once it had spread to distant sites. Early surgery with curative intent was emphasized with the goal of local-regional control. Based on the observation that melanoma initially spreads to regional LNs, Herbert Snow proposed that elective lymphadenectomy (ELND) should be included with WLE to obtain cure (1892).[50] His hypothesis and the work of Dr William Handley (1908) reflected a stochastic model of tumor dissemination in which LNs served as a launching pad for distant metastases. Multiple prospective randomized clinical trials from 1972 onward showed no survival benefit from ELND,[51–53] although the World Health Organization (WHO) trial 13 evaluating immediate LND (ILND) versus delayed LND in 240 patients with a more than 1.5-mm thick truncal melanoma suggested benefits for patients with occult microscopic LN metastases at the time of ILND.[54] The more recent understanding of prognostic factors, such as Breslow thickness, ulceration, mitotic index, and their clinical application alongside technical advances in SLN evaluation, put this controversy to rest.

LN Evaluation

ELND for patients with truncal and head and neck region melanomas proved to be problematic given the ambiguous nature of lymphatic drainage associated with these regions. This technical issue spurred research into technologies to identify lymphatic drainage patterns; in 1977, Morton and colleagues[55] showed that dye and radioactive tracers injected into skin around a melanoma would allow the reliable identification of the draining LNs and basins associated with truncal dermatomes. This novel technique, lymphoscintigraphy, allowed the development of the hypothesis that the SLN could guide prognostic assessment and surgery as well as other therapies for melanoma. This hypothesis postulated that a unique LN is the first to receive lymphatic drainage from a tumor site and, therefore, should also be the first for melanoma metastases. The use of vital blue dye allowed Morton and his colleagues[55] to demonstrate that the procedure accurately identifies and allows selective biopsy of the SLN for the evaluation of potential involvement by tumor metastases. The use of blue dye along with radiotracer coupled with the portability of radiotracer detectors vastly increased the success rate of SLN biopsy. Retrospective analysis by Gershenwald and colleagues[56] demonstrated that SLN status was the most significant prognostic factor for DFS and disease-specific survival in univariate and multiple covariate analyses. They also concluded that the SLN status should guide decisions regarding the pursuit of complete LND (CLND) in those patients ($\sim$20%) whereby the SLN was positive. There is general consensus that SLN biopsy is justified for intermediate-thickness melanoma of more than 1 mm Breslow thickness, given that approximately 20% of these patients will have occult LN involvement.[57] Thinner melanomas have a lower risk of regional and distant metastases. Decisions regarding SLN biopsy among patients with thin melanomas ($\leq$1 mm) are reasonably guided by the presence of adverse prognostic factors: a mitotic rate of 1 or more per square millimeter or the presence of ulceration, tumor lymphocyte infiltration, or a deep margin positive in the original biopsy. Patients with thicker melanomas of 4 mm or more should also undergo SLN evaluation given the prognostic value of SLN involvement and the dependence of adjuvant therapy decision making on accurate staging at the LN station. Also, some patients may be cured with sentinel lymphadenectomy (SLND), especially in the setting of LN micrometastases. Positive SLN involvement is currently an indication for CLND based on the Multicenter Selective Lymphadenectomy Trial (MSLT-1).[57] The implication of MSLT-1 and a subgroup analysis showing that all patients with micrometastatic disease benefit from CLND has generated debate. Even today, CLND remains a morbid procedure. A minority of patients with SLN involvement exhibits non–SLN involvement on CLND. MSLT-I data show that 88% of patients who have a single tumor-containing sentinel node will have no additional nodal metastases when the CLND specimen is examined. The SunBelt Melanoma Trial showed LN involvement to be approximately 16%.[58] Survival benefits were seen only on subgroup analysis of MSLT-1. An argument can be made that the biology of SLN micrometastatic disease in the SLND group may differ from the observation group whereby palpable LN metastases later developed and that these two groups cannot strictly be compared. For most, the evidence that SLND yields critical prognostic information and may be associated with improved morbidity and mortality associated with bulky regional recurrence has led to the adoption of this approach. However, this debate continues; the questions surrounding the reasonable uses and therapeutic implications of the SLN are being pursued further in the MSLT-II trial that is ongoing. This study will randomize patients with positive LNs to either ILND or observation, with CLND reserved for patients with confirmed non–sentinel node metastases.[59] It will also help answer the question of whether SLN biopsy in some patients is both diagnostic and therapeutic. The importance of the immunobiology of melanoma at the regional LN cannot be understated; studies now in progress at the authors' center and others across the world are addressing the molecular profile of the SLN, which may guide the prognosis and future treatment of disease in a more refined manner. These studies are asking questions beyond whether there is tumor in the SLN or not, such as whether the SLN host response is adequate or dysfunctional as it now seems it may be in a significant fraction of patients. The SLN as a forum for biologic study, and as a pivot point for tumor progression, is likely to be a productive focus of studies on the immunobiology of this disease for years to come.

MEDICAL MANAGEMENT

Most patients present with early stages of diseases, so skin examination for early detection is a mandate for all physicians in primary care as well as those who specialize in the management of melanoma from medical as well as surgical and dermatologic disciplines. Data from Germany, where the state of Schleswig Holstein adopted a program of screening among dermatologists, and many primary care practitioners now suggests that routine full-body skin examination significantly reduces the incident thickness of melanoma and the mortality attributable to the disease by up to 50% based on time trends for melanoma incidence and mortality in the state of Schleswig Holstein compared with surrounding German states and neighboring Denmark. These results have already led to the nationwide pursuit of regular skin screening for detection of melanoma across Germany—and health care systems elsewhere in the world are considering the role of screening and secondary prevention on this basis.[60] Although the German model used a day-long training module, simpler Internet-based training modules that require only 1 to 2 hours for primary care physicians[61] may provide more practicable current alternatives; one such primary care educational effort coupled with recommended annual total-body skin screening has been initiated in the University of Pittsburgh Medical Center Health System whereby incident melanoma thickness and melanoma mortality will be followed closely over the next several years. These measures, together with evidence that appropriate surgical management cures most patients with stage IA-IB melanoma, and many with stage IIA disease, are rapidly evolving at this time. The overall 5-year survival rates for early stage disease (AJCC IA-IIA) exceed 80%.[5] The pattern of relapse for operable early melanoma suggests that data for such patients should be judged at longer horizons. The insidious nature of some melanoma relapses and the later distribution of relapses from early stage disease make the issues of surveillance of relapse particularly important.[62] There are wide variations in the recommended frequency, and the utilization of radiologic and biomarker studies across the world. These lie beyond the scope of this overview, except to note that the economic and patient anxiety and overdiagnosis toll of surveillance have not always been factored into recommendations (eg, S3 German, Italian, and other high-intensity programs as compared with Australian, Dutch, British, and more minimalist recommendations). Sadly, there is little rigorous evidence to support the application of interval radiologic or biomarker studies in the follow-up of patients with melanoma. Closer interval follow-ups using imaging and blood testing for biomarkers, such as S1000B, which have been favored in Europe, have not been demonstrated to translate into improved survival outcomes when compared with clinical assessment at wider intervals. The data that are available generally do not account for the enormous fiscal costs and potential for patient and societal harms of the imaging assessments proposed. Because therapies for advanced melanoma are improving rapidly, the data on surveillance for earlier cohorts of patients will not be applicable to the present and future in which therapies may have increased potential for cure of the disease in the adjuvant as well as the metastatic settings. The need to develop evidence-based approaches to the surveillance of low-, intermediate-, and high-risk patients (stage IA-B, IIA-IIIA, and IIIB-C and other resectable disease) is pressing. Evidence that would guide us in regard to which patients are at risk of late relapse is critical to determine which patients are reasonable to consider for surveillance and, ultimately, for adjuvant therapy. The role of medical therapy in reducing the risk of relapse after surgery (ie, adjuvant therapy) has been compartmentalized in relation to low-, intermediate-, and high-risk populations of patients, with variable results. Research using more informative tissue assessment is ongoing to determine the efficacy of neoadjuvant therapy in melanoma. The agents in use today have fulfilled some of the criteria that Paul Ehrlich (1854–1915) articulated more than a century ago for the *Magische Kugel* or "magic bullet"; these will likely change our approach to surveillance for recurrence in intermediate- and high-risk operable disease, as well as inoperable disease, as therapies that can cure metastatic disease become more generally available.

Immunology and Immunotherapy in Melanoma

Burnet and colleagues[63] coined the term *immune surveillance*, which implied surveillance of the host for malignant cells, which were presumed to be recognized and destroyed as they emerged. This idea was supported by the observation of spontaneous regression in human melanoma, the lymphocytic/dendritic infiltrates documented pathologically in and around primary melanoma tumors, and the increased incidence of melanoma among immunosuppressed patients. The regression of melanoma among recipients of blood transfusions whereby the blood was derived from patients with a history of melanoma regression[64] and the presence of tumor-specific T cells and antibodies in patients as demonstrated by Morton and colleagues[65,66] showed the importance of immunology in melanoma pathogenesis. Golub and Morton[67] were able to demonstrate in vitro increased cytotoxic activity of lymphocytes derived from patients with melanoma against melanoma cell lines. Mouse models showed the feasibility and efficacy of adoptive lymphocyte transfusion.[68] The discovery of interleukin 2 (IL-2) as a T-cell growth factor helped pave the way for in vivo studies of immune modulation and its role in advanced melanoma. These observations and studies form the bedrock of vaccine studies, high-dose IL-2 cytokine, interferon α2b (IFNα2b), anti-cytotoxic T lymphocyte-antigen 4 (CTLA4) blocking (ipilimumab, tremelimumab), and anti–programmed death 1 (PD-1) therapies that are discussed as they have revolutionized melanoma therapy (please see later discussion).

Adjuvant Treatment

The goal of adjuvant therapy is to reduce the risk of relapse for patients by treatment at a time when measurable or gross disease is undetectable following surgery. This therapy has been pursued in melanoma as in other solid tumors to target potential micrometastases after patients have been surgically rendered disease free. Given the evidence of the immunogenicity of melanoma, adjuvant therapy has been pursued with each of the successive generations of immunomodulators that have been developed over the past 50 years, beginning with bacterial immunostimulants like Bacillus Calmette-Guerin and Corynebacterium parvum. The wider availability of interferons, first as nonrecombinant crude material purchased from the Finnish Red Cross by the American Cancer Society,[69–71] was followed by the industrial production of recombinant IFN by multiple pharmaceutical firms and the first systematic dose-response evaluations by multiple routes for advanced and then adjuvant settings of disease. Kirkwood and colleagues[70] evaluated IFNα2b in a phase I-II study in patients with metastatic melanoma and other cancers. The results showed response rates (RR) comparable with single-agent chemotherapy and durable responses in one-third of patients who responded. Phase III trials commenced in the 1980s and 1990s evaluating the role of adjuvant IFNα2b in various doses and schedules for patients with resectable deep primary and regional nodal involvement by melanoma. Based on the results of a series of studies of the Eastern Cooperative Oncology Group (ECOG) beginning in 1984, the FDA, in 1995, approved high-dose IFNα2b (HDI) for the adjuvant treatment of stage IIB and stage III melanomas. This randomized multicenter phase III study showed benefits in terms of OS and DFS compared with observation. Low-dose IFNα2b and intermediate-dose IFNα2b were then evaluated in multiple French, Austrian, and European cooperative group trials: WHO Melanoma Programs trial 16; EORTC 18871, 18952, 18991 (pegylated IFNα2b); and Nordic Melanoma Cooperative Group trials whereby a relapse-free survival (RFS) benefit was consistently observed. A recent collective meta-analysis[72] concluded that across all dosages, an RFS benefit is observed with a hazard ratio (HR) of approximately 0.83 and an OS HR of approximately 0.91. Analyses of individual trials have shown OS benefits only with HDI as reported in the E1694 and US Intergroup trial E1694, which evaluated HDI in relation to a vaccine that is now known to have had no significant effect on either RFS or OS.[72–74] Debate continues regarding the effects of alternative regimens in retrospectively identified populations such as those with ulcerated primary tumors and microscopic nodal disease, whereby current trials are prospectively testing the effects of alternative regimes of Pegylated IFN (PegIFN). The FDA based the approval of HDI, originally given for 1 year, on mature 7-year data from E1684. In 2011, the FDA approved the 5-year treatment regimen of PegIFN on data from EORTC 18991 showing overall significant RFS improvement at an early median follow-up of 3.8 years. However, a subsequent more mature analysis at a 7.6-year median follow-up for the pegIFNα2b has shown a lesser RFS benefit with HR 0.87, which on Intention to Treat analysis is of marginal significance. As there has never been any evidence of an OS impact for this regimen, the status of this agent is less clear than that for the original E1684 HDI regimen. The historic observations of early improvement of outcomes with HDI led to a series of studies testing 1 month of therapy versus 1 year, or 1 month of therapy versus observation; but these now[75] have been rigorously tested and demonstrate no evidence of a durable benefit from 1 month alone, so that this article of investigation has been closed. Flaherty and colleagues[76] have conducted the intergroup trial S0008 testing biochemotherapy (BCT) versus HDI and have shown a significant RFS benefit of BCT over HDI for the first time in history but without any evidence of an impact on OS. These findings may not be revisited given the rapid advances in molecularly targeted therapy for the tumor with BRAF, MEK, and possibly ERK inhibitors that have entered adjuvant exploration with results pending and the advances in immunotherapy with immune checkpoint inhibitors, such as anti-CTLA4 blocking antibodies and anti–PD-1 and anti-programmed cell death 1 ligand (PD-L1). Current clinical trials evaluating the role of ipilimumab in the adjuvant setting are enrolling across the US Intergroup and likely to complete accrual by 2014. These trials will evaluate the RFS and OS impact of ipilimumab at 3 or 10 mg/kg in relation to the standard of HDI in more than 1500 patients from ECOG-ACRIN and SWOG as well as other US Cooperative Groups and the NCI-Canada and ICORG.

Neoadjuvant Treatment

Neoadjuvant therapy in multiple solid tumors (breast, bladder, esophageal, and rectal) is associated with better outcomes in terms of survival and surgical outcomes. Given the evidence of immunogenicity and the phenomenon of immune evasion with progression in melanoma, the use of immunomodulatory agents for the neoadjuvant setting has been attractive for the past decade. Phase II trials have evaluated chemotherapy in combination and with immune modulatory agents (BCT) including such agents as IL-2, IFNα2b, cisplatin, dacarbazine (DTIC), and vinblastine. As might be expected, these trials showed a higher RR but were associated with significant toxicities.[77,78] Phase III studies evaluating BCT versus polychemotherapy showed no benefit in terms of RR or progression-free survival (PFS).[79,80]

The use of the neoadjuvant platform to investigate mechanisms of action beyond the response of disease in this earlier setting of potential resectability was first reported from studies at the University of Pittsburgh Cancer Institute (UPCI) in 2006 by Moschos and colleagues.[81] Patients (n = 20) received intravenous (IV) daily IFN as in the first month of the 1-year E1684 regimen, followed by surgery with the goal of evaluating both response and tissue correlates of therapy. Ten percent of patients (n = 2) demonstrated pathologic complete response (CR) and 40% (n = 8) had partial responses (PR). Tumor specimens systematically evaluated before and following therapy showed increased T-cell and dendritic cell populations with radical changes in the level of constitutively expressed STAT3 in the tumor tissue over the month of IV IFN. The same approach undertaken at UPCI with ipilimumab showed increased tumor infiltration by activated T cells with induction/potentiation of memory T cells. The change in Treg observed within the tumor showed an inverse relationship with the clinical benefit and was associated with improved PFS at 1 year.[82] The study of the combination of ipilimumab and IFN is now ongoing in the neoadjuvant setting at UPCI to pave the way for this combination in future phase III trials.

MANAGEMENT OF METASTATIC INOPERABLE (ADVANCED, SYSTEMIC) DISEASE

The helplessness felt by Dr Thomas Fawdington in 1826 at the lack of therapies available for patients with metastatic melanoma has been shared by medical specialists with an interest in melanoma to the present. However, advances in metastatic melanoma have changed in the past few years in ways that few in the field could have predicted a decade ago. These advances notwithstanding, melanoma is still a disease that is incurable for most patients. For the 40% of patients with mutated BRAF V600E who have responded and then relapsed (or less often failed altogether to respond) with molecularly targeted therapies, including the BRAF and MEK inhibitors (MEKi), disease progression is often rapid and options remain palliative in nature. The results with the currently approved immunotherapies IL-2 and ipilimumab benefit 15% to 20% of patients and may be prolonged but do not benefit most patients. Although the results of the anti-PD-1 checkpoint inhibitors have been gratifying and durable in a somewhat larger fraction of patients, these are at best half the population and as yet have not received regulatory approval.

The most common sites of distant spread include the lung, liver, bone, and brain (majority asymptomatic). Local recurrence can range from 1% to 12% for melanomas that are 1 mm or less to 3 mm or more in thickness, respectively.[83] Melanoma, like hormone receptor ER/PR+ breast cancer, renal cell carcinoma, and low-grade lymphomas, presents not infrequently as a late hematogenous relapse. Surgical resection to render patients disease free should be explored for patients with solitary or limited metastasis in a multidisciplinary setting. In trials patients undergoing metastectomy in the setting of long prior DFS and oligometastatic disease showed up to 40% 5 year DFS.[84,85] Local recurrence is treated with resection for negative margins. Medical treatment of melanoma over the past 30 years has evolved from single-agent cytotoxic chemotherapy to immunotherapy and to tailored signaling inhibitor molecularly targeted antitumor agents that in many ways fulfill the proverbial hope for a magic bullet. This coming revolution is likely to be even more paradigm shifting regarding the immunotherapy and checkpoint inhibitors like anti-CTLA4 and anti-PD-1 or PDL-1 and are overviewed here and then detailed in the balance of this issue.

Chemotherapy

The origins of chemotherapy for cancer lie in the World War I exposure of soldiers to mustard gas, which was the precursor of the therapeutic mustard alkylators and nitrosoureas, such as carmustine. Unfortunately, these agents remain toxic and their efficacy has been marginal in melanoma, although DTIC was approved as a nonclassic alkylator and remains on the formulary; oral analogues, such as temozolomide, have been approved for therapy for other solid tumors and have had a role in melanoma over the past generation. The FDA approved DTIC in 1975. Studies in the 1970s[86–88] showed RR of 19% to 28% and OS of approximately 5 months, but larger recent studies suggest RR of approximately 10%.[89] Temozolomide, an oral progenitor of the active agent of DTIC, has demonstrable central nervous system penetration but only small gains over DTIC. Melphalan was systemically used in the 1960s for melanoma[90] but today is only used in isolated limb infusion or perfusion therapy for patients with extensive *in transit* disease of the extremity.[91] Platinating agents, such as cisplatin (RR 16.3%)[92] and carboplatin (RR 19%),[93] have not shown superiority to DTIC. Vinca alkaloids, including vindesine, vinorelbine, and vinflunine, were explored again without significant benefit over DTIC. Nitrosoureas, particularly fotemustine and lomustine, have been explored because of their lipophilic nature; but the hopes that these agents would prove useful for brain metastases have not been substantiated.

The taxanes, including paclitaxel (RR 15.6%–16.4%)[94,95] and docetaxel (RR 17%),[96] have been explored; the first benefit over DTIC has been reported by nab-paclitaxel in a phase III study.[97] PFS, the primary end point, was significantly improved, with nab-paclitaxel (median 4.8 vs 2.5 months, HR 0.79, 95% confidence interval [CI] 0.63–0.99). There was a trend toward improved OS: median 12.8 versus 10.7 months (HR 0.83, 95% CI 0.58–1.20, $P = .09$). Combination chemotherapy has not shown superiority to single-agent DTIC; the commonly used/compared regimens included cisplatin, vinblastine, dacarbazine (CVD), or cisplatin, tamoxifen, carmustine, dacarbazine (DBCT or Dartmouth regimen). CVD was compared with DTIC in a phase III study whereby RR was 19% versus 14%, respectively, without a difference in survival. In phase III, DBCT was not found to be superior to DTIC, with an RR of 18.5% versus 10.2%, respectively, and no difference in OS.[98]

BCT

BCT arose from the effort to achieve durable responses using immunotherapy coupled with the rapidity and magnitude of responses obtained using chemotherapy. Chemotherapy combined with IL-2 and/or IFNα2b have been tested in multiple phase I, II, and III studies. The addition of IFNα2b to single-agent chemotherapy[99–101] or multi-agent chemotherapy[102–104] did not show additional durable benefits despite the high overall RR (up to 50%). Similarly, IL-2 did not show benefits added to chemotherapy.[105–107] In an effort to gain the synergistic effects of IFNα2b and IL-2, the combination was added to CVD in both sequential and concurrent dosing. Both approaches resulted in high overall response rate (ORR) with a 23% CR and 9% durable response.[108] CVD with IFNα2b and IL-2 given concurrently was compared with CVD alone in a phase III study. No clear superiority was discerned between the two arms in terms of ORR and OS.[79] The Dartmouth regimen with IFNα2b and IL-2 compared with DBCT again showed no difference in terms of OS or PFS.[109] Although BCT regimens produced high RR, this did not translate into a survival benefit with the added expense of patient toxicity and inconvenience given the complex delivery schedules in spite of attempts to deliver cytokines subcutaneously.

Immunotherapy

The goal of immunotherapy has been to activate the immune system, to recognize and kill tumor cells. Immune approaches could potentially eliminate the last tumor cells which survived cytotoxics limited by their first order kinetics. Immune agents currently approved for treatment of metastatic melanoma include high-dose IL-2 (HD-IL-2) and ipilimumab. IL-2 was the second cytokine to show significant antitumor activity in patients with metastatic melanoma after IFNα2b in the adjuvant setting. Efforts at the NCI[110–112] demonstrated the effects of IL-2 on T cells and the induction of lymphocyte-activated killer cell (LAK) function, which was associated with cellular tumoricidal functions in vitro. This effect was noted to be dose dependent. Phase II clinical trials of IL-2 as a single agent alone or in combination with LAK cells (adoptive cell therapy) were conducted in the late 1980s and early 1990s.[113–115] Data from these trials (n = 270 patients) showed an overall objective RR of 16% with 17 CR (6%) and 26 PR (10%).[114] Durable responses in these phase II trials were taken to regulatory review with FDA approval of IL-2 in 1998. Lower doses of IL-2 given subcutaneously alone or in combination with other immunotherapies did not show superiority to HD-IL-2.[116,117] Similarly, other cytokines, including IL-12, IL-18, and granulocyte macrophage colony-stimulating factors, did not show superiority to IL-2.[113] A relatively small phase III study (n = 182) combining IL-2 with gp100 peptide vaccine compared with IL-2 showed promise. The combination arm showed greater CR

(16% vs 6%) with increased median OS (17.8 vs 11.1 months, $P = .06$).[118] IL-2 in combination with ipilimumab and anti–PD-1 antibody remains a topic of interest given the perceived synergies between these therapies.

Upregulating the host immune response to achieve therapeutic antitumor responses in melanoma has become a reality in relation to the effector T-cell response to melanoma. CTLA4 is an inhibitory immune checkpoint that downregulates T-cell proliferation. Antibody blockade of CTLA4 leads to T-cell proliferation and IL-2 production, with augmented antitumor cytotoxic activity. Ipilimumab is an immunoglobulin G1 monoclonal antibody directed against CTLA4. In 2011, the FDA approved ipilimumab for therapy for unresectable or metastatic melanoma based on the OS benefit seen with ipilimumab $\pm$ gp100 vaccine compared with gp100 vaccine alone (HR 0.66–0.68, $P = .0004$).[119] This benefit on OS in second-line therapy was confirmed in a further first-line phase III trial comparing ipilimumab plus DTIC to DTIC alone (11.2 vs 9.1 months, HR 0.72, $P<.001$). Trials evaluating ipilimumab in combination with other therapies, including radiation, fotemustine, IFNα2b, bevacizumab, and targeted agents, are under way. However, trials looking at the inhibitory receptor PD-1 expressed by activated T cells, memory T cells, and regulatory T cells have moved forward at an even more rapid pace. Binding of PD-1 to its ligands PDL-1/PDL-2 results in downregulation of T-cell activity. PDL-1 is expressed by melanoma tumor cells and stroma and can be used as a biomarker for anti–PD-1/PDL-1 directed therapies. Nivolumab (BMS936558) is an anti–PD-1 antibody that was evaluated in a phase I/II study in patients with advanced cancers, including 94 patients with melanoma.[120] An ORR of 28% was observed with toxicities that were significantly less than observed with anti–CTLA4-blocking antibodies. BMS936559, an anti–PDL-1 antibody, showed 20% ORR (9 out of 52 evaluable patients with melanoma) in a phase I trial.[121] The anti–PDL-1 antibody has shown similar antitumor activity and modest toxicity.[122] Trials are underway evaluating the Merck anti–PD-1 monoclonal antibody MK-3475; this agent has shown single-agent activity as high as a 53% response that is being pursued in a phase III evaluation against melanoma and lung cancer, along with phase II combinations with IFN and vaccines.

Targeted Therapy

The MAPK and the Akt pathway (PI3K/Akt) are major pathways constitutively activated in a significant proportion of melanomas. The last few years have been an exciting period for targeted therapies in melanoma. Discovery of activating mutations in BRAF V600E/K in 40% to 50% of cutaneous melanomas, and NRAS mutations in another 20% of cutaneous melanomas, coupled with highly active and specific agents that are capable of inhibiting these pathways has translated into a therapeutic revolution with significant palliative effect for many patients with metastatic melanoma and improved survival for patients with metastatic melanoma. The FDA approved BRAF inhibitors (BRAFi)-vemurafenib and dabrafenib (BRAF V600E or E and K mutation positive), and the MEKi trametinib. Vemurafenib was compared with DTIC in a phase III study with superiority in terms of PFS (5.3 vs 1.6 months, HR 0.26, $P<.001$) and OS (HR 0.37, $P<.001$ at 6 months).[123] Similarly, dabrafenib showed superiority when compared with DTIC in a phase III open-label trial that allowed crossover. Median PFS was 5.1 months versus 2.7 months in the DTIC arm (HR 0.30).[124] These agents have also shown promise in patients with melanoma brain metastases, a disease site that was notoriously hard to treat and previously often excluded from new trials. Trametinib was compared with DTIC or paclitaxel (Taxol) in BRAF V600E/K mutant patients. It was found to be superior to chemotherapy in terms of PFS and OS despite the evaluation in a crossover design.[125] MEKi plays a role in patients with BRAF mutations as well as those with the nonoverlapping NRAS mutations found in cutaneous and also in uveal melanomas. In combination with BRAFi, the findings suggest improved anti-tumor effects as well as diminished toxicities; combinations of BRAFi (dabrafenib) and MEKi (trametinib) have received regulatory approval in January 2014 because of the phase II trial results that make it likely this combination will supersede single-agent BRAFi therapy. MEKi continue to be investigated in patients with NRAS mutant disease, and especially uveal (GNAQ/GNA11 mutant) melanoma. The eventual development of resistance to these agents with NRAS or MEK mutations, BRAF truncations and amplification, and increased expression of receptor tyrosine kinases is a problem. Melanoma exhibits a high degree of tumor heterogeneity and a mutational frequency that surpasses all other solid tumors.[28] Current clinical trials are evaluating combination therapy with BRAFi and MEKi with the goal to overcome resistance and deliver sustained durable responses, although this may require ternary or more complex combinations given the mutational landscape of the disease. Sorafenib, a multi-kinase inhibitor, showed RR of less than 10%[126] and no benefit in combination with carboplatin and paclitaxel in phase III studies as the first-line and as second-line therapy.[127] Imatinib has been explored as an agent in cKIT-positive melanomas. Although it showed limited efficacy in phase II trials, it was shown to have impressive response in patients with activating cKIT mutation.[128] It continues to be evaluated in cKIT-mutated patients under the auspices of clinical trials. Temsirolimus showed minimal activity in phase II study.[129]

Approaches to inhibit the angiogenesis observed in melanoma, and the elevated vascular endothelial growth factor (VEGF) levels that may contribute to immunotherapy resistance have been a longstanding quest. Phase II trials of bevacizumab with IFNα2b showed stable disease; studies of other putatively antiangiogenic approaches, including thalidomide and semaxanib, did not show promise. VEGF-trap combined with HDIL-2 is currently under evaluation in a large phase II (NCT01258855) multicenter clinical trial. Heat shock protein 90, a chaperone for BRAF, is upregulated in melanoma. HSP 90–targeted therapy is a potential adjunct to BRAFi therapy to overcome BRAFi resistance.

FUTURE DIRECTIONS

The body of knowledge accumulated over the past decades has served as a strong foundation on which the melanoma community is building on at a feverish pace. Every aspect of this field from prevention to surgery to medical therapies has benefitted from this revolution, which in turn has translated into better patient outcomes. As the understanding of the pathophysiology of melanoma grows, so does the armamentarium of therapeutics. Every decade has held out hope for a cure: IFNα2b in the 1980s, IL-2 in the 1990s, and ipilimumab and BRAFi in the 2000s. The advent of anti–PD-1 therapies and an understanding of tumor evasion, with a series of additional checkpoints, such as TIM1 and BTLA, assure us of exponential improvements in the coming decade. Biomarkers with predictive as well as prognostic utility and combinations of molecularly targeted antitumor therapies and significantly more effective immunotherapy remain the hot topics moving forward. Biomarkers and mutational analysis will form the basis of tailored therapies for patients in terms of both medical therapies and active surveillance. Both lack of and low rates of durable RR with single-agent therapies leads us to think that effective therapy will be a combination of immunologic, targeted agents and possibly chemotherapy. Understanding the manner in which the tumor is able to overcome or subvert the immune response to the tumor at the primary site and in the regional lymphatics is a key challenge. Melanoma has shown its ability to evolve in order to survive as evidenced by the rapid rate of genetic change in this tumor. The only system that can match its ability to adapt and counter the tumor is the human immune system. Ultimately, the cure for advanced melanoma is likely to reside in awaking and modulating this sleeping giant.

REFERENCES

1. Siegel R, Ma J, Zou Z, et al. Cancer statistics. CA Cancer J Clin 2014;64:9–29.
2. Miller AJ, Mihm MC Jr. Melanoma. N Engl J Med 2006;355:51–65.
3. Howlader N, Noone A, Krapcho M, et al. SEER cancer statistics review, 1975-2009 (vintage 2009 populations). Bethesda (MD): National Cancer Institute; 2012. Available at: http://seer.cancer.gov/csr/1975_2009_pops09/. Based on November 2011 SEER data submission, posted to the SEER web site, April 2012.
4. WHO. Skin cancers. Available at: http://www.who.int/uv/faq/skincancer/en/index1.html. Accessed November 2, 2013.
5. Balch CM, Gershenwald JE, Soong SJ, et al. Final version of 2009 AJCC melanoma staging and classification. J Clin Oncol 2009;27:6199–206.
6. Urteaga O, Pack GT. On the antiquity of melanoma. Cancer 1966;19:607–10.
7. Laennec R. Extrait au memoire de M Laennec, sur les melanoses. Paris: Bull L'Ecole Societie de Medicine; 1812. p. 24.
8. Norris W. Case of fungoid disease. Edinburgh Med Surg J 1820;16:562–5.
9. Norris W. Eight cases of melanosis with pathological and therapeutical remarks on that disease. London: Longman; 1857.
10. Fawdington T. A case of melanosis, with general observations on the pathology of the interesting disease. London; Manchester (United Kingdom): Longman; Orme, Rees, Brown & Green; and Robinson & Bent; 1826.
11. Cooper S. The first lines of the theory and practice of surgery. London: Longman; 1840.
12. Lynch HT, Krush AJ. Heredity and malignant melanoma: implications for early cancer detection. Can Med Assoc J 1968;99:17–21.
13. Clark WH Jr, Reimer RR, Greene M, et al. Origin of familial malignant melanomas from heritable melanocytic lesions. 'The B-K mole syndrome'. Arch Dermatol 1978;114:732–8.
14. Naeyaert JM, Brochez L. Clinical practice. Dysplastic nevi. N Engl J Med 2003; 349:2233–40.
15. Lancaster HO. Some geographical aspects of the mortality from melanoma in Europeans. Med J Aust 1956;43:1082–7.
16. Beaumont KA, Wong SS, Ainger SA, et al. Melanocortin MC(1) receptor in human genetics and model systems. Eur J Pharmacol 2011;660:103–10.
17. Holland EA, Schmid H, Kefford RF, et al. CDKN2A (P16(INK4a)) and CDK4 mutation analysis in 131 Australian melanoma probands: effect of family history and multiple primary melanomas. Genes Chromosomes Cancer 1999;25:339–48.
18. Sviderskaya EV, Hill SP, Evans-Whipp TJ, et al. p16(Ink4a) in melanocyte senescence and differentiation. J Natl Cancer Inst 2002;94:446–54.
19. Goldstein AM, Chan M, Harland M, et al. High-risk melanoma susceptibility genes and pancreatic cancer, neural system tumors, and uveal melanoma across GenoMEL. Cancer Res 2006;66:9818–28.
20. Kraemer K. Dysplastic nevi as precursors to hereditary melanoma. J Dermatol Surg Oncol 1983;9:619–22.
21. Haluska FG, Tsao H, Wu H, et al. Genetic alterations in signaling pathways in melanoma. Clin Cancer Res 2006;12:2301s–7s.

22. Malumbres M, Barbacid M. RAS oncogenes: the first 30 years. Nat Rev Cancer 2003;3:459–65.
23. Padua RA, Barrass N, Currie GA. A novel transforming gene in a human malignant melanoma cell line. Nature 1984;311:671–3.
24. Davies H, Bignell GR, Cox C, et al. Mutations of the BRAF gene in human cancer. Nature 2002;417:949–54.
25. Curtin JA, Busam K, Pinkel D, et al. Somatic activation of KIT in distinct subtypes of melanoma. J Clin Oncol 2006;24:4340–6.
26. Van Raamsdonk CD, Bezrookove V, Green G, et al. Frequent somatic mutations of GNAQ in uveal melanoma and blue naevi. Nature 2009;457:599–602.
27. Halaban R, Zhang W, Bacchiocchi A, et al. PLX4032, a selective BRAF(V600E) kinase inhibitor, activates the ERK pathway and enhances cell migration and proliferation of BRAF melanoma cells. Pigment Cell Melanoma Res 2010;23:190–200.
28. Johannessen CM, Johnson LA, Piccioni F, et al. A melanocyte lineage program confers resistance to MAP kinase pathway inhibition. Nature 2013;504:138–42.
29. Westerdahl J, Ingvar C, Masback A, et al. Risk of cutaneous malignant melanoma in relation to use of sunbeds: further evidence for UV-A carcinogenicity. Br J Cancer 2000;82:1593–9.
30. Nordlund JJ, Kirkwood J, Forget BM, et al. Demographic study of clinically atypical (dysplastic) nevi in patients with melanoma and comparison subjects. Cancer Res 1985;45:1855–61.
31. Elder DE, Goldman LI, Goldman SC, et al. Dysplastic nevus syndrome: a phenotypic association of sporadic cutaneous melanoma. Cancer 1980;46:1787–94.
32. Arneja JS, Gosain AK. Giant congenital melanocytic nevi. Plast Reconstr Surg 2007;120:26e–40e.
33. Hemminki K, Zhang H, Czene K. Familial and attributable risks in cutaneous melanoma: effects of proband and age. J Invest Dermatol 2003;120:217–23.
34. Larson AA, Leachman SA, Eliason MJ, et al. Population-based assessment of non-melanoma cancer risk in relatives of cutaneous melanoma probands. J Invest Dermatol 2007;127:183–8.
35. Amundadottir LT, Thorvaldsson S, Gudbjartsson DF, et al. Cancer as a complex phenotype: pattern of cancer distribution within and beyond the nuclear family. PLoS Med 2004;1:e65.
36. Florell SR, Boucher KM, Garibotti G, et al. Population-based analysis of prognostic factors and survival in familial melanoma. J Clin Oncol 2005;23:7168–77.
37. Hisada M, Biggar RJ, Greene MH, et al. Solid tumors after chronic lymphocytic leukemia. Blood 2001;98:1979–81.
38. Monnerat C, Chompret A, Kannengiesser C, et al. BRCA1, BRCA2, TP53, and CDKN2A germline mutations in patients with breast cancer and cutaneous melanoma. Fam Cancer 2007;6:453–61.
39. Bichakjian CK, Halpern AC, Johnson TM, et al. Guidelines of care for the management of primary cutaneous melanoma. American Academy of Dermatology. J Am Acad Dermatol 2011;65:1032–47.
40. Lowe M, Hill N, Page A, et al. The impact of shave biopsy on the management of patients with thin melanomas. Am Surg 2011;77:1050–3.
41. Page AJ, Li A, Hestley A, et al. Increasing age is associated with worse prognostic factors and increased distant recurrences despite fewer sentinel lymph node positives in melanoma. Int J Surg Oncol 2012;2012:456987.
42. Devitt B, Liu W, Salemi R, et al. Clinical outcome and pathological features associated with NRAS mutation in cutaneous melanoma. Pigment Cell Melanoma Res 2011;24:666–72.

43. Handley W. The pathology of melanotic growths in relation to their operative treatment. Lancet 1907;1:927–33.
44. Khayat D, Rixe O, Martin G, et al. Surgical margins in cutaneous melanoma (2 cm versus 5 cm for lesions measuring less than 2.1-mm thick). Cancer 2003;97:1941–6.
45. Veronesi U, Cascinelli N, Adamus J, et al. Thin stage I primary cutaneous malignant melanoma. Comparison of excision with margins of 1 or 3 cm. N Engl J Med 1988;318:1159–62.
46. Balch CM, Urist MM, Karakousis CP, et al. Efficacy of 2-cm surgical margins for intermediate-thickness melanomas (1 to 4 mm). Results of a multi-institutional randomized surgical trial. Ann Surg 1993;218:262–7 [discussion: 267–9].
47. Cohn-Cedermark G, Rutqvist LE, Andersson R, et al. Long term results of a randomized study by the Swedish Melanoma Study Group on 2-cm versus 5-cm resection margins for patients with cutaneous melanoma with a tumor thickness of 0.8-2.0 mm. Cancer 2000;89:1495–501.
48. Thomas JM, Newton-Bishop J, A'Hern R, et al. Excision margins in high-risk malignant melanoma. N Engl J Med 2004;350:757–66.
49. Haigh PI, DiFronzo LA, McCready DR. Optimal excision margins for primary cutaneous melanoma: a systematic review and meta-analysis. Can J Surg 2003;46:419–26.
50. Neuhaus SJ, Clark MA, Thomas JM. Dr Herbert Lumley Snow, MD, MRCS (1847-1930): the original champion of elective lymph node dissection in melanoma. Ann Surg Oncol 2004;11:875–8.
51. Balch CM, Soong SJ, Bartolucci AA, et al. Efficacy of an elective regional lymph node dissection of 1 to 4 mm thick melanomas for patients 60 years of age and younger. Ann Surg 1996;224:255–63 [discussion: 263–6].
52. Balch CM, Soong S, Ross MI, et al. Long-term results of a multi-institutional randomized trial comparing prognostic factors and surgical results for intermediate thickness melanomas (1.0 to 4.0 mm). Intergroup Melanoma Surgical Trial. Ann Surg Oncol 2000;7:87–97.
53. Veronesi U, Adamus J, Bandiera DC, et al. Delayed regional lymph node dissection in stage I melanoma of the skin of the lower extremities. Cancer 1982;49: 2420–30.
54. Cascinelli N, Morabito A, Santinami M, et al. Immediate or delayed dissection of regional nodes in patients with melanoma of the trunk: a randomised trial. WHO Melanoma Programme. Lancet 1998;351:793–6.
55. Morton DL, Wen DR, Wong JH, et al. Technical details of intraoperative lymphatic mapping for early stage melanoma. Arch Surg 1992;127:392–9.
56. Gershenwald JE, Thompson W, Mansfield PF, et al. Multi-institutional melanoma lymphatic mapping experience: the prognostic value of sentinel lymph node status in 612 stage I or II melanoma patients. J Clin Oncol 1999;17:976–83.
57. Morton DL, Thompson JF, Cochran AJ, et al. Sentinel-node biopsy or nodal observation in melanoma. N Engl J Med 2006;355:1307–17.
58. McMasters KM, Noyes RD, Reintgen DS, et al. Lessons learned from the Sunbelt Melanoma Trial. J Surg Oncol 2004;86:212–23.
59. Morton DL. Overview and update of the phase III Multicenter Selective Lymphadenectomy Trials (MSLT-I and MSLT-II) in melanoma. Clin Exp Metastasis 2012; 29:699–706.
60. Katalinic A, Waldmann A, Weinstock MA, et al. Does skin cancer screening save lives?: an observational study comparing trends in melanoma mortality in regions with and without screening. Cancer 2012;118:5395–402.

61. Markova A, Weinstock MA, Risica P, et al. Effect of a web-based curriculum on primary care practice: basic skin cancer triage trial. Fam Med 2013;45:558–68.

62. Leiter U, Buettner PG, Eigentler TK, et al. Hazard rates for recurrent and secondary cutaneous melanoma: an analysis of 33,384 patients in the German Central Malignant Melanoma Registry. J Am Acad Dermatol 2012;66:37–45.

63. Burnet FM. Cancer a biological approach. Br Med J 1957;1(5023):841–7.

64. Sumner WC, Foraker AG. Spontaneous regression of human melanoma: clinical and experimental studies. Cancer 1960;13:79–81.

65. Morton DL, Malmgren RA, Holmes EC, et al. Demonstration of antibodies against human malignant melanoma by immunofluorescence. Surgery 1968; 64:233–40.

66. Morton DL, Eilber FR, Joseph WL, et al. Immunological factors in human sarcomas and melanomas: a rational basis for immunotherapy. Ann Surg 1970; 172:740–9.

67. Golub SH, Morton DL. Sensitisation of lymphocytes in vitro against human melanoma-associated antigens. Nature 1974;251:161–3.

68. Smith HG, Harmel RP, Hanna MG Jr, et al. Regression of established intradermal tumors and lymph node metastases in guinea pigs after systemic transfer of immune lymphoid cells. J Natl Cancer Inst 1977;58:1315–22.

69. Krown SE. Interferons in malignancy: biological products or biological response modifiers? J Natl Cancer Inst 1988;80:306–9.

70. Kirkwood JM, Ernstoff MS, Davis CA, et al. Comparison of intramuscular and intravenous recombinant alpha-2 interferon in melanoma and other cancers. Ann Intern Med 1985;103:32–6.

71. Kirkwood JM, Harris JE, Vera R, et al. A randomized study of low and high doses of leukocyte alpha-interferon in metastatic renal cell carcinoma: the American Cancer Society collaborative trial. Cancer Res 1985;45:863–71.

72. Mocellin S, Pasquali S, Rossi CR, et al. Interferon alpha adjuvant therapy in patients with high-risk melanoma: a systematic review and meta-analysis. J Natl Cancer Inst 2010;102:493–501.

73. Wheatley K, Ives N, Hancock B, et al. Interferon as adjuvant treatment for melanoma. Lancet 2002;360:878.

74. Lens MB, Dawes M. Interferon alfa therapy for malignant melanoma: a systematic review of randomized controlled trials. J Clin Oncol 2002;20:1818–25.

75. Flaherty LE, Moon J, Atkins MB, et al. Phase III trial of high-dose interferon alpha-2b versus cisplatin, vinblastine, DTIC plus IL-2 and interferon in patients with high-risk melanoma (SWOG S0008): An intergroup study of CALGB, COG, ECOG, and SWOG. J Clin Oncol 2012;30(Suppl) [Abstract 8504].

76. Pectasides D, Dafni U, Bafaloukos D, et al. Randomized phase III study of 1 month versus 1 year of adjuvant high-dose interferon alfa-2b in patients with resected high-risk melanoma. J Clin Oncol 2009;27:939–44.

77. Buzaid AC, Colome M, Bedikian A, et al. Phase II study of neoadjuvant concurrent biochemotherapy in melanoma patients with local-regional metastases. Melanoma Res 1998;8:549–56.

78. Shah GD, Socci ND, Gold JS, et al. Phase II trial of neoadjuvant temozolomide in resectable melanoma patients. Ann Oncol 2010;21:1718–22.

79. Atkins MB, Hsu J, Lee S, et al. Phase III trial comparing concurrent biochemotherapy with cisplatin, vinblastine, dacarbazine, interleukin-2, and interferon alfa-2b with cisplatin, vinblastine, and dacarbazine alone in patients with metastatic malignant melanoma (E3695): a trial coordinated by the Eastern Cooperative Oncology Group. J Clin Oncol 2008;26:5748–54.

80. Keilholz U, Punt CJ, Gore M, et al. Dacarbazine, cisplatin, and interferon-alfa-2b with or without interleukin-2 in metastatic melanoma: a randomized phase III trial (18951) of the European Organisation for Research and Treatment of Cancer Melanoma Group. J Clin Oncol 2005;23:6747–55.

81. Moschos SJ, Edington HD, Land SR, et al. Neoadjuvant treatment of regional stage IIIB melanoma with high-dose interferon alfa-2b induces objective tumor regression in association with modulation of tumor infiltrating host cellular immune responses. J Clin Oncol 2006;24:3164–71.

82. Tarhini AA, Edington H, Butterfield LH, et al. Immune monitoring of the circulation and the tumor microenvironment in patients with regionally advanced melanoma receiving neoadjuvant ipilimumab. PLoS One 2014;9:e87705.

83. Moehrle M, Kraemer A, Schippert W, et al. Clinical risk factors and prognostic significance of local recurrence in cutaneous melanoma. Br J Dermatol 2004; 151:397–406.

84. Howard JH, Thompson JF, Mozzillo N, et al. Metastasectomy for distant metastatic melanoma: analysis of data from the first multicenter selective lymphadenectomy trial (MSLT-I). Ann Surg Oncol 2012;19:2547–55.

85. Wasif N, Bagaria SP, Ray P, et al. Does metastasectomy improve survival in patients with stage IV melanoma? A cancer registry analysis of outcomes. J Surg Oncol 2011;104:111–5.

86. Luce JK, Thurman WG, Isaacs BL, et al. Clinical trials with the antitumor agent 5-(3,3-dimethyl-1-triazeno)imidazole-4-carboxamide(NSC-45388). Cancer Chemother Rep 1970;54:119–24.

87. Nathanson L, Wolter J, Horton J, et al. Characteristics of prognosis and response to an imidazole carboxamide in malignant melanoma. Clin Pharmacol Ther 1971;12:955–62.

88. Costanza ME, Nathanson L, Lenhard R, et al. Therapy of malignant melanoma with an imidazole carboxamide and bis-chloroethyl nitrosourea. Cancer 1972; 30:1457–61.

89. Patel PM, Suciu S, Mortier L, et al. Extended schedule, escalated dose temozolomide versus dacarbazine in stage IV melanoma: final results of a randomised phase III study (EORTC 18032). Eur J Cancer 2011;47:1476–83.

90. Bodenham DC. A study of 650 observed malignant melanomas in the South-West region. Ann R Coll Surg Engl 1968;43:218–39.

91. Kroon HM, Thompson JF. Isolated limb infusion: a review. J Surg Oncol 2009; 100:169–77.

92. Glover D, Ibrahim J, Kirkwood J, et al. Phase II randomized trial of cisplatin and WR-2721 versus cisplatin alone for metastatic melanoma: an Eastern Cooperative Oncology Group Study (E1686). Melanoma Res 2003;13:619–26.

93. Evans LM, Casper ES, Rosenbluth R. Phase II trial of carboplatin in advanced malignant melanoma. Cancer Treat Rep 1987;71:171–2.

94. Bedikian AY, Plager C, Papadopoulos N, et al. Phase II evaluation of paclitaxel by short intravenous infusion in metastatic melanoma. Melanoma Res 2004;14: 63–6.

95. Wiernik PH, Einzig AI. Taxol in malignant melanoma. J Natl Cancer Inst Monogr 1993;(15):185–7.

96. Aamdal S, Wolff I, Kaplan S, et al. Docetaxel (Taxotere) in advanced malignant melanoma: a phase II study of the EORTC Early Clinical Trials Group. Eur J Cancer 1994;30A:1061–4.

97. Hersh E, Vecchio M, Brown M, et al. Phase 3, randomized, open-label multicenter trial of nab-paclitaxel vs dacarbazine in previously untreated patients

with metastatic malignant melanoma [abstract]. Pigment Cell Melanoma Res 2012;25:863.

98. Chapman PB, Einhorn LH, Meyers ML, et al. Phase III multicenter randomized trial of the Dartmouth regimen versus dacarbazine in patients with metastatic melanoma. J Clin Oncol 1999;17:2745–51.

99. Middleton MR, Lorigan P, Owen J, et al. A randomized phase III study comparing dacarbazine, BCNU, cisplatin and tamoxifen with dacarbazine and interferon in advanced melanoma. Br J Cancer 2000;82:1158–62.

100. Garcia M, del Muro XG, Tres A, et al. Phase II multicentre study of temozolomide in combination with interferon alpha-2b in metastatic malignant melanoma. Melanoma Res 2006;16:365–70.

101. Margolin KA, Doroshow JH, Akman SA, et al. Phase II trial of cisplatin and alpha-interferon in advanced malignant melanoma. J Clin Oncol 1992;10:1574–8.

102. Bafaloukos D, Pavlidis N, Fountzilas G, et al. Recombinant interferon ALFA-2A in combination with carboplatin, vinblastine, and bleomycin in the treatment of advanced malignant melanoma. Am J Clin Oncol 1996;19:296–300.

103. Stein ME, Bernstein Z, Tsalic M, et al. Chemoimmunohormonal therapy with carmustine, dacarbazine, cisplatin, tamoxifen, and interferon for metastatic melanoma: a prospective phase II study. Am J Clin Oncol 2002;25:460–3.

104. Daponte A, Ascierto PA, Gravina A, et al. Cisplatin, dacarbazine, and fotemustine plus interferon alpha in patients with advanced malignant melanoma. A multicenter phase II study of the Italian Cooperative Oncology Group. Cancer 2000;89:2630–6.

105. Dummer R, Gore ME, Hancock BW, et al. A multicenter phase II clinical trial using dacarbazine and continuous infusion interleukin-2 for metastatic melanoma. Clinical data and immunomonitoring. Cancer 1995;75:1038–44.

106. Isacson R, Kedar E, Barak V, et al. Chemo-immunotherapy in patients with metastatic melanoma using sequential treatment with dacarbazine and recombinant human interleukin-2: evaluation of hematologic and immunologic parameters and correlation with clinical response. Immunol Lett 1992;33:127–34.

107. Guida M, Latorre A, Mastria A, et al. Subcutaneous recombinant interleukin-2 plus chemotherapy with cisplatin and dacarbazine in metastatic melanoma. Eur J Cancer 1996;32A:730–3.

108. Legha SS, Ring S, Bedikian A, et al. Treatment of metastatic melanoma with combined chemotherapy containing cisplatin, vinblastine and dacarbazine (CVD) and biotherapy using interleukin-2 and interferon-alpha. Ann Oncol 1996;7:827–35.

109. Atzpodien J, Neuber K, Kamanabrou D, et al. Combination chemotherapy with or without s.c. IL-2 and IFN-alpha: results of a prospectively randomized trial of the Cooperative Advanced Malignant Melanoma Chemoimmunotherapy Group (ACIMM). Br J Cancer 2002;86:179–84.

110. Mazumder A, Grimm EA, Zhang HZ, et al. Lysis of fresh human solid tumors by autologous lymphocytes activated in vitro with lectins. Cancer Res 1982;42:913–8.

111. Lotze MT, Grimm EA, Mazumder A, et al. Lysis of fresh and cultured autologous tumor by human lymphocytes cultured in T-cell growth factor. Cancer Res 1981;41:4420–5.

112. Rosenberg SA, Lotze MT, Muul LM, et al. Observations on the systemic administration of autologous lymphokine-activated killer cells and recombinant interleukin-2 to patients with metastatic cancer. N Engl J Med 1985;313:1485–92.

113. Atkins MB. Cytokine-based therapy and biochemotherapy for advanced melanoma. Clin Cancer Res 2006;12:2353s–8s.
114. Atkins MB, Lotze MT, Dutcher JP, et al. High-dose recombinant interleukin 2 therapy for patients with metastatic melanoma: analysis of 270 patients treated between 1985 and 1993. J Clin Oncol 1999;17:2105–16.
115. Parkinson DR, Abrams JS, Wiernik PH, et al. Interleukin-2 therapy in patients with metastatic malignant melanoma: a phase II study. J Clin Oncol 1990;8: 1650–6.
116. Eton O, Rosenblum MG, Legha SS, et al. Phase I trial of subcutaneous recombinant human interleukin-2 in patients with metastatic melanoma. Cancer 2002; 95:127–34.
117. Karp SE. Low-dose intravenous bolus interleukin-2 with interferon-alpha therapy for metastatic melanoma and renal cell carcinoma. J Immunother 1998;21: 56–61.
118. Schwartzentruber DJ, Lawson DH, Richards JM, et al. gp100 peptide vaccine and interleukin-2 in patients with advanced melanoma. N Engl J Med 2011; 364:2119–27.
119. Hodi FS, O'Day SJ, McDermott DF, et al. Improved survival with ipilimumab in patients with metastatic melanoma. N Engl J Med 2010;363:711–23.
120. Topalian SL, Hodi FS, Brahmer JR, et al. Safety, activity, and immune correlates of anti-PD-1 antibody in cancer. N Engl J Med 2012;366:2443–54.
121. Brahmer JR, Tykodi SS, Chow LQ, et al. Safety and activity of anti-PD-L1 antibody in patients with advanced cancer. N Engl J Med 2012;366:2455–65.
122. Hamid O, Sosman JA, Lawrence DP, et al. Clinical activity, safety, and biomarkers of MPDL3280A, an engineered PD-L1 antibody in patients with locally advanced or metastatic melanoma (mM). J Clin Oncol 2013;31(Suppl) [abstract: 9010].
123. Chapman PB, Hauschild A, Robert C, et al. Improved survival with vemurafenib in melanoma with BRAF V600E mutation. N Engl J Med 2011;364:2507–16.
124. Hauschild A, Grob JJ, Demidov LV, et al. Dabrafenib in BRAF-mutated metastatic melanoma: a multicentre, open-label, phase 3 randomised controlled trial. Lancet 2012;380:358–65.
125. Flaherty KT, Robert C, Hersey P, et al. Improved survival with MEK inhibition in BRAF-mutated melanoma. N Engl J Med 2012;367:107–14.
126. Eisen T, Ahmad T, Flaherty KT, et al. Sorafenib in advanced melanoma: a phase II randomised discontinuation trial analysis. Br J Cancer 2006;95:581–6.
127. Hauschild A, Agarwala SS, Trefzer U, et al. Results of a phase III, randomized, placebo-controlled study of sorafenib in combination with carboplatin and paclitaxel as second-line treatment in patients with unresectable stage III or stage IV melanoma. J Clin Oncol 2009;27:2823–30.
128. Hodi FS, Friedlander P, Corless CL, et al. Major response to imatinib mesylate in KIT-mutated melanoma. J Clin Oncol 2008;26:2046–51.
129. Margolin K, Longmate J, Baratta T, et al. CCI-779 in metastatic melanoma: a phase II trial of the California Cancer Consortium. Cancer 2005;104:1045–8.

Understanding the Biology of Melanoma and Therapeutic Implications

Ryan J. Sullivan, MD[a], David E. Fisher, MD, PhD[b],*

KEYWORDS

- BRAF • NRAS • Immunotherapy • Targeted therapy • MITF

KEY POINTS

- Melanomagenesis is a complex process that involves carcinogenic exposure (eg, ultraviolet B radiation) and genetic predisposition (MCR1 polymorphisms).
- Microphthalmia-associated transcription factor, the "master regulator of melanocyte development," functions as an oncogene when dysregulated, leading to the upregulation of cell cycle progression and favorable metabolic changes, and the inhibition of apoptosis.
- Mutations of oncogenes (BRAF, NRAS, CKIT, GNAQ, GNA11) and a tumor suppressor gene (NF1) are present in most melanomas, although the rate of each type of mutation varies according to anatomic site subset (eg, mucosal vs cutaneous vs uveal).
- The mitogen-activated protein kinase (MAPK) pathway is upregulated in nearly all melanomas and is susceptible to small molecule inhibition.
- The interplay among the MAPK pathway, tumor antigen expression, and immune infiltration predicts therapeutic synergy with combined molecular and immune targeting.

INTRODUCTION

Over the past 3 decades, several breakthroughs have greatly expanded what is known about melanocyte biology, relevant oncogenic mutations and deletions and amplifications in melanoma, the influence of molecular signaling pathways on melanomagenesis, and the interaction of aberrant signaling pathways with host immune elements. This increased understanding has led to a remarkable number of improvements in the diagnosis, classification, and treatment of this disease. This advancement is an amazing achievement with great relevance, because the number of new cases of and deaths from melanoma continues to increase. A hallmark of this recent success

[a] Center for Melanoma, Massachusetts General Hospital Cancer Center, Harvard Medical School, 55 Fruit Street, Boston, MA 02114, USA; [b] Department of Dermatology, Massachusetts General Hospital Cancer Center, Harvard Medical School, Bartlett 6, 55 Fruit Street, Boston, MA 02114, USA
* Corresponding author.
E-mail address: dfisher3@partners.org

Hematol Oncol Clin N Am 28 (2014) 437–453
http://dx.doi.org/10.1016/j.hoc.2014.02.007
0889-8588/14/$ – see front matter © 2014 Elsevier Inc. All rights reserved.

is the regulatory approval of 4 therapeutic agents over the past 3 years, with at least another 6 promising agents that have just entered or completed phase III clinical trials.[1-5] Still, most patients diagnosed with metastatic melanoma will die of their disease within a few years of diagnosis.[6,7] To achieve the goal of successfully treating metastatic melanoma for nearly all afflicted, continued breakthroughs will be required to provide clinicians with diagnostic tools to identify subsets of patients most likely to benefit from a specific line of therapy, and improved treatment strategies for these identified subsets. This article reviews the relevant discoveries regarding melanocyte and melanoma biology that have been or are beginning to be translated into transformative therapies.

MELANOMA DEVELOPMENT
Melanocyte Formation in Development

Melanocytes are neural crest–derived cells that develop as a branch of alternative differentiation programs that include the closely related lineages of sympathetic neurons, Schwann cells, or melanocytes. In addition to residing in the basal epidermis and in hair follicles, other melanocyte populations can be found along mucosal surfaces and in the meninges, choroidal layer of the eye, and stria vascularis within the cochlea. The pigments produced by melanocytes are composed of numerous chemical species that have been broadly classified as red/blond pigments (pheomelanin) and brown/black pigments (eumelanin). Although brown/black pigment has a measureable (albeit modest) ultraviolet protective capability, pheomelanin has been associated with increased reactive oxygen species in the skin.[8]

Two forms of skin pigmentation exist: constitutive and adaptive. The constitutive or basal skin pigment level is associated with the type of pigment synthesized and the maturation process of the melanin-containing vesicles (called melanosomes). People of varying constitutive pigmentation are thought to have a constant number of melanocytes but variations in relative pigment production per cell. The adaptive pigmentation response typically reflects melanin synthesis triggered by ultraviolet radiation. This pigment has been shown to be initiated by ultraviolet-induced DNA damage in overlying epidermal melanocytes followed by p53 stabilization and transcriptional activation of the proopiomelanocortin (POMC) gene.[9,10] POMC is posttranslationally cleaved into various small peptides, one of which is the melanocyte-stimulating hormone (MSH) that is secreted and stimulates its receptor (melanocortin receptor 1 [MC1R]) on underlying melanocytes. Activation of MC1R by MSH peptide results in cyclic adenosine monophosphate induction within melanocytes, followed by stimulation of the gene encoding a transcription factor called microphthalmia-associated transcription factor (MITF), which activates expression of all known pigment-producing enzymes and nearly all of the machinery required for the packaging, maturation, and secretion of pigment-laden melanosomes. Nonfunctional polymorphic variants of MC1R are frequently responsible for the red hair/fair skin/freckling phenotype in numerous species, including humans.

Role of Ultraviolet Radiation

Ultraviolet radiation is deeply implicated in the formation of common forms of cutaneous melanoma in man. Ultraviolet wavelengths residing within the ultraviolet B portion of the spectrum produce stereotypical nucleotide adducts known as cyclobutane pyrimidine dimers, which in turn result in formation of pyrimidine dimer mutations, in which a cytosine located in a dipyrimidine sequence becomes mutated to thymidine. These "ultraviolet signature mutations" are easily recognizable within irradiated DNA. Exomic deep sequencing of human melanomas has been performed recently, and clearly reveals a striking abundance of these ultraviolet-derived genomic mutations within melanomas.[11] Still, features of melanoma suggest contributions in addition to ultraviolet radiation, such as red/blond pigment, that may provide new opportunities to improve prevention strategies.[8]

Role of MITF

Microphthalmia-associated transcription factor is a transcriptional regulator of the pigment pathway in melanocytes. However, MITF deficiency affects melanocytes more profoundly than purely affecting pigment synthesis. MITF deficiency produces Waardenburg syndrome type 2A in man and complete absence of the melanocyte lineage in numerous species.[12] This vital role for MITF in melanocyte development has led to its being dubbed a "master regulator of melanocyte development." In contrast to consequences of MITF deficiency, more recent studies showed that genomic amplification of MITF, a recurrent activating germline point mutation, activates melanoma oncogenes in man.[13,14] The recurrent point mutation in MITF was identified in cases of familial melanoma, and resulted in disruption of a SUMO-modification consensus sequence, thereby modestly increasing transcriptional activity of MITF protein. The means through which MITF dysregulation contributes to melanocytic transformation to malignancy is still being determined. It is unlikely that MITF's oncogenic activity is related to its production of eumelanin (dark eumelanin pigment is likely to be protective against melanoma and nonmelanoma skin cancers). However, MITF has also been seen to directly regulate expression of antiapoptotic genes (BCL2, BCL2A1), the cell cycle regulator CDK2, the metabolic regulator PGC1α, and numerous others.[15-17] Because of the role of MITF as a lineage survival factor, its role as an active regulator of melanoma proliferation/survival is likely to occur in most melanomas regardless of whether it is also an amplified or mutated oncogene. Its direct phosphorylation by mitogen activated protein kinase (MAPK) and subsequent ubiquitin-dependent proteolysis link MITF activity to the common melanoma oncogenes BRAF and NRAS.[18,19]

MOLECULAR SIGNALING IN MELANOMA
MAPK Signaling

The MAPK signaling pathway is critical to the pathobiology of several malignancies, including melanoma.[20] Canonical signaling (**Fig. 1**) through the pathway begins with ligand–receptor, either receptor tyrosine kinase (RTK) or G-protein–coupled receptor (GPCR) activation, engagement at the cell surface that ultimately triggers recruitment and activation of 1 of 3 (H-, K-, and N-) RAS isoforms.[21] Once activated, RAS binds to the RAS-binding domain on 1 of 3 (A-, B-, C-) RAF isoforms, triggering RAF homodimerization or heterodimerization and activation of its serine-threonine kinase domain.[22-24] Phosphorylation of MAPK kinase (MEK) by RAF leads its activation, which then leads to the activation of its only known substrate, MAPK otherwise known as the extracellular signal-regulated kinase (ERK).[25,26] The activation of ERK then leads to a host of downstream events that promote cell cycle progression and cell survival.

Deregulation of cell cycle progression is a critical consequence of MAPK activation in melanoma, and can occur through genomic mutations and amplifications (discussed later) or through hyperactivation of ERK. ERK phosphorylation and cyclin D1 expression, measured by immunohistochemistry staining, have been correlated in the analysis of primary melanomas.[27] Additionally, in uveal and acral melanoma,

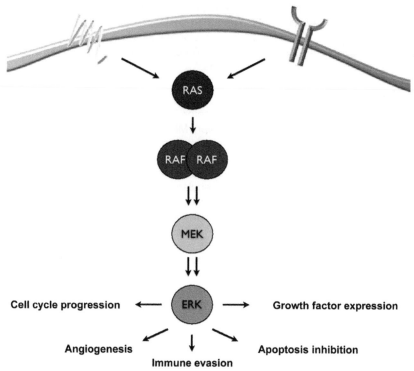

Fig. 1. Canonical mitogen-activated protein kinase (MAPK) pathway signaling. ERK, extracellular signal-regulated kinase; MEK, MPAK kinase.

increased MAPK signaling has been shown to be associated with cyclin D expression in the absence of oncogenic mutations of either BRAF or NRAS.[28,29] In the setting of oncogenic BRAF mutations, the cyclin-dependent kinase (CDK) inhibitor p27[KIP1] is downregulated and cyclin D1, is constitutively activated, both in an ERK-dependent manner, leading to enhanced proliferation.[30,31] In the setting of oncogenic NRAS mutations, cyclin D1 also seems to be regulated through ERK phosphorylation and plays an important role in driving proliferation.[32,33]

MAPK signaling also leads to the inhibition of apoptosis in melanoma cells. This process likely occurs through several mechanisms, although most of its effects seem to be in the regulation of various proapoptotic and antiapoptotic B-cell lymphoma 2 (BCL2) family members, including BIM, BAD, BMF, MCL-1, BAX, NOXA, and PUMA.[34–39] The preponderance of evidence suggests that the most critical effects of MAPK hyperactivation, particularly via oncogenic BRAF, on apoptosis are exerted through inhibition/downregulation of the proapoptotic BH3-protein BIM.[34,36,38] This effect may occur through several mechanisms, including decreased RNA expression, increased antiapoptotic BCL2 family member expression, or alterations in the BIM splicing machinery.[40]

Phosphoinositol-3-Kinase Signaling

The phosphoinositol-3-kinase (PI3K) pathway is the second major signaling pathway involved in melanoma pathogenesis.[41] Canonical activation of the PI3K pathway begins, much like the MAPK pathway activation, with cell surface receptor–ligand engagement, thereby triggering conversion of PIP2 to PIP3 that then binds to and activates Akt. Activated Akt leads to several cellular processes that promote cell proliferation, cell survival, and angiogenesis. In melanoma, the PI3K pathway may be activated via several mechanisms, including NRAS activation, either through mutation or loss of neurofibromatosis 1 (NF1) function, which can activate PI3K in a receptor-independent mechanism, loss of function of the PI3K regulator, phosphatase and tensin homologue (PTEN), or oncogenic mutation of Akt3.[20,42–45] One of the key downstream events of Akt activation is the activation of the mammalian target of rapamycin complexes 1 and 2 (mTORC1 and mTORC 2) through the inhibition of the tuberous sclerosis complex 1 and 2 (TSC1/TSC2), a tumor suppressor protein that regulates mTOR. mTORC1 and mTORC2 activation then lead to several cellular events, often hallmarked by the phosphorylation of the ribosomal protein S6 (phosphor-S6), that lead to proliferation, angiogenesis, and resistance to apoptosis.

TSC1/TSC2 expression is regulated by several molecules, including AMP kinase 1 (AMPK1), which is turn is activated by liver kinase B1 (LKB1). This pathway seems to be important in melanoma, particularly BRAF-mutant melanoma, because oncogenic BRAF is associated with downregulation of LKB1, and LKB1 expression is increased in the setting of BRAF inhibitor therapy.[46] This mechanism serves as a critical connection between the MAPK and PI3K signaling pathways that may have prognostic and therapeutic implications. Specifically, a recent analysis of patients treated with BRAF inhibitors showed that outcome of therapy was significantly improved when on-treatment phospho-sS6 was absent compared with when it was preserved.[47] It is conceivable that incorporating an "early look" at phospho-S6 expression in patients treated with BRAF inhibitors could help clinicians switch to a broader molecular-targeted regimen that incorporates PI3K pathway inhibition.

Oncogenic Mutations

The transformation of melanocytes into melanoma cells is a complex process that involves the acquisition of multiple molecular aberrations. These aberrations include genetic mutations and amplifications of well-described oncogenes that lead to hyperactivation of signal transduction pathways that promote cell growth, angiogenesis, survival, and immune evasion. The pattern of mutations varies depending on where the melanoma arises (**Fig. 2**).

BRAF

Oncogenic mutations in the kinase domain of the serine/threonine kinase BRAF are present in nearly 50% of melanomas.[48,49] These mutations most commonly involve the valine at the 600 position (V600), whereby this is exchanged for a glutamic acid (V600E) or an arginine (V600K). Other mutations have also been described in BRAF, but the V600 mutations dominate, representing most (>95%) of the BRAF mutations identified in melanoma, and are associated with constitutive activation of the MAPK pathway.[49] In the setting of oncogenic BRAF mutations, RAS-RAF engagement and RAF dimerization is not required for RAF-induced activation of MEK and ERK.[50,51]

BRAF[V600E] mutations are the most common BRAF mutations and occur more commonly in women, younger patients, and non–sun exposed areas.[52] In contrast, BRAF[V600K] mutations occur more frequently in older patients and men in sun-exposed areas.[53] These mutations seem to be more frequent in geographic locations with more intense sun exposure, such as Australia and Texas, and less common in the Northeast. Both mutations lead to a constitutively activated kinase that signals in monomeric form and is susceptible to inhibition with small molecules. Three such

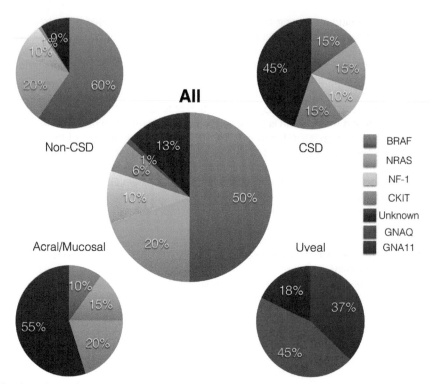

Fig. 2. Estimated oncogenic-driving mutation rate by anatomic subtype. CSD, cutaneous, chronic sun damaged skin; non-CSD, cutaneous, nonchronic sun damaged skin.

agents, vemurafenib, dabrafenib, and LGX818 have shown significant clinical activity, with both vemurafenib and dabrafenib having achieved regulatory approval for the treatment of patients with BRAF$^{V600E/K}$-mutant melanoma.[1,3,54]

NRAS/NF1

The N-isoform of RAS is mutated in 15% to 25% of patients with melanoma, and seems to be represented in similar frequencies in all anatomic subsets of the disease.[20] NRAS mutations seem to be mutually exclusive to BRAF mutations in most cases (dual positivity is seen at an incidence of <0.5%), and direct oncogenic signaling through the MAPK and PI3K pathways.[43,55] In addition, the tumor suppressor gene neurofibromatosis 1 (NF1), a potent regulator of NRAS, is dysfunctional in another 10% to 15% of cases, which leads to upregulation of NRAS signaling.[45] These recently identified loss-of-function mutations of NF1 are probably associated with similar activation of the MAPK and PI3K pathways as are activating NRAS mutations, and may be susceptible to the same treatment approaches.

CKIT

The tyrosine kinase receptor CKIT provides growth-pathway activation after interaction with and activation by its ligand stem cell factor. This pathway is critical in several normal cellular processes, including melanocyte pigment production.[18,56] However, mutations and genomic amplifications in the kinase or transmembrane domains lead to constitutive activation of the receptor and are associated with several malignancies, including melanoma and gastrointestinal stromal tumor (GIST).[57,58] In melanoma, mutations are typically seen in the transmembrane domains coded in exons 11 and 13, are more commonly found in acral/lentiginous and mucosal melanomas, and may be sensitive to small molecule inhibition with CKIT inhibitors, such as imatinib.[58–61]

GNAQ/GNA11

G-protein coupled receptors are 7-transmembrane domain receptors that transduce signals from several types of ligands, including hormones, growth factors, cytokines, and chemokines. Mutations in the 1 of 2 G-proteins, GNAQ and GNA11, have been identified in most patients with uveal melanoma.[62,63] In this setting, these constitutively activated proteins lead to the activation of protein kinase C, which triggers MAPK pathway activity through MEK phosphorylation, and renders these cells susceptible to MEK and PKC inhibitor therapy.[64–69]

Other mutations

Although BRAF, NRAS, CKIT, GNAQ/GNA11, and NF1 mutations are primary mutations that are typically mutually exclusive of each other, several other mutations or genetic aberrations affect the oncogenic phenotype in melanoma.

Cell cycle regulation Dysregulation of the cell cycle at the genomic level is common in melanoma.[11,70] The most commonly aberrant cell cycle–regulating gene in melanoma is CDNK2A, which codes for p16^{INK4A}, a CDK inhibitor, and is either deleted or mutated in at least 50% to 60% of tumors.[71,72] Additionally, loss of p16 can occur through promoter methylation in up to 10% to 20% of cases; thus up to 60% to 80% of patients may have disruption of p16^{INK4A} expression or function.[73] These aberrations lead to deregulation and overexpression of CDK4, which contributes to oncogenesis in the setting of other oncogenic drivers, such as NRAS and BRAF mutations.[70]

Most melanomas are sporadic; however, germline mutations of CDNK2A are the most commonly inherited mutation associated with hereditary melanoma.[74–77] Affected individuals have an approximately two-thirds lifetime risk of developing melanoma. A second, heritable form of melanoma involves germline-activating mutations of CDK4.[78] Although these are not as common as CDNK2A mutations, they are similarly associated with multiple nevi, early-onset melanoma, and the development of multiple primary melanomas.

Mutations in the tumor suppressor p53 are common in human malignancies, although they are infrequently seen in patients with melanoma.[11,79] However, amplification and overexpression of MDM2, a protein that ubiquitinates p53 therapy, leading to its jettisoning from the nucleus and proteasomal degradation, is present in more than 10% and 50% of patients with melanoma, respectively.[80,81]

PTEN loss PTEN is a tumor suppressor gene/protein and the major regulator of PI3K activation. Mutations leading to a truncated and/or nonfunctional protein and deletion of PTEN (so-called PTEN loss) are seen in approximately 25% of patients with melanoma.[11] These mutations are most commonly seen concomitant with BRAF mutations, although they rarely occur in the setting of NRAS mutations or BRAF and NRAS wild-type melanomas.[11,42,43,82] In the context of oncogenic BRAF mutations, PTEN loss is associated with PI3K pathway signaling and reduced effectiveness of BRAF inhibitors.[83,84] Recent data suggest that PTEN loss is specifically associated with PI3Kβ signaling, and the first PI3Kβ inhibitors currently are being tested in a clinical trial (ClinicalTrials.gov identifier: NCT01673737).[85] Dual targeting of the MAPK pathway and PI3Kβ is expected to be explored early in the development of these agents.

ONCOGENE-DIRECTED TREATMENTS

The identification of targetable mutations in melanoma, as with other malignancies such as chronic myelogenous leukemia, non–small cell lung cancer, and GIST, has led to a robust clinical development effort of small molecule inhibitors for the treatment of melanoma. As depicted in **Fig. 3**, several potential types of agents are being tested in patients with molecularly defined subtypes of melanoma. The most success to date has involved inhibitors of BRAF and MEK in BRAF-mutant melanoma and, to a lesser extent, MEK and KIT inhibitors in NRAS-mutant and CKIT-mutant melanoma, respectively. Although the clinical data from these studies is addressed elsewhere in this issue, 2 key principles of targeted therapy development in melanoma are addressed here.

The first principle of targeted therapy drug development is to use effective inhibitors of the target. With the identification of oncogenic BRAF mutations in almost all patients, inhibitors of RAF generally and BRAF specifically were brought quickly to the clinic.[49] The first 2 RAF inhibitors to make it to early-phase clinical trials were sorafenib and RAF265. Both are pan-RAF inhibitors, meaning they inhibit BRAF and CRAF, and the mutant forms of BRAF.[86,87] In preclinical studies, these agents had broad activity against BRAF mutant and wild-type cell lines.[86–91] Although some initial enthusiasm was shown for sorafenib in combination with chemotherapy, it was proven ineffective as a single agent and in combination with chemotherapy in numerous phase I, II, and III trials.[92–98] Additionally, RAF265 has been shown to be similarly ineffective.[99] With each agent, both on- and off-target toxicity limited the drug exposures predicted for efficient RAF inhibition, and likely explains the relative ineffectiveness of these agents compared with the more selective BRAF inhibitors that either have been approved or are in clinical development.[93,99] The first of these to demonstrate effectiveness in patients with melanoma was vemurafenib, a more selective RAF inhibitor that has nearly 10-fold greater inhibition of mutant BRAF versus wild-type BRAF.[100] In dose-escalation of this agent, drug exposure was lower than predicted and not dose-dependent; treatment with this formulation was associated with minimal activity.[101] With reformulation, drug exposure was dose-dependent, and most patients with BRAF mutations experienced disease regression.[101] Clinical activity was confirmed in phase II and III trials, leading to its approval by the U.S. Food and Drug Administration (FDA) in 2011.[1,102]

The second principle of effective drug development is careful patient selection. The development of the KIT inhibitor imatinib for the treatment of melanoma provides an excellent example of this principle. In fact, the clinical development of imatinib in melanoma was nearly permanently derailed by 2 phase II trials[103] performed in patients with stage IV melanoma.[104] The genesis of these trials was that KIT expression, measured through immunohistochemistry testing, was seen in most patients with melanoma; although no responses were seen in these trials of 18 and 29 patients, survival was poor and toxicity high, and although immunohistochemistry expression was seen in only greater than 50% of samples that were available, this did not seem to correlate to outcome. Since the completion of these trials, mutations and amplifications of CKIT have been identified (as described earlier), and in 3 phase II trials enriched with patients with either CKIT mutation or amplification, response rates have ranged from 17% to 29% in all patients and 30% to 54% in patients with mutation or amplification.[58–61] This example highlights the concept that an inhibitor will only be effective

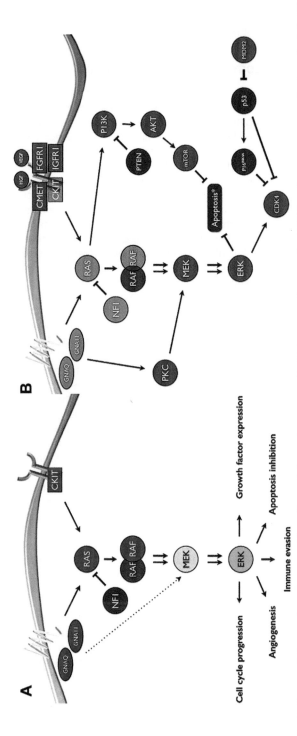

Fig. 3. Targeted therapy in melanoma. The effects of the major oncogenic driving mutations on the MAPK pathway are summarized on the left (A). Secondary molecular targets are shaded in purple and antitumor proteins are shaded in gray (B). In each instance, inhibitors of these secondary targets are either approved (eg, the MEK inhibitor for BRAF mutant melanoma) or in clinical development. * Additionally, agents that promote apoptosis are in development.

when given to the patients most likely to benefit. As targeted therapy development continues in melanoma, appropriate definition of molecular subsets remains one of the most critical factors to get right.

INTERACTION OF IMMUNOLOGY AND MOLECULAR SIGNALING

Therapies that modulate the immune system to overcome tumor-mediated immune anergy have been used to treat melanoma for decades. Initially, this consisted of using nonspecific immunogenic agents, such as Coley's toxin and Bacillus Calmette-Guérin (BCG), with the latter delivered via direct tumor injection.[105,106] The next generation of immunotherapies involved the use of several different cytokines, including interferon-alpha and interleukin-2 (IL-2), which received FDA-approval for high-risk stages II/III and IV melanoma, respectively.[107,108] Although these treatments help only a subset of patients, they provide an important "proof-of-principle" that immunotherapy can lead to potential cures in a predictable percentage of patients. For example, the use of high-dose IL-2 is associated with durable remission in 5% to 10% of patients with stage IV melanoma.[109] More recently, several newer agents that inhibit checkpoints of T-cell activation and regulation, such as cytotoxic T-lymphocyte antigen 4 (CTLA4) and programed death 1 (PD1) and its ligands (PDL1 and PDL2), have been shown to have amazing clinical activity. Included among these agents are the anti-CTLA4 antibody ipilimumab, which is associated with a doubling of survival at 2 and 3 years and has been approved by the FDA since 2011, and the anti-PD1 antibodies nivolumab and MK3475, which have been associated with response rates ranging from 30% to 40% and 1-year survival rates ranging from 60% to 80%.[4,5,110,111]

With the concomitant development of oncogene-targeted therapies, there has been a major push to combine small molecule target therapies with immunotherapy in an attempt to get the best of both worlds: frequent (oncogene-targeted therapy) and durable responses (immunotherapies). In melanoma, emerging evidence suggests that combining these treatment modalities not only is practical (because of the availability of these agents) but also makes sound biologic sense.[112] In particular, oncogenic BRAF mutations reduce MITF activity, and BRAF/MAPK inhibition is associated with increased MITF activity.[15] Several groups now have shown, in paired patient samples, that BRAF inhibitor therapy is associated with increased tumor expression of melanocyte-derived antigens (MDAs) and leads to an increase in CD-8 and cytotoxic T lymphocyte (CTL) in tumors.[113–115] Ex vivo studies of these tumor-infiltrating lymphocytes suggest that these CTLs are able to recognize MDAs.[113] Finally, MEK inhibitor therapy seems to impair lymphocyte function, whereas treatment with a BRAF inhibitor, if anything, enhances lymphocyte function.[114,116,117] Based on these data, combined modality treatment with a BRAF inhibitor and an immunotherapy, such as IL-2 or immune checkpoint inhibitors, may be associated with better outcomes. To date, the results from only one such trial, involving the combination of vemurafenib and ipilimumab, has been reported.[118] In this study, the degree of hepatic toxicity was very high and precluded further development of the combination. Whether this is a sign of things to come with combined targeted and immunotherapy or just a particular problem with these specific agents is unclear. Several other studies are ongoing combining BRAF (with or without MEK inhibitors), with several cytokines (interferon and IL-2) and checkpoint inhibitors (ClinicalTrails.gov identifiers: NCT01940809, NCT01767454, NCT01943422, NCT01683188, NCT01656642, NCT01959633, NCT01659151, NCT01603212, and NCT01754376).

The mere presence of a BRAF mutation does not seem to be associated with outcome with immunotherapy. Specifically, in retrospective studies of IL-2 and ipilimumab, patients with BRAF mutants had similar response rates to patients without BRAF mutations.[119,120] However, emerging evidence suggests that patients with NRAS mutations may be associated with higher response rates than those with BRAF mutations and those who have BRAF and NRAS wild-type melanoma. In a retrospective analysis of 208 consecutive patients treated with IL-2 in whom 103 had BRAF and NRAS typing, the 15 patients with NRAS mutations had a higher response rate (45%) than those treated with either a BRAF mutation (22%) or no identifiable mutation in BRAF or NRAS (12%).[119] This has been followed up by a retrospective analysis of 173 patients treated with either high-dose IL-2, ipilimumab, the PD1 antibodies MK3475 or nivolumab, or the anti-PDL1 antibody MPDL3280A. In this series, patients treated with NRAS mutations (59/173; 34%) had a 2-fold higher response rate to any immunotherapy than those without a BRAF or NRAS mutation (114/173; 66%); the response rate for patients with BRAF mutations was not calculated for this study, because a large number of these patients were treated after BRAF inhibitor therapy (a scenario associated with a poor response to immunotherapy).[121] Although the mechanism of this association has not been determined, it likely involves molecular signaling pathways mediated by NRAS mutations. If this is true, then pharmacologic manipulation of molecular signaling pathways may improve immunotherapy outcomes.

SUMMARY

The elucidation of melanoma biology has led to the identification of therapeutic targets and the development of effective treatments. Continued laboratory and translational research efforts focused on describing the interplay among molecular biology, immunology, and melanoma is expected lead to further advances and, ultimately, transformative therapies.

REFERENCES

1. Chapman PB, Hauschild A, Robert C, et al. Improved survival with vemurafenib in melanoma with BRAF V600E mutation. N Engl J Med 2011;364(26): 2507–16.
2. Flaherty KT, Robert C, Hersey P, et al. Improved survival with MEK inhibition in BRAF-mutated melanoma. N Engl J Med 2012;367(2):107–14.
3. Hauschild A, Grob JJ, Demidov LV, et al. Dabrafenib in BRAF-mutated metastatic melanoma: a multicentre, open-label, phase 3 randomised controlled trial. Lancet 2012;380(9839):358–65.
4. Hodi FS, O'Day SJ, McDermott DF, et al. Improved survival with ipilimumab in patients with metastatic melanoma. N Engl J Med 2010;363(8):711–23.
5. Robert C, Thomas L, Bondarenko I, et al. Ipilimumab plus dacarbazine for previously untreated metastatic melanoma. N Engl J Med 2011;364(26):2517–26.
6. Balch CM, Gershenwald JE, Soong SJ, et al. Final version of 2009 AJCC melanoma staging and classification. J Clin Oncol 2009;27(36):6199–206.
7. Siegel R, Naishadham D, Jemal A. Cancer statistics, 2013. CA Cancer J Clin 2013;63(1):11–30.
8. Mitra D, Luo X, Morgan A, et al. An ultraviolet-radiation-independent pathway to melanoma carcinogenesis in the red hair/fair skin background. Nature 2012; 491(7424):449–53.

9. D'Orazio JA, Nobuhisa T, Cui R, et al. Topical drug rescue strategy and skin protection based on the role of Mc1r in UV-induced tanning. Nature 2006; 443(7109):340–4.

10. Cui R, Widlund HR, Feige E, et al. Central role of p53 in the suntan response and pathologic hyperpigmentation. Cell 2007;128(5):853–64.

11. Hodis E, Watson IR, Kryukov GV, et al. A landscape of driver mutations in melanoma. Cell 2012;150(2):251–63.

12. Price ER, Fisher DE. Sensorineural deafness and pigmentation genes: melanocytes and the Mitf transcriptional network. Neuron 2001;30(1):15–8.

13. Garraway LA, Widlund HR, Rubin MA, et al. Integrative genomic analyses identify MITF as a lineage survival oncogene amplified in malignant melanoma. Nature 2005;436(7047):117–22.

14. Yokoyama S, Woods SL, Boyle GM, et al. A novel recurrent mutation in MITF predisposes to familial and sporadic melanoma. Nature 2011;480(7375): 99–103.

15. Haq R, Shoag J, Andreu-Perez P, et al. Oncogenic BRAF regulates oxidative metabolism via PGC1alpha and MITF. Cancer Cell 2013;23(3):302–15.

16. Haq R, Yokoyama S, Hawryluk EB, et al. BCL2A1 is a lineage-specific antiapoptotic melanoma oncogene that confers resistance to BRAF inhibition. Proc Natl Acad Sci U S A 2013;110(11):4321–6.

17. McGill GG, Horstmann M, Widlund HR, et al. Bcl2 regulation by the melanocyte master regulator MITF modulates lineage survival and melanoma cell viability. Cell 2002;109(6):707–18.

18. Hemesath TJ, Price ER, Takemoto C, et al. MAP kinase links the transcription factor Microphthalmia to c-Kit signalling in melanocytes. Nature 1998;391(6664): 298–301.

19. Wu M, Hemesath TJ, Takemoto CM, et al. c-Kit triggers dual phosphorylations, which couple activation and degradation of the essential melanocyte factor Mi. Genes Dev 2000;14(3):301–12.

20. Omholt K, Platz A, Kanter L, et al. NRAS and BRAF mutations arise early during melanoma pathogenesis and are preserved throughout tumor progression. Clin Cancer Res 2003;9(17):6483–8.

21. Sullivan RJ, Flaherty K. MAP kinase signaling and inhibition in melanoma. Oncogene 2012;32(19):2373–9.

22. Chong H, Guan KL. Regulation of Raf through phosphorylation and N terminus-C terminus interaction. J Biol Chem 2003;278(38):36269–76.

23. Moodie SA, Willumsen BM, Weber MJ, et al. Complexes of Ras.GTP with Raf-1 and mitogen-activated protein kinase kinase. Science 1993;260(5114): 1658–61.

24. Winkler DG, Cutler RE Jr, Drugan JK, et al. Identification of residues in the cysteine-rich domain of Raf-1 that control Ras binding and Raf-1 activity. J Biol Chem 1998;273(34):21578–84.

25. Garnett MJ, Rana S, Paterson H, et al. Wild-type and mutant B-RAF activate C-RAF through distinct mechanisms involving heterodimerization. Mol Cell 2005;20(6):963–9.

26. Terai K, Matsuda M. The amino-terminal B-Raf-specific region mediates calcium-dependent homo- and hetero-dimerization of Raf. EMBO J 2006;25(15): 3556–64.

27. Oba J, Nakahara T, Abe T, et al. Expression of c-Kit, p-ERK and cyclin D1 in malignant melanoma: an immunohistochemical study and analysis of prognostic value. J Dermatol Sci 2011;62(2):116–23.

28. Takata M, Goto Y, Ichii N, et al. Constitutive activation of the mitogen-activated protein kinase signaling pathway in acral melanomas. J Invest Dermatol 2005; 125(2):318–22.

29. Calipel A, Mouriaux F, Glotin AL, et al. Extracellular signal-regulated kinase-dependent proliferation is mediated through the protein kinase A/B-Raf pathway in human uveal melanoma cells. J Biol Chem 2006;281(14):9238–50.

30. Bhatt KV, Hu R, Spofford LS, et al. Mutant B-RAF signaling and cyclin D1 regulate Cks1/S-phase kinase-associated protein 2-mediated degradation of p27Kip1 in human melanoma cells. Oncogene 2007;26(7):1056–66.

31. Bhatt KV, Spofford LS, Aram G, et al. Adhesion control of cyclin D1 and p27Kip1 levels is deregulated in melanoma cells through BRAF-MEK-ERK signaling. Oncogene 2005;24(21):3459–71.

32. Eskandarpour M, Huang F, Reeves KA, et al. Oncogenic NRAS has multiple effects on the malignant phenotype of human melanoma cells cultured in vitro. Int J Cancer 2009;124(1):16–26.

33. Eskandarpour M, Kiaii S, Zhu C, et al. Suppression of oncogenic NRAS by RNA interference induces apoptosis of human melanoma cells. Int J Cancer 2005; 115(1):65–73.

34. Wang YF, Jiang CC, Kiejda KA, et al. Apoptosis induction in human melanoma cells by inhibition of MEK is caspase-independent and mediated by the Bcl-2 family members PUMA, Bim, and Mcl-1. Clin Cancer Res 2007;13(16):4934–42.

35. Verhaegen M, Bauer JA, Martin de la Vega C, et al. A novel BH3 mimetic reveals a mitogen-activated protein kinase-dependent mechanism of melanoma cell death controlled by p53 and reactive oxygen species. Cancer Res 2006; 66(23):11348–59.

36. Sheridan C, Brumatti G, Martin SJ. Oncogenic B-RafV600E inhibits apoptosis and promotes ERK-dependent inactivation of Bad and Bim. J Biol Chem 2008;283(32):22128–35.

37. Panka DJ, Cho DC, Atkins MB, et al. GSK-3beta inhibition enhances sorafenib-induced apoptosis in melanoma cell lines. J Biol Chem 2008;283(2):726–32.

38. Cartlidge RA, Thomas GR, Cagnol S, et al. Oncogenic BRAF(V600E) inhibits BIM expression to promote melanoma cell survival. Pigment Cell Melanoma Res 2008;21(5):534–44.

39. Smalley KS, Xiao M, Villanueva J, et al. CRAF inhibition induces apoptosis in melanoma cells with non-V600E BRAF mutations. Oncogene 2009;28(1): 85–94.

40. Jiang CC, Lai F, Tay KH, et al. Apoptosis of human melanoma cells induced by inhibition of B-RAFV600E involves preferential splicing of bimS. Cell Death Dis 2010;1:e69.

41. Kwong LN, Davies MA. Navigating the therapeutic complexity of PI3K pathway inhibition in melanoma. Clin Cancer Res 2013;19(19):5310–9.

42. Tsao H, Zhang X, Fowlkes K, et al. Relative reciprocity of NRAS and PTEN/MMAC1 alterations in cutaneous melanoma cell lines. Cancer Res 2000;60(7): 1800–4.

43. Tsao H, Goel V, Wu H, et al. Genetic interaction between NRAS and BRAF mutations and PTEN/MMAC1 inactivation in melanoma. J Invest Dermatol 2004; 122(2):337–41.

44. Davies MA, Stemke-Hale K, Tellez C, et al. A novel AKT3 mutation in melanoma tumours and cell lines. Br J Cancer 2008;99(8):1265–8.

45. Maertens O, Johnson B, Hollstein P, et al. Elucidating distinct roles for NF1 in melanomagenesis. Cancer Discov 2013;3(3):338–49.

46. Zheng B, Jeong JH, Asara JM, et al. Oncogenic B-RAF negatively regulates the tumor suppressor LKB1 to promote melanoma cell proliferation. Mol Cell 2009; 33(2):237–47.

47. Corcoran RB, Rothenberg SM, Hata AN, et al. TORC1 suppression predicts responsiveness to RAF and MEK inhibition in BRAF-mutant melanoma. Sci Transl Med 2013;5(196):196ra98.

48. Brose MS, Volpe P, Feldman M, et al. BRAF and RAS mutations in human lung cancer and melanoma. Cancer Res 2002;62(23):6997–7000.

49. Davies H, Bignell GR, Cox C, et al. Mutations of the BRAF gene in human cancer. Nature 2002;417(6892):949–54.

50. Heidorn SJ, Milagre C, Whittaker S, et al. Kinase-dead BRAF and oncogenic RAS cooperate to drive tumor progression through CRAF. Cell 2010;140(2): 209–21.

51. Poulikakos PI, Zhang C, Bollag G, et al. RAF inhibitors transactivate RAF dimers and ERK signalling in cells with wild-type BRAF. Nature 2010; 464(7287):427–30.

52. Long GV, Menzies AM, Nagrial AM, et al. Prognostic and clinicopathologic associations of oncogenic BRAF in metastatic melanoma. J Clin Oncol 2011; 29(10):1239–46.

53. Menzies AM, Haydu LE, Visintin L, et al. Distinguishing clinicopathologic features of patients with V600E and V600K BRAF-mutant metastatic melanoma. Clin Cancer Res 2012;18(12):3242–9.

54. Dummer R, Robert C, Nyakas M, et al. Initial results from a phase I, open-label, dose escalation study of the oral BRAF inhibitor LGX818 in patients with BRAF V600 mutant advanced or metastatic melanoma [abstract]. J Clin Oncol 2013; 31(Suppl). Abstract 9028.

55. Kwong LN, Costello JC, Liu H, et al. Oncogenic NRAS signaling differentially regulates survival and proliferation in melanoma. Nat Med 2012;18(10): 1503–10.

56. Funasaka Y, Boulton T, Cobb M, et al. c-Kit-kinase induces a cascade of protein tyrosine phosphorylation in normal human melanocytes in response to mast cell growth factor and stimulates mitogen-activated protein kinase but is down-regulated in melanomas. Mol Biol Cell 1992;3(2):197–209.

57. Wardelmann E, Merkelbach-Bruse S, Pauls K, et al. Polyclonal evolution of multiple secondary KIT mutations in gastrointestinal stromal tumors under treatment with imatinib mesylate. Clin Cancer Res 2006;12(6):1743–9.

58. Curtin JA, Busam K, Pinkel D, et al. Somatic activation of KIT in distinct subtypes of melanoma. J Clin Oncol 2006;24(26):4340–6.

59. Carvajal RD, Antonescu CR, Wolchok JD, et al. KIT as a therapeutic target in metastatic melanoma. JAMA 2011;305(22):2327–34.

60. Guo J, Si L, Kong Y, et al. Phase II, open-label, single-arm trial of imatinib mesylate in patients with metastatic melanoma harboring c-Kit mutation or amplification. J Clin Oncol 2011;29(21):2904–9.

61. Hodi FS, Corless CL, Giobbie-Hurder A, et al. Imatinib for melanomas harboring mutationally activated or amplified KIT arising on mucosal, acral, and chronically sun-damaged skin. J Clin Oncol 2013;31(26):3182–90.

62. Van Raamsdonk CD, Bezrookove V, Green G, et al. Frequent somatic mutations of GNAQ in uveal melanoma and blue naevi. Nature 2009;457(7229): 599–602.

63. Van Raamsdonk CD, Griewank KG, Crosby MB, et al. Mutations in GNA11 in uveal melanoma. N Engl J Med 2010;363(23):2191–9.

64. Chen X, Wu Q, Tan L, et al. Combined PKC and MEK inhibition in uveal melanoma with GNAQ and GNA11 mutations. Oncogene 2013. http://dx.doi.org/10.1038/onc.2013.418.

65. Wu X, Li J, Zhu M, et al. Protein kinase C inhibitor AEB071 targets ocular melanoma harboring GNAQ mutations via effects on the PKC/Erk1/2 and PKC/NF-kappaB pathways. Mol Cancer Ther 2012;11(9):1905–14.

66. von Euw E, Atefi M, Attar N, et al. Antitumor effects of the investigational selective MEK inhibitor TAK733 against cutaneous and uveal melanoma cell lines. Mol Cancer 2012;11:22.

67. Khalili JS, Yu X, Wang J, et al. Combination small molecule MEK and PI3K inhibition enhances uveal melanoma cell death in a mutant GNAQ- and GNA11-dependent manner. Clin Cancer Res 2012;18(16):4345–55.

68. Selumetinib shows promise in metastatic uveal melanoma. Cancer Discov 2013;3(7):OF8.

69. Selumetinib increases the efficacy of first-line dacarbazine. Cancer Discov 2013;3(7):OF16.

70. Sheppard KE, McArthur GA. The cell cycle regulator CDK4 an emerging therapeutic target in melanoma. Clin Cancer Res 2013;19:5320–8.

71. McArthur GA, Young RJ, Sheppard KE, et al. Clinical significance of genomic alterations of the CDK4-pathway and sensitivity to the CDK4 inhibitor PD 0332991 in melanoma [abstract]. J Clin Oncol 2012;30(Suppl). Abstract 8520.

72. Castellano M, Pollock PM, Walters MK, et al. CDKN2A/p16 is inactivated in most melanoma cell lines. Cancer Res 1997;57(21):4868–75.

73. Jonsson A, Tuominen R, Grafstrom E, et al. High frequency of p16(INK4A) promoter methylation in NRAS-mutated cutaneous melanoma. J Invest Dermatol 2010;130(12):2809–17.

74. Fargnoli MC, Chimenti S, Keller G, et al. CDKN2a/p16INK4a mutations and lack of p19ARF involvement in familial melanoma kindreds. J Invest Dermatol 1998;111(6):1202–6.

75. Liu L, Dilworth D, Gao L, et al. Mutation of the CDKN2A 5' UTR creates an aberrant initiation codon and predisposes to melanoma. Nat Genet 1999;21(1):128–32.

76. Liu L, Lassam NJ, Slingerland JM, et al. Germline p16INK4A mutation and protein dysfunction in a family with inherited melanoma. Oncogene 1995;11(2):405–12.

77. Ranade K, Hussussian CJ, Sikorski RS, et al. Mutations associated with familial melanoma impair p16INK4 function. Nat Genet 1995;10(1):114–6.

78. Puntervoll HE, Yang XR, Vetti HH, et al. Melanoma prone families with CDK4 germline mutation: phenotypic profile and associations with MC1R variants. J Med Genet 2013;50(4):264–70.

79. Lubbe J, Reichel M, Burg G, et al. Absence of p53 gene mutations in cutaneous melanoma. J Invest Dermatol 1994;102(5):819–21.

80. Muthusamy V, Hobbs C, Nogueira C, et al. Amplification of CDK4 and MDM2 in malignant melanoma. Genes Chromosomes Cancer 2006;45(5):447–54.

81. Polsky D, Bastian BC, Hazan C, et al. HDM2 protein overexpression, but not gene amplification, is related to tumorigenesis of cutaneous melanoma. Cancer Res 2001;61(20):7642–6.

82. Tsao H, Zhang X, Benoit E, et al. Identification of PTEN/MMAC1 alterations in uncultured melanomas and melanoma cell lines. Oncogene 1998;16(26):3397–402.

83. Nathanson KL, Martin AM, Wubbenhorst B, et al. Tumor genetic analyses of patients with metastatic melanoma treated with the BRAF inhibitor dabrafenib (GSK2118436). Clin Cancer Res 2013;19(17):4868–78.

84. Shi H, Hugo W, Kong X, et al. Acquired resistance and clonal evolution in melanoma during BRAF inhibitor therapy. Cancer Discov 2014;4(1):80–93.

85. Wee S, Wiederschain D, Maira SM, et al. PTEN-deficient cancers depend on PIK3CB. Proc Natl Acad Sci U S A 2008;105(35):13057–62.

86. Su Y, Vilgelm AE, Kelley MC, et al. RAF265 inhibits the growth of advanced human melanoma tumors. Clin Cancer Res 2012;18(8):2184–98.

87. Wilhelm SM, Adnane L, Newell P, et al. Preclinical overview of sorafenib, a multikinase inhibitor that targets both Raf and VEGF and PDGF receptor tyrosine kinase signaling. Mol Cancer Ther 2008;7(10):3129–40.

88. Beeram M, Patnaik A, Rowinsky EK. Raf: a strategic target for therapeutic development against cancer. J Clin Oncol 2005;23(27):6771–90.

89. Smalley KS, Flaherty KT. Development of a novel chemical class of BRAF inhibitors offers new hope for melanoma treatment. Future Oncol 2009;5(6):775–8.

90. Wilhelm S, Carter C, Lynch M, et al. Discovery and development of sorafenib: a multikinase inhibitor for treating cancer. Nat Rev Drug Discov 2006;5(10):835–44.

91. Chen J, Shen Q, Labow M, et al. Protein kinase D3 sensitizes RAF inhibitor RAF265 in melanoma cells by preventing reactivation of MAPK signaling. Cancer Res 2011;71(12):4280–91.

92. Amaravadi RK, Schuchter LM, McDermott DF, et al. Phase II trial of temozolomide and sorafenib in advanced melanoma patients with or without brain metastases. Clin Cancer Res 2009;15(24):7711–8.

93. Eisen T, Ahmad T, Flaherty KT, et al. Sorafenib in advanced melanoma: a Phase II randomised discontinuation trial analysis. Br J Cancer 2006;95(5):581–6.

94. Flaherty KT, Lee SJ, Zhao F, et al. Phase III trial of carboplatin and paclitaxel with or without sorafenib in metastatic melanoma. J Clin Oncol 2013;31(3):373–9.

95. Flaherty KT, Schiller J, Schuchter LM, et al. A phase I trial of the oral, multikinase inhibitor sorafenib in combination with carboplatin and paclitaxel. Clin Cancer Res 2008;14(15):4836–42.

96. Hauschild A, Agarwala SS, Trefzer U, et al. Results of a phase III, randomized, placebo-controlled study of sorafenib in combination with carboplatin and paclitaxel as second-line treatment in patients with unresectable stage III or stage IV melanoma. J Clin Oncol 2009;27(17):2823–30.

97. Margolin KA, Moon J, Flaherty LE, et al. Randomized phase II trial of sorafenib with temsirolimus or tipifarnib in untreated metastatic melanoma (S0438). Clin Cancer Res 2012;18(4):1129–37.

98. McDermott DF, Sosman JA, Gonzalez R, et al. Double-blind randomized phase II study of the combination of sorafenib and dacarbazine in patients with advanced melanoma: a report from the 11715 Study Group. J Clin Oncol 2008;26(13):2178–85.

99. Sharfman WH, Hodi FS, Lawrence DP, et al. Results from the first-in-human (FIH) phase I study of the oral RAF inhibitor RAF265 administered daily to patients with advanced cutaneous melanoma [abstract]. J Clin Oncol 2011;29(Suppl). Abstract 8508.

100. Joseph EW, Pratilas CA, Poulikakos PI, et al. The RAF inhibitor PLX4032 inhibits ERK signaling and tumor cell proliferation in a V600E BRAF-selective manner. Proc Natl Acad Sci U S A 2010;107(33):14903–8.

101. Flaherty KT, Puzanov I, Kim KB, et al. Inhibition of mutated, activated BRAF in metastatic melanoma. N Engl J Med 2010;363(9):809–19.

102. Sosman JA, Kim KB, Schuchter L, et al. Survival in BRAF V600-mutant advanced melanoma treated with vemurafenib. N Engl J Med 2012;366(8):707–14.

103. Ugurel S, Hildenbrand R, Zimpfer A, et al. Lack of clinical efficacy of imatinib in metastatic melanoma. Br J Cancer 2005;92(8):1398–405.
104. Wyman K, Atkins MB, Prieto V, et al. Multicenter phase II trial of high-dose imatinib mesylate in metastatic melanoma: significant toxicity with no clinical efficacy. Cancer 2006;106(9):2005–11.
105. Morton D, Eilber FR, Malmgren RA, et al. Immunological factors which influence response to immunotherapy in malignant melanoma. Surgery 1970;68(1): 158–63 [discussion: 63–4].
106. Morton DL, Eilber FR, Holmes EC, et al. BCG immunotherapy of malignant melanoma: summary of a seven-year experience. Ann Surg 1974;180(4):635–43.
107. Atkins MB, Lotze MT, Dutcher JP, et al. High-dose recombinant interleukin 2 therapy for patients with metastatic melanoma: analysis of 270 patients treated between 1985 and 1993. J Clin Oncol 1999;17(7):2105–16.
108. Kirkwood JM, Strawderman MH, Ernstoff MS, et al. Interferon alfa-2b adjuvant therapy of high-risk resected cutaneous melanoma: the Eastern Cooperative Oncology Group Trial EST 1684. J Clin Oncol 1996;14(1):7–17.
109. Atkins MB, Kunkel L, Sznol M, et al. High-dose recombinant interleukin-2 therapy in patients with metastatic melanoma: long-term survival update. Cancer J Sci Am 2000;6(Suppl 1):S11–4.
110. Hamid O, Robert C, Daud A, et al. Safety and tumor responses with lambrolizumab (anti-PD-1) in melanoma. N Engl J Med 2013;369(2):134–44.
111. Topalian SL, Hodi FS, Brahmer JR, et al. Safety, activity, and immune correlates of anti-PD-1 antibody in cancer. N Engl J Med 2012;366(26):2443–54.
112. Sullivan RJ, Lorusso PM, Flaherty KT. The intersection of immune-directed and molecularly targeted therapy in advanced melanoma: where we have been, are, and will be. Clin Cancer Res 2013;19(19):5283–91.
113. Frederick DT, Piris A, Cogdill AP, et al. BRAF inhibition is associated with enhanced melanoma antigen expression and a more favorable tumor microenvironment in patients with metastatic melanoma. Clin Cancer Res 2013;19(5):1225–31.
114. Hong DS, Vence L, Falchook G, et al. BRAF(V600) inhibitor GSK2118436 targeted inhibition of mutant BRAF in cancer patients does not impair overall immune competency. Clin Cancer Res 2012;18(8):2326–35.
115. Wilmott JS, Long GV, Howle JR, et al. Selective BRAF inhibitors induce marked T-cell infiltration into human metastatic melanoma. Clin Cancer Res 2012;18(5):1386–94.
116. Boni A, Cogdill AP, Dang P, et al. Selective BRAFV600E inhibition enhances T-cell recognition of melanoma without affecting lymphocyte function. Cancer Res 2010;70(13):5213–9.
117. Comin-Anduix B, Chodon T, Sazegar H, et al. The oncogenic BRAF kinase inhibitor PLX4032/RG7204 does not affect the viability or function of human lymphocytes across a wide range of concentrations. Clin Cancer Res 2010;16(24):6040–8.
118. Ribas A, Hodi FS, Callahan M, et al. Hepatotoxicity with combination of vemurafenib and ipilimumab. N Engl J Med 2013;368(14):1365–6.
119. Joseph RW, Sullivan RJ, Harrell R, et al. Correlation of NRAS mutations with clinical response to high-dose IL-2 in patients with advanced melanoma. J Immunother 2012;35(1):66–72.
120. Shahabi V, Whitney G, Hamid O, et al. Assessment of association between BRAF-V600E mutation status in melanomas and clinical response to ipilimumab. Cancer Immunol Immunother 2012;61(5):733–7.
121. Johnson DB, Lovly CM, Flavin M, et al. NRAS mutation: a potential biomarker of clinical response to immune-based therapies in metastatic melanoma (MM) [abstract]. J Clin Oncol 2013;31(Suppl). Abstract 9019.

Surgical Management of Melanoma

Vernon K. Sondak, MD[a,b,c,*], Geoffrey T. Gibney, MD[a,b]

KEYWORDS

- Melanoma • Surgery • Sentinel node biopsy • Lymphadenectomy
- Metastasectomy

KEY POINTS

- Management of the primary melanoma: wide excision is well established for the management of primary melanoma of any stage and thickness, using guidelines based on numerous randomized clinical trials.

- Management of clinically negative regional nodes: sentinel node biopsy reliably identifies occult nodal metastases and provides important prognostic information that is unavailable through any other modality. Available data indicate that it should be routinely used in otherwise healthy patients with clinically node-negative melanomas greater than or equal to 0.76 mm in thickness.

- Management of node-positive melanoma: optimum strategies for managing node-positive melanoma are being developed, and should be individualized based on the tumor burden within the node. Although radical lymphadenectomy should be the mainstay of treatment of any patient with macroscopic nodal disease, some patients with small-volume microscopic disease in the sentinel node(s) do well without completion lymphadenectomy. The role of postlymphadenectomy radiation in patients with macroscopic nodal involvement, particularly when multiple nodes are involved and/or extranodal extension is present, remains controversial but randomized trial data provide strong evidence that radiation can decrease regional recurrence inside the treatment field.

- Management of oligometastatic melanoma: resection of limited stage IV melanoma is associated with long-term survival in a small but significant percentage of cases. As systemic therapy options improve, increasing use of preoperative therapy to improve resectability rates should be considered. Surgery also plays an important role in controlling individual lesions that have failed to respond to, or that have escaped from, treatment while other tumors in the same patient have responded or even disappeared.

Financial Disclosures: Dr V.K. Sondak is a compensated consultant for Bristol Myers Squibb, Glaxo Smith-Kline, Merck, Navidea, Novartis, and Provectus. Dr G.T. Gibney is a compensated consultant for Genentech-Roche.

[a] Department of Cutaneous Oncology, Moffitt Cancer Center, 12902 Magnolia Drive, Tampa, FL 33612, USA; [b] Department of Oncologic Sciences, University of South Florida Morsani College of Medicine, Tampa, FL, USA; [c] Department of Surgery, University of South Florida Morsani College of Medicine, Tampa, FL, USA
* Corresponding author. 12902 Magnolia Drive, Tampa, FL 33612.
E-mail address: vernon.sondak@moffitt.org

INTRODUCTION

The medical management of metastatic cutaneous melanoma has changed greatly over the past several years, spurred on by progress in the understanding of the molecular biology of melanoma and of the human antitumor immune response. These scientific advances led to the development of new drugs, which proved their value in large clinical trials. In comparison, little has changed in the surgical management of localized and metastatic melanoma in the past decade, but the fundamental principles on which that surgical management is based were also established in large clinical trials and have withstood the test of time. Even with the introduction of more effective drugs for the treatment of metastatic melanoma, surgery remains the mainstay of treatment of every patient in whom complete excision of all disease is feasible, even those with regionally advanced or oligometastatic disease. In view of the rapid advances of the past few years, treatment decisions regarding the surgical and medical management of melanoma should ideally be made by a multidisciplinary team of specialists working together. For optimum results, it behooves each member of that team to understand the fundamental principles and key supporting clinical data underlying the various available management options. This article summarizes the fundamental principles and key supporting clinical data underlying the modern surgical approach to treating cutaneous melanoma of all stages. Although many of the principles described also apply to treatment of melanoma arising on mucosal surfaces, a detailed discussion of the treatment of those forms of melanoma is beyond the scope of this article.

SURGICAL TREATMENT OF LOCALIZED DISEASE
Surgical Treatment of Primary Melanoma

Radical wide excision (often referred to as wide local excision, a term with no intrinsic meaning because there is no such thing as a nonlocal excision) is the standard-of-care treatment of all forms of localized, biopsy-proven primary cutaneous melanoma (stages 0–III), including cases in which there is clinical evidence of regional nodal metastasis. There are 2 fundamental aspects to the radical wide excision procedure: wide excision refers to the planned removal of a predefined and measured amount of normal-appearing skin beyond the visible edge of any residual pigmentation, lesional tissue, or biopsy scar. This wide excision contrasts with the narrow excision used to biopsy suspect pigmented skin lesions, wherein the lesion is removed with only a millimeter or two (nonmeasured) of adjacent normal skin to provide the pathologist with the opportunity to examine the entirety of the clinical lesion. Radical excision indicates that the removal of normal tissue extends down to the level of the underlying muscular fascia, in contrast with the more limited amount of subcutaneous tissue that is normally excised in treatment of a typical nonmelanoma skin cancer–like basal or squamous cell carcinoma. It has never been shown that removing the muscular fascia is necessary for the success of the procedure,[1,2] and practice patterns differ in whether to always, never, or selectively remove the underlying fascia.[3]

The width of excision for an invasive primary melanoma is based on data derived from a series of randomized controlled trials,[4] and the recommended width of excision increases for thick primary tumors within the limits of anatomic constraints.[5] **Table 1** summarizes the recommendations for invasive cutaneous melanoma by thickness and tumor location used by most surgical oncologists, and in keeping with the current National Comprehensive Cancer Network guidelines. Although these guidelines are based on data from randomized trials, there are still unanswered

Table 1
Recommended margins of wide excision for invasive cutaneous melanoma based on primary tumor thickness and location

Breslow Thickness (mm)	Primary Site	Recommended Excision Margin (cm)
0.01–1.00	Anywhere on the skin	1
1.01–2.00	Head/neck, distal extremity[a]	1
	Trunk or proximal extremity[b]	2
>2.00	Head/neck, distal extremity[a]	1
	Trunk or proximal extremity	2

Note: Local anatomic constraints and specific patient factors may justify minor deviations from the standard margin recommendations.
[a] Subungual primary tumors may require distal digital amputation.
[b] If a skin graft would be required to reconstruct the excision defect, it is acceptable to take a 1-cm excision margin.

questions about the optimum management of primary melanoma in several clinical situations, including melanoma in situ, desmoplastic melanoma, and subungual primary tumors.[6]

The obvious goal of radical wide excision is to remove all visible tumor as well as microscopic extensions and any microscopic or macroscopic satellites within 1 to 2 cm of the primary site. The excision margins are measured intraoperatively on the skin; it is not expected that there will be 1 or 2 cm of histologically normal tissue beyond the last melanoma cell, only a histologically negative final margin. Histologic involvement of the resected margins sometimes necessitates further excision. Persistent positive margins after maximal excision can be a vexing problem; radiation and topical therapy with imiquimod have each been advocated but have never been proved to be effective in prospective trials. For desmoplastic melanomas, evidence is emerging that postoperative radiation can decrease local recurrence rates and should be considered in at least a subset of patients.[7,8]

Local recurrence after radical wide excision occurs more commonly for thick tumors; those with ulceration, angiolymphatic invasion, and/or satellitosis; and for primary tumors situated on the head and neck, palms, and soles. In a large prospective clinical trial for patients with melanoma 1 to 4 mm in thickness, patients with tumors on the trunk or proximal extremity were randomized to either a 2-cm or a 4-cm margin of excision, whereas patients with tumors on the head and neck or distal extremity were allocated to a 1-cm margin of excision.[9] Overall local recurrence rates were 1.1% for the proximal extremity, 3.1% for the trunk, 5.3% for the distal extremity, and 9.4% for the head and neck. Ulceration had a major impact on local recurrence that was statistically significant after adjusting for other prognostic factors: local recurrence was 1.1% for nonulcerated melanomas versus 6.6% for ulcerated melanomas in the randomized arms (trunk and proximal extremity) with no significant difference for those randomized to 2-cm or 4-cm margins, but was 2.1% for nonulcerated melanomas versus 16.2% for ulcerated melanomas in the nonrandomized group (distal extremity and head and neck) receiving only a 1-cm margin.[9]

Most guidelines call for narrower margins of excision for melanoma in situ (usually 0.5 cm) than for invasive melanoma,[5] but this recommendation is not based on any prospective trial data. Lentigo maligna melanoma on the head and neck is particularly likely to be undertreated by a 0.5-cm margin,[10] and is often best approached using a staged technique that allows for careful histologic evaluation of the margins before proceeding with reconstruction. For melanoma in situ arising outside the head and neck area, the difference in morbidity between a 0.5-cm margin and a 1.0-cm margin is often small enough to justify using the wider margin, especially if there is any suspicion that residual invasive melanoma might be present.

Staging of the Clinically Negative Regional Lymph Nodes

After the achievement of local disease control, the next objective of surgical management of primary melanoma is frequently the staging of the regional lymph nodes. The absence or presence of microscopic tumor deposits within clinically negative lymph nodes is the most impactful predictor of long-term patient survival in clinical stage I and II melanoma,[11] and, unlike the postulated situation in breast cancer, there is strong evidence that even tiny nodal micrometastases have clinical relevance.[12,13] Melanoma micrometastases in the regional lymph nodes cannot reliably be detected by positron emission tomography (PET)/computed tomography (CT) scanning[14,15] or even ultrasonography,[16,17] but sentinel lymph node biopsy provides a low-morbidity technique for identifying these micrometastases with a high degree of accuracy.[18] In 2012, an evidence-based assessment of the indications for sentinel lymph node biopsy in melanoma was issued as a joint effort of the American Society of Clinical Oncology (ASCO) and the Society of Surgical Oncology (SSO).[19] Their key recommendations are:

- Sentinel lymph node biopsy is recommended for patients with cutaneous melanomas with Breslow thickness of 1 to 4 mm at any anatomic site
- Sentinel lymph node biopsy may be recommended for staging purposes and to facilitate regional disease control for patients with melanomas that are greater than 4 mm in Breslow thickness
- There is insufficient evidence to support routine sentinel lymph node biopsy for patients with melanomas that are less than 1 mm in Breslow thickness, although it may be considered in selected high-risk patients
- Completion lymph node dissection is recommended for all patients with a positive sentinel lymph node biopsy

(*Modified from* Wong and colleagues.[19])

The joint ASCO-SSO guideline panel found the strongest published evidence to support sentinel node biopsy for patients with intermediate-thickness melanomas, based on data provided by the interim analysis of the randomized evaluation of sentinel node biopsy, the Multicenter Selective Lymphadenectomy Trial I (MSLT-1), published in 2006.[11] The final analysis of the MSLT-1 trial has been completed, and confirms and extends the findings from that interim publication (**Table 2**).[20] These results, as well as data from large institutional series, provide support for a recommendation that sentinel lymph node biopsy be routinely used for patients with clinically node-negative thick melanomas (>4 mm) as well.[21–23] The most controversial area regarding the use of sentinel node biopsy is with regard to thin melanomas (<1 mm), which were not adequately assessed in the MSLT-1 study or included in the prospective but nonrandomized Sunbelt Melanoma Trial.[24]

Most newly diagnosed cutaneous melanomas are currently in the T1 category (≤1 mm in thickness), and overall survival at 10 years for patients with T1 melanoma in the American Joint Committee on Cancer (AJCC) melanoma database was 92%.[25] Performing sentinel node biopsy on all patients with thin melanomas would clearly not be cost-effective,[26] so the ASCO-SSO recommendation that it may be considered in selected cases with high-risk features makes sense.[19] The most widely accepted

Table 2
Summary of selected final results of the MSLT-1

	Result	Comment
Feasibility	A sentinel node was identified in 99.5% of 943 patients with melanomas ≥1.2 mm randomized to sentinel node biopsy	The procedure proved highly feasible worldwide
Yield and false-positives	The sentinel node was positive in 19% of 938 patients with melanomas ≥1.2 mm undergoing sentinel node biopsy; 16% for melanomas 1.2–3.5 mm, and 33% for melanomas >3.5 mm. Nodal recurrence occurred in 5.9% of 763 patients with a negative sentinel node; 4.8% for melanomas 1.2–3.5 mm and 10.3% for melanomas >3.5 mm	Sentinel node biopsy is an effective staging procedure with an acceptable false-negative rate; true-positive and false-negative cases are more common for thick melanomas
Prognostic significance	A positive sentinel node was associated with ~2.5-fold increases in disease recurrence and death from melanoma for melanomas 1.2–3.5 mm; 10-year melanoma-specific survival was 85% for patients with a negative sentinel node vs 62% for patients with a positive sentinel node	Sentinel node status is the strongest available prognostic indicator in clinically node-negative intermediate-thickness melanoma
Survival impact of sentinel node biopsy	There was a nonsignificant 3% increase in 10-year melanoma-specific survival for patients with intermediate-thickness melanoma randomized to sentinel node biopsy vs observation	Sentinel node biopsy does not significantly affect survival for all patients subjected to the procedure
Relapse-free survival impact	Patients randomized to sentinel node biopsy had a statistically significant improvement in relapse-free survival compared with observation	Sentinel node biopsy significantly reduces melanoma recurrence for intermediate and thick melanomas, mostly by markedly decreasing subsequent nodal relapse
Impact on node-positive patients	Patients with intermediate-thickness melanoma and positive nodes who were randomized to sentinel node biopsy (with completion lymphadenectomy) had a statistically significant improvement in distant metastasis-free survival and melanoma-specific survival compared with observation arm patients who had positive nodes; there was no significant difference for patients with thick melanomas and positive nodes	Early treatment of intermediate-thickness node-positive melanoma by complete lymphadenectomy improves outcomes significantly; patients with thick node-positive melanomas may be at such high risk of distant disease that timing of lymphadenectomy loses importance

Adapted from Morton DL, Thompson JF, Cochran AJ, et al. Sentinel node biopsy or nodal observation in melanoma: final trial report. N Engl J Med 2014;370: 599–609.

high-risk features for selecting patients with thin melanoma for sentinel lymph node biopsy are listed below, along with an estimate of the impact of that factor on the likelihood of finding a positive sentinel node.

Thickness 0.76 to 0.99 mm

In a registry series of 1250 patients with melanomas less than or equal to 1 mm selected by a wide variety of criteria to undergo sentinel node biopsy, metastases were detected in 6.3% of 891 melanomas greater than or equal to 0.76 mm but in only 2.5% of 359 melanomas less than or equal to 0.75 mm. No metastases were detected in sentinel nodes from patients with melanomas less than 0.5 mm.[27] In a large contemporary single-institution experience from a center in which sentinel node biopsy was routinely offered to patients with melanoma greater than or equal to 0.76 mm without requiring any other high-risk feature to be present, 8.4% of patients had a positive sentinel node.[28]

Ulceration

A positive sentinel node was present in 18.3% of patients in a registry series[27] and 23.5% of patients in a single-institution series[28] who had ulcerated T1 melanomas, making this rare finding (present in 8.9% and 6.6% of cases in the two series respectively) perhaps the highest risk factor for sentinel node positivity in thin melanoma.

Mitotic count

The presence of even 1 dermal mitosis in a T1 melanoma upstages the tumor from T1a to T1b in the current AJCC staging system. In general, increasing mitotic counts correlate with a poorer prognosis[25] and a greater likelihood of nodal metastasis for patients with cutaneous melanoma.[29] The exact impact of mitotic count on the likelihood of a positive node in patients with T1 melanoma is less clear, with 1 series involving 181 cases showing that only those patients with mitotic counts greater than 0 had positive sentinel nodes, whereas other studies have found either no significant association between mitotic count and nodal status[27] or have found that even cases without identified mitoses still have a 5% risk of having a positive node.[28]

Other factors that have been used to select patients for sentinel node biopsy include patient age, because younger patients have a higher risk of positive sentinel nodes across all tumor thickness categories[29] as well as more years at risk for nodal recurrence, and Clark level greater than III.[27] The latter criterion is most contentious because, within the T1 melanoma spectrum, Clark level IV melanomas are more likely to be at the thicker end (≥0.76 mm) where most nodal metastases are encountered.

Until more evidence regarding optimum criteria for selecting patients with thin melanomas for sentinel node biopsy can be accumulated, decision making regarding this procedure should be individualized. In an editorial accompanying the ASCO-SSO sentinel node biopsy guidelines publication, Gershenwald and colleagues[30] concluded that, "a rational result of this process is a recommendation for [sentinel lymph node] biopsy for many patients with melanomas 0.76–1.00 mm in thickness, but not for the overwhelming majority of patients with melanomas <0.76 mm in thickness." This opinion reflects our current practice, with patient age and comorbidities representing the main factors in addition to Breslow thickness that are used, in conjunction with patient preference, to personalize the decision-making process so that the yield in terms of positive sentinel nodes justifies the risks of the procedure. From a practical standpoint, this leads to the following basic algorithm for selecting patients with melanomas less than 1 mm in thickness for sentinel node biopsy:

- Tumor thickness 0.76 to 0.99 mm; patient age less than or equal to 70 years with no comorbidities: recommend sentinel lymph node biopsy (expected rate of positive nodes ≥5%).
- Tumor thickness 0.76–0.99 mm; patient age 70 to 80 years, or patients with minor comorbidities not representing a contraindication to general anesthesia: recommend sentinel lymph node biopsy if tumor ulcerated or with mitotic count greater than 0 (expected rate of positive nodes ≥10%).
- Tumor thickness <0.76 mm or patient age greater than 80 years or any patient with significant comorbidities: do not recommend sentinel lymph node biopsy.

A few other situations have created sufficient controversy regarding sentinel lymph node biopsy to deserve mention. Desmoplastic melanomas have been purported to have a lower risk of nodal metastases, and some investigators have advocated abandoning sentinel lymph node biopsy in this histologic type.[31] We and others have found that pure desmoplastic melanomas do have a significantly lower risk of nodal metastases compared with tumors of mixed or nondesmoplastic histology,[32,33] but we think that the risk of nodal metastases is still high enough to justify routine consideration of the procedure in all patients with desmoplastic melanomas greater than or equal to 1 mm in thickness.[33] Pediatric patients with melanoma have a higher incidence of nodal metastases but an apparent better overall prognosis compared with adults, and the role of sentinel node biopsy in these patients remains contentious, especially for so-called atypical melanocytic proliferations of childhood.[34] We think that sentinel lymph node biopsy has an important role in these patients, and recommend it routinely for pediatric melanomas greater than or equal to 1 mm in thickness and for those atypical melanocytic tumors in which melanoma is in the differential diagnosis.[35,36]

SURGICAL TREATMENT OF REGIONAL LYMPH NODE METASTASES

Once diagnosed, standard management of regional lymph node metastases in melanoma is radical lymphadenectomy. This procedure is referred to as a completion lymphadenectomy when it is performed after a positive sentinel lymph node biopsy (and hence completing the removal of the remaining nonsentinel lymph nodes), as an elective lymphadenectomy when it is performed on a clinically negative nodal basin in the absence of any histologic proof of nodal involvement, and as a therapeutic lymphadenectomy when it is performed on a clinically positive nodal basin after histologic confirmation of nodal involvement. In the modern era of sentinel lymph node biopsy, elective lymphadenectomy should no longer routinely be performed. In contrast, therapeutic lymphadenectomy is virtually always indicated for clinically evident nodal metastasis; adjuvant systemic therapy and/or radiation is not an adequate substitute for surgical treatment of the clinically positive nodal basin, although it may be used in conjunction with surgery.[37] The most controversial area in the management of melanoma nodal metastases concerns the role and indications for completion lymphadenectomy after a positive sentinel lymph node biopsy.

Arguments in Favor of Routine Completion Lymphadenectomy

- To date, no subsets of patients with a positive sentinel node have been identified who have a 0 or even less than a 5% chance of having involved nonsentinel nodes.[24,38]

- The histopathologic analysis of nonsentinel nodes is almost always less intensive than that performed on sentinel nodes, so estimates of nonsentinel node involvement by tumor routinely understate the risk of residual tumor. Moreover, the finding of nonsentinel node involvement by standard histopathologic techniques seems to have prognostic significance.[39]
- Recurrent disease in the nodal basin after prior sentinel node biopsy may be advanced at presentation, potentially jeopardizing the ability to achieve regional disease control.
- Findings of the MSLT-1 randomized trial indicate that sentinel node–positive patients on the sentinel node biopsy arm who underwent completion (early) lymphadenectomy had less morbidity than patients on the observation arm who underwent therapeutic (delayed) lymphadenectomy at the time of nodal recurrence.[40]
- Findings of the MSLT-1 randomized trial indicate that sentinel node–positive patients on the sentinel node biopsy arm who underwent completion (early) lymphadenectomy had better survival outcomes than patients on the observation arm who underwent therapeutic (delayed) lymphadenectomy at the time of nodal recurrence, particularly for patients with intermediate-thickness melanomas.[11,20]

Arguments Against Routine Completion Lymphadenectomy

- To date, no study has shown that completion lymphadenectomy improves survival compared with nodal observation after a positive sentinel node biopsy. Furthermore, serial follow-up of the nodal basin with ultrasonography could allow detection of in-basin recurrence early enough to permit therapeutic lymphadenectomy with similar rates of regional disease control and morbidity to those achieved after completion lymphadenectomy.
- Not all patients with a positive sentinel node develop clinical evidence of regional recurrence. In some cases, this is because of the prior development of widespread metastatic disease, whereas in others the sentinel lymph node biopsy may have removed the only foci of nodal involvement. Hence, with routine use of completion lymphadenectomy, all sentinel node–positive patients are subjected to the morbidity of lymph node removal but not all patients benefit from it.

The uncertainty regarding completion lymphadenectomy will likely remain until the premise that nodal observation in conjunction with serial ultrasonography is an acceptable alternative has been prospectively tested in the randomized MSLT-2 trial for patients with positive sentinel nodes. This large trial recently completed accrual with over 1900 sentinel node-positive patients randomized, but will require many additional years of follow-up before mature results are available. Even then, it is likely that the patients entered onto this trial will represent a selected subset of patients with lower risk of having nonsentinel nodes because of patient and physician biases that are nearly impossible to avoid. For now, the joint ASCO-SSO guideline panel's conclusion that completion lymphadenectomy is recommended for all patients with a positive sentinel lymph node biopsy remains the standard-of-care recommendation,[19] and patients who decline lymphadenectomy should be carefully followed to allow detection and treatment of nodal recurrence as early as feasible.

ROLE OF POSTOPERATIVE RADIATION AFTER LYMPHADENECTOMY

When patients undergo completion lymphadenectomy after a positive sentinel lymph node biopsy, the risk of recurrence within the dissected lymph node basin is low.[24] The risk of recurrence within the lymph node basin after lymphadenectomy is highest for patients with multiple macroscopically involved lymph nodes, particularly if extracapsular extension is present. Adjuvant postoperative radiation has been shown in a prospective randomized trial to decrease the risk of recurrence within the treated lymph node basin field in these high-risk patients.[37] However, relapse-free and overall survival were not significantly improved for the radiation arm. It may be that salvage therapy for nodal basin recurrence with surgery and radiation ultimately achieves the same benefit (regional control of disease) while sparing some patients the morbidity of unnecessary treatment, so for now adjuvant postoperative radiation remains controversial but may have a role in selected patients at very high risk of regional recurrence.

SURGICAL TREATMENT OF METASTATIC MELANOMA

Patients with isolated, resectable metastatic melanoma (stage IV), with or without a known cutaneous primary site, are appropriate candidates for aggressive surgical management. Identifying which patients will benefit from metastasectomy requires good clinical judgment and a thorough radiologic evaluation to identify the extent of disease. Patients presenting with metastatic disease who are being considered for surgery should undergo a preoperative evaluation including whole-body PET-CT scanning and brain magnetic resonance imaging, as well as cross-sectional imaging studies to delineate the local extent of the lesions to be removed.[41] If the radiologic evaluation suggests that one or more metastases may not be amenable to complete removal or that there are additional small lesions consistent with unresectable metastases, then alternative approaches such as systemic therapy should be strongly considered. Tumor biology ultimately determines the success of intervention. A long disease-free interval before the development of the resectable metastasis, and even measured tumor-doubling times of the metastatic disease, have been shown to predict potential benefit from metastasectomy.[42] When surgery is performed, complete resection should routinely be the goal. Incomplete resection can be used for symptom palliation in highly selected cases, particularly for symptomatic gastrointestinal and central nervous system metastases.[43]

Incidence of Resectable Metastatic Melanoma

The frequency with which patients present with limited metastatic disease potentially amenable to resection has not been well defined. There is evidence that presentation with oligometastatic disease amenable to resection may be more common than most oncologists surmise. Of 291 patients who developed stage IV melanoma after enrolling onto MSLT-1 in whom complete data regarding postrecurrence treatment were available, 161 (55%) underwent surgery alone or with systemic therapy as a component of the initial treatment of their metastatic disease.[44] This high rate of surgical use on recurrence is likely to reflect a selected population of patients (all of whom initially presented with clinically node-negative melanoma) who were being closely followed by surgical oncologists with frequent laboratory and imaging studies as required by the clinical trial protocol. In contrast, a review of 70 consecutive patients presenting with metastatic melanoma to a European center over an 18-month period found that most (78.6%) were not candidates for complete resection.[45] Most of the patients had at least 7 distinct metastatic foci at presentation; only 18.6% presented with a single metastasis. In that unselected experience, only 6 patients, or 8.6% of the total group, had a complete resection, whereas in another 9 patients incomplete surgery was performed. Even this experience, which seems more representative of what a modern, multidisciplinary melanoma team would encounter, still indicates a substantial role for surgery in the front-line management of stage IV melanoma.

Outcomes with Surgery

For the aforementioned cohort of MSLT-1 patients who developed stage IV melanoma, the selected group of patients receiving surgery with or without systemic therapy had a median survival of 15.8 months, as opposed to 6.9 months for those receiving systemic therapy alone.[44] Four years after surgery, 69.3% of patients were still alive. Surgery was associated with better survival for patients regardless of M substage: M1a, median greater than 60 months versus 12.4 months (P = .01); M1b, median 17.9 versus 9.1 months (P = .11); and M1c, median 15.0 versus 6.3 months (P<.0001).[44] It must be stressed that the results in this surgically treated cohort represent a highly selected subpopulation of patients, and should not be considered to represent what can be achieved with surgery in unselected patients with stage IV melanoma.

There has only been 1 prospective (albeit nonrandomized) trial evaluating surgery for patients with stage IV melanoma: trial S9430 conducted by the Southwest Oncology Group.[46] Patients with stage IV melanoma were enrolled as soon as the determination of potential resectability was made, before undergoing surgery, which allowed the investigators to estimate resectability rate as well as to define relapse-free and overall survival after complete resection. Over a 10-year period, a total of 77 patients were enrolled. This low annual accrual rate suggests that patients with potentially resectable metastases are not common in most oncologic practices. Among the 77 study patients, 3 patients had no evidence of melanoma in the resected specimen (the suspected metastatic deposit was either a second primary malignancy or a benign finding) and 2 patients had only stage III disease. An additional 8 patients were not able to have their disease completely resected. Therefore, 64 patients (88.9% of eligible patients with stage IV melanoma) who were deemed resectable before surgery were resected to a disease-free state. Among these 64 patients, after a median follow-up of 5 years, all but 6 (9.4%) had recurred, with a median relapse-free survival of approximately 5 months. Overall survival was longer than relapse-free survival, at a median of 21 months, with an estimated 12-month survival of 75%. Survival at 4 years was 31%.[46] The resectability and survival rates reported in S9430 were prospectively derived from otherwise unselected patient populations and are the most representative data currently available for comparing surgical and nonsurgical approaches to stage IV melanoma. The key outcome parameters from S9430 compared with contemporary results achievable with systemic therapy are discussed here.

Complete response rate and duration of response

The S9430 data indicated that nearly 90% of surgical candidates achieved a complete response; that is, were rendered disease-free by surgery.[46] No therapies currently available can achieve a complete response in such a high percentage of treated patients. Although the duration of response is short at a median of 5 months, about half of patients can be reinduced into another complete response with a second or subsequent surgery.[44,46]

Progression-free survival

The median progression-free survival of 5 months seen among resected patients in S9430 is higher than that observed in 2 phase III randomized trials of ipilimumab[47,48] but similar to that observed in 2 phase III randomized trials of single-agent BRAF inhibitors.[49,50] The median progression-free survival time after surgery is shorter than the progression-free survival seen in the phase II experience with anti-Programmed Death 1 (PD1) antibody therapy (>7 months for MK-3475)[51] or with combined BRAF and MEK inhibitors (9.4 months)[52] in unselected (and clearly less favorable) patients.

Overall survival
In the S9430 trial and other multi-institutional reports of surgery for stage IV melanoma, survival times for resected patients have been longer (median 15.8 months and 21 months),[44,46] with more patients alive at 1 year than were seen with conventional (pre-2011) therapies as assessed in cooperative group trials.[53] Overall survival data for patients treated with the BRAF inhibitors vemurafenib and dabrafenib showed median times of 13.6 and 18.2 months, respectively. In the phase III ipilimumab data, median overall survival was 10.1 and 11.2 months.[47,48] However, pooled data on patients treated with ipilimumab showed 17% alive at 7 years,[54] which is similar to the overall survival rate seen in the S9430 trial. Long-term follow-up of newer systemic therapy strategies, such as combined BRAF plus MEK inhibitors,[52] single-agent anti-PD1/anti-Programmed Death Ligand 1 therapy,[51] and combined nivolumab plus ipilimumab, are expected to show further gains in overall survival,[55] potentially exceeding the results obtained with surgery.

Integration of Surgery and Systemic Therapy in Patients with Metastatic Melanoma

New systemic therapy approaches to metastatic melanoma are becoming so effective that a reconsideration of the role of surgery in front-line management may be appropriate. If phase III results with BRAF plus MEK inhibitors or anti-PD1 antibodies alone or with ipilimumab match or exceed the outcomes seen in phase II trials, then that will likely be the case. For now, the high rate with which complete eradication of all known disease can be achieved continues to argue for resection whenever feasible.

Preoperative use of systemic therapy, or neoadjuvant therapy, to enhance resectability or to improve long-term outcomes in metastatic melanoma is still evolving. Previous neoadjuvant studies with chemotherapy, interferon, and biochemotherapy in patients with resectable stage III disease showed clinical activity,[56–58] but it remains unclear from these nonrandomized trials whether there were long-term survival gains. Given the high response rate and rapid time to response associated with BRAF and MEK inhibitors in metastatic *BRAF*-mutant melanoma, selected patients may benefit from neoadjuvant BRAF targeted therapy. These patients include those considered borderline resectable or in whom unfavorable clinicopathologic characteristics argue against surgery (eg, those with multiple metastases and a short disease-free interval and/or an increased serum lactate dehydrogenase level). Multiple case reports and a case series have now described the successful application of BRAF targeted therapy before resection of regionally advanced or distant metastatic melanoma.[59–62] When single-agent BRAF inhibitors are used, we reevaluate patients about 2 to 4 months after initiation of therapy, in hopes of scheduling the operation before drug resistance emerges and leads to clinically evident tumor progression. Neoadjuvant treatment with combined BRAF and MEK inhibitors might allow a longer time on therapy before resistance can emerge, and in so doing perhaps induce complete responses that remove the need for surgery altogether. For patients who undergo successful resection after kinase inhibitor treatment, it is unclear whether maintenance BRAF inhibition offers further clinical benefit compared with reserving further systemic therapy for subsequent unresectable recurrence. Individualized decision making is appropriate in this scenario, recognizing that a minority of patients (about 10% in the S9430 trial)[46] are long-term survivors after surgery without any additional systemic treatment.

The role of adjuvant systemic therapy after metastasectomy remains to be defined. The use of adjuvant interferon has largely been evaluated in high-risk stage II and III patients, and even in those patients it remains controversial. Long-term follow-up of multiple studies has shown that adjuvant interferon consistently improves relapse-free survival in stage II and III patients,[63] and meta-analyses have shown improved overall survival as well.[64,65] Adjuvant interferon has not been thoroughly evaluated in resected stage IV patients. The immune checkpoint inhibitors ipilimumab and nivolumab have now been evaluated in phase II studies of resected patients with stage IV melanoma.[66,67] The ongoing phase III E1609 trial comparing interferon with ipilimumab includes both high-risk stage III and stage IV (M1a and M1b) patients. At this time, use of adjuvant therapy after metastasectomy is generally limited to clinical investigation.

SUMMARY

Surgery remains the primary treatment of patients with localized and regionally metastatic melanoma. The use of defined excision margins (1–2 cm) for resection of primary cutaneous melanoma and sentinel lymph node biopsy for primary lesions greater than or equal to 1 mm in depth (and in selected patients with thinner lesions) have become standard approaches worldwide. Completion lymphadenectomy after positive sentinel lymph node biopsy reduces regional recurrence, and evidence from the MSLT-1 randomized trial indicates that this approach improves survival in patients with intermediate-thickness melanoma compared with nodal observation. The results of the MSLT-2 randomized trial are eagerly awaited to determine whether completion lymphadenectomy can be delayed until signs of lymph node recurrence are detected on physical examination or by ultrasonography. Until then, lymphadenectomy remains the standard-of-care treatment of any patient with positive nodes, but it bears special emphasis that therapeutic lymphadenectomy is virtually always indicated in patients with macroscopic lymph node involvement.

With the major recent advances seen in the development of systemic therapies for metastatic melanoma, the incorporation of BRAF targeted and immune-based therapies into surgical plans is now best accomplished using a multidisciplinary team approach involving both surgical and medical oncologists. This team approach often includes the use of neoadjuvant BRAF inhibition for cytoreduction and to increase resectability, and should test the ability of adjuvant immunotherapy after metastasectomy to decrease recurrence rates and increase the percentage of patients achieving long-term survival by supporting clinical trials already underway and in development. As more patients are achieving durable partial and complete responses with systemic therapies, the role of metastasectomy is being challenged, but for now it remains a well-accepted and valuable approach. Furthermore, metastasectomy in patients showing mixed responses to systemic therapies may provide prolonged clinical benefit as well as palliation of symptoms.

REFERENCES

1. Kenady DE, Brown BW, McBride CM. Excision of underlying fascia with a primary malignant melanoma: effect on recurrence and survival rates. Surgery 1982;92:615–8.
2. Grotz TE, Glorioso JM, Pockaj BA, et al. Preservation of the deep muscular fascia and locoregional control in melanoma. Surgery 2013;153:535–41.
3. DeFazio JL, Marghoob AA, Pan Y, et al. Variation in the depth of excision of melanoma: a survey of US physicians. Arch Dermatol 2010;146:995–9.

4. Lens MB, Dawes M, Goodacre T, et al. Excision margins in the treatment of primary cutaneous melanoma: a systematic review of randomized controlled trials comparing narrow vs. wide excision. Arch Surg 2001;137:1101–5.

5. Coit DG, Thompson JA, Andtbacka R, et al. NCCN clinical practice guidelines in oncology: melanoma. Version 2. 2014. Available at: http://www.nccn.org/professionals/physician_gls/pdf/melanoma.pdf. Accessed February 1, 2014.

6. Wong JY, Sondak VK. Cutaneous melanoma: unanswered questions about margin recommendations for primary cutaneous melanoma. J Natl Compr Canc Netw 2012;10:357–65.

7. Guadagnolo BA, Prieto V, Weber R, et al. The role of adjuvant radiotherapy in the local management of desmoplastic melanoma. Cancer 2013. [Epub ahead of print].

8. Strom T, Caudell JJ, Han D, et al. Radiotherapy influences local control in patients with desmoplastic melanoma. Cancer 2013. [Epub ahead of print].

9. Balch CM, Soong SJ, Smith T, et al. Long-term results of a prospective surgical trial comparing 2 cm vs. 4 cm excision margins for 740 patients with 1-4 mm melanomas. Ann Surg Oncol 2001;8:101–8.

10. Möller MG, Pappas-Politis E, Zager JS, et al. Surgical management of melanoma-in-situ using a staged marginal and central excision technique. Ann Surg Oncol 2009;16:1526–36.

11. Morton DL, Thompson JF, Cochran AJ, et al. Sentinel-node biopsy or nodal observation in melanoma. N Engl J Med 2006;355:1307–17.

12. Scheri RP, Essner R, Turner RR, et al. Isolated tumor cells in the sentinel node affect long-term prognosis of patients with melanoma. Ann Surg Oncol 2007; 14:2861–6.

13. Murali R, DeSilva C, McCarthy SW, et al. Sentinel lymph nodes containing very small (<0.1 mm) deposits of metastatic melanoma cannot be safely regarded as tumor-negative. Ann Surg Oncol 2012;19:1089–99.

14. Wagner JD, Schauwecker D, Davidson D, et al. Inefficacy of F-18 fluorodeoxy-D-glucose-positron emission tomography scans for initial evaluation in early-stage cutaneous melanoma. Cancer 2005;104:570–9.

15. El-Maraghi RH, Kielar AZ. PET vs sentinel lymph node biopsy for staging melanoma: a patient intervention, comparison, outcome analysis. J Am Coll Radiol 2008;5:924–31.

16. Sanki A, Uren RF, Moncrieff M, et al. Targeted high-resolution ultrasound is not an effective substitute for sentinel lymph node biopsy in patients with primary cutaneous melanoma. J Clin Oncol 2009;27:5614–9.

17. Chai CY, Zager JS, Szabunio MM, et al. Preoperative ultrasound is not useful for identifying nodal metastasis in melanoma patients undergoing sentinel node biopsy: preoperative ultrasound in clinically node-negative melanoma. Ann Surg Oncol 2012;19:1100–6.

18. Valsecchi ME, Silbermins D, de Rosa N, et al. Lymphatic mapping and sentinel lymph node biopsy in patients with melanoma: a meta-analysis. J Clin Oncol 2011;29:1479–87.

19. Wong SL, Balch CM, Hurley P, et al. Sentinel lymph node biopsy for melanoma: American Society of Clinical Oncology and Society of Surgical Oncology joint clinical practice guideline. J Clin Oncol 2012;30:2912–8.

20. Morton DL, Thompson JF, Cochran AJ, et al. Sentinel node biopsy or nodal observation in melanoma: final trial report. N Engl J Med 2014;370:599–609.

21. Cherpelis BS, Haddad F, Messina J, et al. Sentinel lymph node micrometastasis and other histologic factors that predict outcome in patients with thicker melanomas. J Am Acad Dermatol 2001;44:762–6.

22. Rondelli F, Vedovati MC, Becattini C, et al. Prognostic role of sentinel node biopsy in patients with thick melanoma: a meta-analysis. J Eur Acad Dermatol Venereol 2012;26:560–5.

23. Pasquali S, Haydu LE, Scolyer RA, et al. The importance of adequate primary tumor excision margins and sentinel node biopsy in achieving optimal locoregional control for patients with thick primary melanomas. Ann Surg 2013;258: 152–7.

24. McMasters KM, Noyes RD, Reintgen DS, et al. Lessons learned from the Sunbelt Melanoma Trial. J Surg Oncol 2004;86:212–23.

25. Balch CM, Gershenwald JE, Soong SJ, et al. Final version of 2009 AJCC melanoma staging and classification. J Clin Oncol 2009;27:6199–206.

26. Agnese DM, Abdessalam SF, Burak WE Jr, et al. Cost-effectiveness of sentinel lymph node biopsy in thin melanomas. Surgery 2003;134:542–7.

27. Han D, Zager JS, Shyr Y, et al. Clinicopathologic predictors of sentinel lymph node metastasis in thin melanoma. J Clin Oncol 2013;31:4387–93.

28. Han D, Yu D, Zhao X, et al. Sentinel node biopsy is indicated for thin melanomas $\geq$0.76 mm. Ann Surg Oncol 2012;19:3335–42.

29. Sondak VK, Taylor JM, Sabel MS, et al. Mitotic rate and younger age are predictors of sentinel lymph node positivity: lessons learned from the generation of a probabilistic model. Ann Surg Oncol 2004;11:247–58.

30. Gershenwald JE, Coit D, Sondak VK, et al. The challenge of defining guidelines for sentinel lymph node biopsy in patients with thin primary cutaneous melanomas. Ann Surg Oncol 2012;19:3301–3.

31. Pawlik TM, Ross MI, Prieto VG, et al. Assessment of the role of sentinel lymph node biopsy for primary cutaneous desmoplastic melanoma. Cancer 2006; 106:900–6.

32. Murali R, Shaw HM, Lai K, et al. Prognostic factors in cutaneous desmoplastic melanoma: a study of 252 patients. Cancer 2010;116:4130–8.

33. Han D, Zager JS, Yu D, et al. Desmoplastic melanoma: is there a role for sentinel lymph node biopsy? Ann Surg Oncol 2013;20:2345–51.

34. Reed D, Kudchadkar R, Zager JS, et al. Controversies in the evaluation and management of atypical melanocytic proliferations in children, adolescents and young adults. J Natl Compr Canc Netw 2013;11:679–86.

35. Han D, Zager JS, Han G, et al. The unique clinical characteristics of melanoma diagnosed in children. Ann Surg Oncol 2012;19:3888–95.

36. Mills OL, Marzban S, Zager JS, et al. Sentinel node biopsy in atypical melanocytic neoplasms in childhood: a single institution experience in 24 patients. J Cutan Pathol 2012;39:331–6.

37. Burmeister BH, Henderson MA, Ainslie J, et al. Adjuvant radiotherapy versus observation alone for patients at risk of lymph-node field relapse after therapeutic lymphadenectomy for melanoma: a randomised trial. Lancet Oncol 2012;13: 589–97.

38. van der Ploeg AP, van Akkooi AC, Haydu LE, et al. The prognostic significance of sentinel node tumour burden in melanoma patients: an international, multicenter study of 1539 sentinel node-positive melanoma patients. Eur J Cancer 2014;50:111–20.

39. Leung AM, Morton DL, Ozao-Choy J, et al. Staging of regional lymph nodes in melanoma: a case for including nonsentinel lymph node positivity in the American Joint Committee on Cancer staging system. JAMA Surg 2013;148:879–84.

40. Faries MB, Thompson JF, Cochran A, et al. The impact on morbidity and length of stay of early versus delayed complete lymphadenectomy in melanoma: results

of the Multicenter Selective Lymphadenectomy Trial (I). Ann Surg Oncol 2010;17: 3324–9.

41. Bronstein Y, Ng CS, Rohren E, et al. PET/CT in the management of patients with stage IIIC and IV metastatic melanoma considered candidates for surgery: evaluation of the additive value after conventional imaging. AJR Am J Roentgenol 2012;198:902–8.

42. Leung AM, Hari DM, Morton DL. Surgery for distant melanoma metastasis. Cancer J 2012;18:176–84.

43. McLoughlin JM, Zager JS, Sondak VK, et al. Treatment options for limited or symptomatic metastatic melanoma. Cancer Control 2008;15:239–47.

44. Howard JH, Thompson JF, Mozzillo N, et al. Metastasectomy for distant metastatic melanoma: analysis of data from the First Multicenter Selective Lymphadenectomy Trial (MSLT-I). Ann Surg Oncol 2012;19:2547–55.

45. Wevers KP, Hoekstra HJ. Stage IV melanoma: completely resectable patients are scarce. Ann Surg Oncol 2013;20:2352–6.

46. Sosman JA, Moon J, Tuthill RJ, et al. A phase II trial of complete resection for stage IV melanoma: results of Southwest Oncology Group (SWOG) clinical trial S9430. Cancer 2011;117:4740–6.

47. Hodi FS, O'Day SJ, McDermott DF, et al. Improved survival with ipilimumab in patients with metastatic melanoma. N Engl J Med 2010;363:711–23.

48. Robert C, Thomas L, Bondarenko I, et al. Ipilimumab plus dacarbazine for previously untreated metastatic melanoma. N Engl J Med 2011;364:2517–26.

49. Chapman PB, Hauschild A, Robert C, et al. Improved survival with vemurafenib in melanoma with BRAF V600E mutation. N Engl J Med 2011;364: 2507–16.

50. Hauschild A, Grob JJ, Demidov LV, et al. Dabrafenib in BRAF-mutated metastatic melanoma: a multicentre, open-label, phase 3 randomised controlled trial. Lancet 2012;380:358–65.

51. Hamid O, Robert C, Daud A, et al. Safety and tumor responses with lambrolizumab (anti-PD-1) in melanoma. N Engl J Med 2013;369:134–44.

52. Flaherty K, Infante JR, Daud A, et al. Combined BRAF and MEK inhibition in melanoma with BRAF V600 mutations. N Engl J Med 2012;367:1694–703.

53. Korn EL, Liu PY, Lee SJ, et al. Meta-analysis of phase II cooperative group trials in metastatic stage IV melanoma: determining progression-free and overall survival benchmarks for future phase II trials. J Clin Oncol 2008;26: 527–34.

54. Schadendorf D, Hodi FS, Robert C, et al. Pooled analysis of long-term survival data from phase II and phase III trials of ipilimumab in metastatic or locally advanced, unresectable melanoma [abstract]. European Cancer Congress 2013. Abstract 24.

55. Wolchok JD, Kluger H, Callahan MK, et al. Nivolumab plus ipilimumab in advanced melanoma. N Engl J Med 2013;369:122–33.

56. Shah GD, Socci ND, Gold JS, et al. Phase II trial of neoadjuvant temozolomide in resectable melanoma patients. Ann Oncol 2010;21:1718–22.

57. Moschos SJ, Edington HD, Land SR, et al. Neoadjuvant treatment of regional stage IIIB melanoma with high-dose interferon alfa-2b induces objective tumor regression in association with modulation of tumor infiltrating host cellular immune responses. J Clin Oncol 2006;24:3164–71.

58. Lewis KD, Robinson WA, McCarter M, et al. Phase II multicenter study of neoadjuvant biochemotherapy for patients with stage III malignant melanoma. J Clin Oncol 2006;24:3157–63.

59. Fadaki N, Cardona-Huerta S, Martineau L, et al. Inoperable bulky melanoma responds to neoadjuvant therapy with vemurafenib. BMJ Case Rep 2012;2012. pii:bcr2012007034.

60. Koers K, Francken AB, Haanen JB, et al. Vemurafenib as neoadjuvant treatment for unresectable regional metastatic melanoma. J Clin Oncol 2013;31:e251–3.

61. Kolar GR, Miller-Thomas MM, Schmidt RE, et al. Neoadjuvant treatment of a solitary melanoma brain metastasis with vemurafenib. J Clin Oncol 2013;31:e40–3.

62. Zager JS, Gibney GT, Kudchadkar R, et al. Neoadjuvant BRAF inhibition for locally or regionally advanced melanoma [abstract]. Pigment Cell Melanoma Res 2012;25:901 abstract 37.

63. Kirkwood JM, Manola J, Ibrahim J, et al. A pooled analysis of Eastern Cooperative Oncology Group and intergroup trials of adjuvant high-dose interferon for melanoma. Clin Cancer Res 2004;10:1670–7.

64. Mocellin S, Pasquali S, Rossi CR, et al. Interferon alpha adjuvant therapy in patients with high-risk melanoma: a systematic review and meta-analysis. J Natl Cancer Inst 2010;102:493–501.

65. Mocellin S, Lens MB, Pasquali S, et al. Interferon alpha for the adjuvant treatment of cutaneous melanoma. Cochrane Database Syst Rev 2013;(6):CD008955.

66. Sarnaik AA, Yu B, Yu D, et al. Extended dose ipilimumab with a peptide vaccine: immune correlates associated with clinical benefit in patients with resected high-risk stage IIIc/IV melanoma. Clin Cancer Res 2011;17:896–906.

67. Gibney GT, Weber JS, Kudchadkar RR, et al. Safety and efficacy of adjuvant anti-PD1 therapy (nivolumab) in combination with vaccine in resected high-risk metastatic melanoma [abstract]. J Clin Oncol 2013;31(Suppl). abstract 9056.

Melanoma Adjuvant Therapy

Ahmad A. Tarhini, MD, PhD[a],*, Prashanth M. Thalanayar, MD[b]

KEYWORDS

- Adjuvant • Melanoma • Interferon • Ipilimumab

KEY POINTS

- Adjuvant interferon-alfa is the current standard of care with demonstrable relapse-free survival and overall survival (high-dose regimen) benefit for high-risk melanoma.
- New agents like immune checkpoint inhibitors and targeted therapies are being actively investigated.
- Therapeutic predictive biomarker studies may further refine patient selection.

INTRODUCTION

Malignant melanoma is increasing in incidence at a faster rate than any other malignancy in the United States, where it currently represents the fifth most common cancer in men and the seventh most common cancer in women. In 2014, it is estimated that 76,100 patients will be diagnosed with melanoma in the United States, and about 9710 will die from this disease.[1] Careful surveillance in high-risk individuals, early diagnosis, and prompt surgical removal remain the mainstay of management of operable melanoma. For high-risk melanoma, adjuvant therapy targets micrometastatic disease, which is the source of future mortality from melanoma recurrence and presents an opportunity for curing this disease. Various modalities, including immunologic therapy, chemotherapy, and radiation therapy, have been tested in the adjuvant setting over the past 3 decades.

Clinical Predictors of Risk in Patients with Melanoma

The 2002 American Joint Committee on Cancer (AJCC) tumor, lymph node, and metastasis (TNM) staging system was updated in 2009 and new prognostic factors

Disclosure: Dr A.A. Tarhini has research grant funding from Merck and BMS, and he is a consultant (Advisory Board participation) for Merck, BMS, and Genentech.
[a] Department of Medicine, Division of Hematology-Oncology, University of Pittsburgh Cancer Institute, UPMC Cancer Pavilion, 5150 Centre Avenue (555), Pittsburgh, PA 15232, USA;
[b] Department of Internal Medicine, University of Pittsburgh Medical Center, 200 Lothrop Street, Pittsburgh, PA 15213, USA
* Corresponding author.
E-mail address: tarhiniaa@upmc.edu

Hematol Oncol Clin N Am 28 (2014) 471–489
http://dx.doi.org/10.1016/j.hoc.2014.02.004
0889-8588/14/$ – see front matter © 2014 Elsevier Inc. All rights reserved.

that have practical implications were added.[2] Stages I and II are grouped as localized melanoma that is restricted to the skin. Stage III is characterized by the presence of lymph node involvement and/or in-transit metastases, whereas stage IV comprises distant metastatic spread.

A vital factor for primary melanoma is the depth of the primary tumor (Breslow tumor thickness). Tumor thickness increases by every millimeter, and the survival rate declines (**Table 1**). In the presence of ulceration of the primary tumor, survival rates become proportionately lower than nonulcerated melanoma of equivalent T category but are similar to those of patients with a nonulcerated melanoma of the subsequent T category. Increased mitotic rate (at least 1 mitosis/mm^2) is strongly correlated with diminished survival rates. It has replaced the Clark level of invasion as a complementary criterion to ulceration for differentiating T1a versus T1b primary tumor.[2]

Involvement of regional lymph nodes or the presence of intralymphatic (satellite or in-transit) metastasis comprises stage III. The seventh edition of the AJCC staging system has no minimum threshold of lymphatic tumor burden defining the presence of regional nodal metastases. In particular, lymph node tumors of less than 0.2 mm that were ignored in the 2002 staging version were included because minute lymph node deposits (including detection by immunohistochemical staining) are thought to be relevant to recurrence and mortality. For the same T stage, the nodal subclassification N1a (micrometastasis) and N1b (macrometastasis) constitute stage IIIA and stage IIIB, respectively (**Table 2**). In-transit lymphatic metastases without and with metastatic lymph nodes correspond with N2c and N3, respectively.[2] This population of patients without distant spread of primary melanoma who are at high risk for recurrence and death is 3 times the size of the population with metastatic disease.

For advanced disease with metastasis to distant sites with specific attention to number and location, lactate dehydrogenase (LDH) blood levels are key to prognosis. One-year survival of patients with M1c disease (visceral metastases or any distant metastasis with high LDH) is 33%, compared with 62% for M1a melanomas (distant skin, subcutaneous, and lymph node metastases) and 53% for M1b melanomas (lung metastases).[2] Oligometastatic melanoma that is amenable to surgical removal may still have good survival rates if chosen appropriately.[3]

Indications for Adjuvant Therapy

Adjuvant therapy has been tested primarily in AJCC stages IIB, IIC, and III, in which maximal benefit has been proved. These patients have an estimated risk of recurrence

Table 1
Melanoma prognosis based on primary tumor depth and ulceration as derived from the seventh edition of the AJCC melanoma staging system

T Classification[2]	10-y Survival (%)
T1 = thickness ≤ 1 mm	92
T2 = thickness 1–2 mm	80
T3 = thickness 2–4 mm	63
T4 = thickness >4 mm	50
T4a = T4 nonulcerated (IIB)	71
T3b = T3 ulcerated (IIB)	68 (ulceration despite lesser tumor size affects prognosis)
T4b = T4 ulcerated (IIC)	53

Data from Balch CM, Gershenwald JE, Soong SJ, et al. Final version of 2009 AJCC melanoma staging and classification. J Clin Oncol 2009;27:6201.

Table 2
The impact of lymphatic metastases on melanoma survival as derived from the seventh edition of the AJCC melanoma staging system

Nodal Staging[2]	5-y Survival (%)
Any N1 (single metastatic node)	70
Any N2 (2–3 nodes)	30–50
Any N3 (>4 nodes/matted nodes/in-transit metastases/satellites with metastatic nodes)	39
IIIA	78
IIIB	59
IIIC	40

Data from Balch CM, Gershenwald JE, Soong SJ, et al. Final version of 2009 AJCC melanoma staging and classification. J Clin Oncol 2009;27:6203.

that exceeds 30% (ranging from 30% chance of recurrence for IIB to 60% chance of recurrence for IIIC).[2]

Immunotherapy with Interferon-alfa

The type I interferon (IFN) family includes IFN-α, IFN-beta, IFN-epsilon, IFN-kappa, and IFN-omega, whereas IFN-gamma alone constitutes the family of type II IFN. Among the IFNs, IFN-α2 has been the most widely studied clinically.

Mechanism

The IFN molecule is thought primarily to induce an immunomodulatory effect and less of a directly cytotoxic or antiangiogenic effect.[4] Research in IFN-α in the neoadjuvant setting has shown significant influence of IFN-α on signal transducer and activator of transcription (STAT) signaling and the histopathologic course of events that take place in the tumor. An influx of dendritic cells (DCs) and T lymphocytes into the tumor tissue was noted. The tumor upregulates STAT3 and there is subsequent elaboration of vascular endothelial growth factor (VEGF), tumor growth factor beta, and interleukin (IL)-10 among other mediators of immune tolerance. IFN-α downregulated STAT3 expression in tumor cells. Also, simultaneous induction of STAT1 in the lymph nodes was observed and this correlated with a reversal in T-cell signaling defects.[5]

IFN-α: Regimens Testing High-dose IFN-α

The impetus to study IFN-α in the adjuvant setting for high-risk resected melanomas was derived from the evidence of activity of IFN-α in the metastatic setting. **Table 3** summarizes phase II trials of IFN-α in metastatic melanoma. The first 2 randomized trials that studied the benefits of postsurgical adjuvant therapy for high-risk melanoma were the North Central Cancer Treatment Group (NCCTG) trial[6] and the Eastern Cooperative Group (ECOG) trial E1684.[7] Both trials tested high-dose IFN-α (HDI) (>10 million units [MU]/dose).

The ECOG E1684 trial was initiated in 1984 using a regimen consisting of intravenous (IV) HDI at 20 MU/m² for 5 consecutive days a week for 4 weeks as the induction phase followed by subcutaneous (SC) administration at 10 MU/m² thrice weekly for 48 weeks as maintenance. At a median follow-up of 6.9 years, 287 patients were studied in total, showing a statistically significant difference in relapse-free survival (RFS) and overall survival (OS) in favor of HDI compared with the observation arm. The estimated 5-year RFS in the treatment arm was 37% (95% confidence interval [CI], 30%–46%) versus 26% (95% CI, 19%–34%) in the control group. The 5-year OS

Table 3
Phase II trials of IFN-α for metastatic melanoma

Study Reference	Number of Enrolled Patients (Follow-up)	Therapy and IFN Subspecies	Dose: Treatment Arm (MU/m²)	Schedule: Treatment Arm	ORR	CR	PR
Ernstoff, 1983	17	IFN-α2b	10–100	5 d/wk × 1 mo	NA	NA	2
Creagan, 1984	23	IFN-α2a	50	Thrice weekly × 12 wk	20	1	5
Creagan, 1985	350	IFN-α2a + cimetidine	50	Thrice weekly × 12 wk	23	0	8
Creagan, 1984	31	IFN-α2a	12	Thrice weekly × 12 wk	23	3	4
Legha, 1987	62	IFN-α2a	First arm: escalating (3–36 × 10⁶ U/d) Second arm: fixed dose (18 × 10⁶ U/d)	First arm: daily during induction followed by thrice weekly Second arm: thrice weekly	First: 12.9% Second: 16.1%	First: 0 Second: 0	First: 9.7% Second: 6.5%
Hersey, 1985	200	IFN-α2a	15–50	Thrice weekly	10	2	0
Dorval, 1986	22	IFN-α2b	10	Thrice weekly	24	2	4
Neefe, 1990	97	IFN-α2a	Escalating: 3 to 36 × 10⁶ U	Daily for 10 d then 70 d total	8	6	2
Coates, 1986	15	IFN-α2a	20	5 d/wk every 2 wk	0	0	0

Abbreviations: CR, complete response; MU, million units; NA, not available; ORR, objective response rates; PR, partial response.

was 46% (95% CI, 39%–55%) versus 37% (95% CI, 30%–46%) in the treatment and observation arms, respectively. The greatest impact on survival was observed in patients with clinically node-negative but pathologically positive nodes (N1 disease). The outcomes of this trial led to regulatory approval by the United States Food and Drug Administration (FDA) in 1995.[7]

IFN-α: Other ECOG and Intergroup Trials Testing HDI

When weighed against these survival benefits, the toxicity profile of HDI as observed in E1684, with a 67% incidence for grade 3 toxicity, 9% incidence for grade 4 toxicity, and 2 early therapy-related hepatotoxic deaths, raised concerns over patients' endurance and adherence to this regimen. These concerns motivated investigators to study other forms or regimens that varied by dose level, route of administration, or duration of IFN-α therapy. **Table 4** lists the phase III adjuvant trials of IFN-α conducted in high-risk melanoma.

E1690

This trial conducted by the ECOG and the US Intergroup followed suit using the E1684 HDI regimen and compared its benefit with a low-dose regimen of IFN-α2b (LDI) at 3 MU SC thrice weekly for 2 years and a third arm consisting of patients who were observed without therapy (Obs). Accrual of patients in E1690 was completed between 1991 and 1995, and at 4.3 years median follow-up the 5-year estimated RFS rates were 44% for HDI, 40% for LDI, and 35% for the Obs arm.[8] The effect of HDI on RFS alone reached significance ($P = .03$). Neither HDI nor LDI established OS benefit compared with Obs (52% high dose vs 53% low dose vs 55% observation). However, improved OS of the E1690 Obs arm was notable compared with E1684 Obs arm (median 6 years vs 2.8 years). Although, unlike E1684, E1690 did not require elective lymph node dissection, a retrospective analysis showed evidence of crossover from the observation arm at regional nodal recurrence to IFN-α salvage therapy that may have affected the survival analysis in E1690.

E1694

This trial conducted by the US Intergroup compared HDI with a ganglioside vaccine, which was considered the optimal vaccine candidate at the time. The GMK vaccine consisted of purified ganglioside GM2 coupled to keyhole limpet hemocyanin (KLH) and combined with the QS-21 adjuvant. It was hypothesized that vaccination kindled antibodies against GM2 capable of exclusively attaching to GM2 and knocking off malignant melanocytes in vitro via complement or antibody-based cell-medicated cytotoxicity. HDI was superior compared with GMK with improved RFS (hazard ratio [HR], 1.47; $P = .001$) and OS (HR, 1.52; $P = .009$).[9]

E2696

E2696 was an ECOG-led, randomized, phase II that recruited 107 patients with surgically resected stage IIB, III, and IV disease that was conducted between 1998 and 2000.[10] The intent was to study the anti-GM2 antibody response to GMK vaccine in the presence versus absence of IFN. The study compared 3 arms: arm A (GMK plus concurrent HDI), arm B (GMK plus sequential HDI), and arm C (GMK alone). The combined approach reduced the risk of recurrence compared with GMK alone (HR 1.96 for C vs B and HR 1.75 for C vs A).

IFN-α: Other Doses, Routes and Durations Tested

The search for less toxic and more efficacious regimens led to multiple trials using other dosing ranges, routes of administration, durations of therapy, and formulations.

Table 4
Phase III studies of IFN-α for high-risk melanoma

Study Reference	Number of Patients Eligible for Analysis	TNM Stage	Therapy and IFN Subspecies	IFN Dose and Schedule: Treatment Arm	Median Follow-up at Time of Reporting (y)	DFS	OS	% Node Positive
High Dose								
NCCTG 83-7052 Creagan et al[6]	262	II–III (T2–T4N0M0/ T$_{any}$N+M0)	IFN-α2a vs observation	IM 20 MU/m² thrice weekly for 4 mo	6.1	NS	NS	61
ECOG E1684 Kirkwood et al[7]	287	II–III (T4N0M0/ T$_{any}$N+M0)	IFN-α2b: high dose (HDI) vs observation	IV 20 MU/m² 5 d a week for 4 wk and then SC 10MU/m² 3 d a week for 48 wk	6.9, 12.1	S	S (S at 6.9 y, NS at 12.1 y)	89
ECOG E1690 Kirkwood et al[8]	642	II–III (T4N0M0/ T$_{any}$N+M0)	IFN-α2b: high dose (HDI) vs low dose vs observation	High dose: IV 20 MU/m² 5 d a week for 4 wk and then SC 10 MU/m² 3 d a week for 48 wk. Low dose: SC 3 MU/m² 2 d a week for 2 y	4.3, 6.6	S	NS	75
ECOG E1694 Kirkwood et al[9]	774	II–III (T4N0M0/ T$_{any}$N+M0)	IFN-α2b: high dose (HDI) vs GMK vaccine	IV 20 MU/m² 5 d a week for 4 wk and then SC 10 MU/m² 2 d a week for 48 wk	1.3, 2.1	S	S	77
Italian Melanoma Intergroup Chiarion-Sileni et al[12]	330	III (T$_{any}$N1–N3M0)	Intensified IFN-α2b (IHDI) every other month vs IFN-α2b high dose (HDI) for 1 y	IHDI: IV 20 MU/m² 5 d/wk for 4 wk every other month for 4 cycles. Standard HDI: IV 20 MU/m² 5 d/wk for 4 wk then SC 10 MU/m² 3 d/wk for 48 wk	5.0	NS	NS	100
Intermediate Dose								
EORTC 18952 Eggermont et al[20]	1388	II–III (T4N0M0/ T$_{any}$N+M0)	IFN-α2b for 1 y vs 2 y vs observation	IV 10 MU 5 d a week for 4 wk and then SC 10 MU 3 d a week for 1 y Or SC 5 MU 3 d a week for 2 y	4.65	NS	NS	74

Trial	N	Stage	Comparison	Schedule	Follow-up (y)	DFS	OS	%
EORTC 18991 Eggermont et al[21]	1256	III (T_any N+M0)	PEG–IFN-α2b vs observation	SC 6 μg/kg/wk for 8 wk and then SC 3 μg/kg/wk for 5 y	3.8	S	NS	100
Low Dose								
Austrian Melanoma Cooperative Group Pehamberger et al[24]	311	II (T2–T4N0M0)	IFN-α2a vs observation	SC 3 MU 7 d a week for 3 wk and then SC 3 MU 3 d a week for 1 y	3.4 (mean)	S	NS	0
French Melanoma Cooperative Group Grob et al[22]	499	II (T2–T4N0M0)	IFN-α2a vs observation	SC 3 MU 3 d a week for 3 y	>3	0.74 (HR), S	0.70 (HR), S	0
WHO-16 Cascinelli et al[16]	444	III (T_any N+M0)	IFN-α2a vs observation	SC 3 MU 3 d a week for 3 y	7.3	NS	NS	100
Scottish Melanoma Cooperative Group Cameron et al[18]	96	II–III (T3–T4N0M0/ T_any N+M0)	IFN-α2a vs observation	SC 3 MU 3 d a week for 6 mo	6.5	NS	NS	NA
EORTC 18871/DKG-80 Kleeberg et al[15]	728	II–III (T3–T4N0M0/ T_any N+M0)	IFN-α2b vs IFN-γ vs ISCADOR M vs observation	IFN-α2b: SC 1 MU every other day for 12 mo; IFN-γ: SC 0.2 mg every other day for 12 mo; ISCADOR M®	8.2	NS; NS; NS	NS; NS; NS	58
UKCCCR/AIM-HIGH Hancock et al[17]	674	II–III (T3–T4N0M0/ T_any N+M0)	IFN-α2a vs observation	SC 3 MU 3 d a week for 2 y	3.1	NS	NS	70
DeCOG Hauschild et al[19]	840	III (T3_any N+M0)	IFN-α2a for 18 mo (A) vs 3 y (B)	SC 3 MU 3 d a week for 18 mo vs 3 y	4.3	NS	NS	18
DeCOG Garbe et al[23]	441	III (T_any N+M0)	IFN-α2a (A) vs IFN-α2a + DTIC (B) vs observation (C)	SC 3 MU 3 d a week for 24 mo (A) vs SC 3 MU 3 d a week for 24 mo + DTIC 850 mg/m² every 4–8 wk for 24 mo (B) vs	3.9	S	NS	100

Abbreviations: DFS, disease-free survival; NA, not available; NS, not significant.

Although the Sunbelt Melanoma Trial studied lymph node dissection (LND) versus LND plus standard HDI,[11] the Italian Melanoma Group trial studied a shorter duration of a more intense course of IFN than the standard regimen,[12] with no statistically significant differences seen.

Hellenic trial

The Hellenic Oncology Group intended to test the hypothesis that the IV induction phase of the HDI regimen was the most important part of the regimen and was sufficient in exerting the therapeutic impact of HDI in high-risk melanoma.[13] In the phase III He 13A/98 study, patients were randomized between 1998 and 2004 to a modified induction phase of 15 MU/m^2 HDI only versus the same induction phase followed by a modified maintenance phase of 10 MU (not per square meter) thrice weekly for a year. With 182 patients per arm, and a median follow-up of 5.25 years, the analysis in 2009 revealed no statistically significant difference in either median RFS or OS. However, the study was criticized for the modified regimen used and the small sample size to allow it to show a clinically significant difference.

E1697

US Intergroup study E1697 tested a similar hypothesis among patients with resectable intermediate risk melanoma ($\geq$T3 or any thickness with microscopic nodal disease N1a–N2a). Between 1998 and 2010, the study recruited 1150 patients and randomized them to either 4 weeks of HDI (20 MU/m^2/d for 5 days weekly) or observation.[14] In 2010, a third interim analysis deemed the study futile and the study was closed. When presented to American Society of Clinical Oncology (ASCO) in 2011, the study reported no impact on either RFS or OS with this 4-week regimen. The results of this trial supported the E1684 HDI 1-year regimen as the standard for high-risk melanoma.

Other trials have investigated less intensive regimens for the dosing of IFN-α. These trials included low-doses (1 MU SC every other day) tested in the European Organization for Research and Treatment of Cancer (EORTC) 18871 trial (stage IIB, IIIA),[15] low doses ($\leq$3 MU SC thrice weekly) tested in the World Health Organization (WHO) Melanoma Trial 16 (stage III),[16] E1690 (T4, N1),[8] the UKCCCR AIM-HIGH trial (stage IIB/III),[17] a Scottish trial (stage IIB, III),[18] and the 2010 German Dermatologic Cooperative Group (DeCOG) study (T3$_{any}$N).[19] Intermediate dose regimens (5–10 MU/m^2) were tested in the EORTC 18952 (T4 N1-2)[20] and EORTC 18991 (TxN1)[21] studies. Although these trials showed benefit in RFS for the IFN arms, this impact was lost with time. Support for this observation also comes from the French multicenter trial, which indicated that the effect of IFN-α on RFS was lost on cessation of treatment.[22]

EORTC 18952

This trial[20] enrolled 1388 patients with stage IIB/III disease to 4 weeks of induction with 10 MU IV 5 times a week, followed by one of 2 maintenance regimens" SC 10 MU 3 days a week for 1 year versus SC 5 MU 3 days a week for 2 years. The third arm was an observation control arm. The study was conducted from 1996 to 2000. At 4.65 years median follow-up, the results showed a statistically insignificant 7.2% increase in distant metastasis-free interval (47% vs 43% and 40% respectively) and a 5.4% increase in OS (53% in the 2-year arm compared with 48% each in the 1-year and observation arms). The increase in OS was observed only in patients treated for 25 months with 5 MU IFN-α2b and not in those treated for 13 months with 10 MU IFN-α2b. These results suggest that the duration of therapy might be more important than the dose.

DeCOG

In 2008, a randomized phase III DeCOG trial[23] studied a combination of LDI/dacarbazine (DTIC) versus LDI alone. Analysis at 4 years median follow-up revealed that the low-dose IFN group showed an improvement in disease-free survival (DFS) (HR, 0.69) and OS (HR, 0.62). However, the trial was designed to find whether DTIC adds any benefit to IFN-α and not whether LDI was superior to observation. These results do not match the earlier trials that tested LDI (ie, the Austrian Melanoma Cooperative Group trial and French Melanoma Cooperative Group trial[22,24]), which showed no OS benefit for LDI. Unlike in North America, LDI therapy has been approved as an adjuvant therapy for stage II patients by the European Medicines Agency in Europe. Regional differences exist in Europe in the adjuvant use of IFN. High-dose IFN regimens are not used in Europe as commonly as in the United States.

Pegylated IFN

EORTC 18991

Pegylated (peg) IFN-α as tested in this trial achieved regulatory approval for use as adjuvant therapy for high-risk melanoma with lymph node metastases.[21] The covalent bonding of the IFN molecule with a polyethylene glycol moiety results in sustained absorption and longer half-life. The EORTC 18991 trial studied the efficacy and safety of peg–IFN-α2b versus observation among 1256 patients recruited from 2000 to 2002 with resected AJCC stage III melanoma. The regimen comprised an induction dose of peg-IFN SC 6 μg/kg a week for 8 weeks followed by maintenance dose of once-weekly SC injections at 3 μg/kg for up to 5 years. At 7.6 years median follow-up, the group released data that showed an improved RFS in the treatment arm (HR, 0.87; 95% CI, 0.76–1.00; $P = .05$) with no difference in OS/distant metastases free survival (DMFS) between observation and treatment groups. Subset analysis indicated that subjects with microscopic nodal metastasis and ulcerated primary tumor had the greatest benefit in terms of RFS, OS, and DMFS. During the study, peg-IFN was discontinued for toxicity in 37% of patients.

IFN-α: Meta-analyses

At least 4 different systematic reviews and meta-analyses on adjuvant therapy have been published from 2002 to 2010. The largest was a 2010 meta-analysis from Mocellin and colleagues[25] that included randomized controlled trials published between 1990 and 2008 covering 8122 patients, of whom 4362 subjects had received IFN-α. In 12 of the 14 studies included, IFN-α was tested against observation, and 17 different comparisons were established. In subgroup analysis, no specific regimen, dosing, formulation, study design, or staging provided any difference in overall HR estimates. Four of 14 comparators revealed a statistically significant OS benefit with IFN-α. The review concluded that adjuvant IFN-α therapy showed a statistically significant 18% risk reduction for recurrence (HR, 0.82; 95% CI, 0.77–0.87; $P<.001$) and 11% risk reduction for death (HR, 0.89; 95% CI, 0.83–0.96; $P = .002$).

Predictors of Benefit and Prognostic Markers

The consistent but modest beneficial effect of adjuvant IFN-α has been well shown, but it also comes at the expense of significant toxicity and cost. Hence, there is a need to focus treatment on patients who are most likely to benefit from adjuvant IFN-α therapy, as was noted in some of the trials. After the Wheatley meta-analysis and later a subset analysis of EORTC 18991 revealed specific benefit among patients with ulcerated primary tumors, some focus has been placed on targeting such patient groups in clinical trials including the ongoing EORTC 18081.[25] This trial will study adjuvant peg-IFN for 2 years versus observation in patients with an ulcerated primary cutaneous melanoma with T(2–4)b, N0, M0 melanoma.[26]

Gogas and colleagues[27] in 2006 reported a prospectively validated analysis of autoimmunity as a biomarker associated with IFN-α benefit. Also, our group at the University of Pittsburgh and ECOG studied these data from the E2696 and E1694 trials to further understand the newly found association between autoimmune-related side effects and improved outcomes with IFN-α. A landmark analysis of E1694 revealed a trend toward a survival advantage associated with HDI-induced autoimmunity in stage III patients treated with HDI. In both trials, the presence of autoantibodies in sera of patients was significantly more frequent in the HDI arm compared with the vaccine arm. However, the development of autoimmunity occurs over a period of up to 1 year and therefore cannot be used as a baseline or early on-treatment predictor of IFN-α therapeutic benefit.[28] We are currently testing the immunogenic predictors of autoimmunity associated with IFN-α in the context of the E1697 trial as potential predictors of IFN-α therapeutic benefits. The expression of methylthioadenosine phosphorylase, which plays a significant role in the activity of STAT1, has shown an association with improved OS and RFS, as noted in a retrospective study from Meyer and colleagues.[29] Accumulating data reinforce the importance of the relative balance of phosphoSTAT1 (pSTAT1)/pSTAT3 in the tumor microenvironment. Serum markers of interest include S100B, melanoma-inhibiting activity, and tumor-associated antigen 90 immune complex (TA90IC).[4] Tarhini and colleagues,[28] showed that a high or increasing serum level of S100B is an independent prognostic marker of risk for mortality in patients with high-risk disease, as tested in the context of the E1694 trial.

ADJUVANT RADIATION THERAPY

In melanoma, radiotherapy (RT) is rarely indicated in the primary tumor setting. Contrary to past belief that melanoma is a radio-resistant tumor, in vitro studies of melanoma cell lines have showcased radiation responsiveness, although this may widely differ within the same tumor, and that melanoma may require higher-than-standard doses per radiation fraction for effective cytodestruction.[30]

Despite wide excision of primary tumor and complete LND, the risk of local relapse for stage III is 15% to 20% and it is even higher, at about 30% to 50%, for patients with high-risk features: extracapsular lymph node extension, positive margins, involvement of 4 or more nodes, bulky disease (exceeding 3 cm in size), cervical lymph node location, and recurrent disease.[30] In these cases, adjuvant RT may be valuable for local disease control. Data from multiple nonrandomized trials are available but inconsistent. Nevertheless, a few have shown some positive progress in the adjuvant setting and have generally indicated that adjuvant RT was associated with improved local and regional control rates without OS benefit. As in prostate and breast cancer, hypofractionation of radiation therapy seems to be as efficacious as standard radiation dosing in melanoma.[30]

A retrospective study published in 2003 by Ballo and colleagues,[31] from MD Anderson Cancer Center involving 160 patients who had surgery followed by radiotherapy (30 Gy in 6-Gy fractions 2 times per week) showed 10-year local, regional, and locoregional control rates of 94%, 94%, and 91%, respectively. Other results were 10-year disease-specific, disease-free, and distant metastasis-free survival rates of 48%, 42%, and 43%, respectively. Another retrospective study was published by Agrawal and colleagues[32] in 2009, who studied patients from Roswell Park and MDACC with clinically advanced, regional lymph node–metastatic disease (n = 615). It compared surgery plus adjuvant radiotherapy with surgery alone and showed a reduction in the regional recurrence rate (10.2% vs 40.6%); furthermore, adjuvant radiotherapy was significantly associated with 5-year regional control (P<.0001), distant metastasis-free survival (P = .0006), and disease-specific survival (P<.0001). Retrospective data from Strojan and colleagues[33] published in 2010 showed considerable improvement in local relapse control at 2 years by using adjuvant radiotherapy (60 Gy in 2-Gy fractions 5 times a week) compared with surgery alone (78% vs 56%; P = .015) among patients with regionally advanced melanoma to the neck and/or parotid. A more recent randomized trial, ANZMTG 01.01/TROG 02.01 (Australia New Zealand Melanoma Trial Group/Trans-Tasman Oncology Group)[34] compared adjuvant radiotherapy (48 Gy in 20 fractions) with observation, following lymphadenectomy among 217 patients with nodal metastases and a high risk of recurrence (based on number of nodes involved, extranodal spread, and maximum size of involved nodes). After a median follow-up of 40 months, the risk of lymph node field relapse was reduced in the adjuvant radiotherapy group (20 relapses in RT vs 34 in observation; HR, 0.56; 95% CI, 0.32–0.98; P = .041). However, there were no statistically significant differences in RFS or OS. **Table 5** lists various retrospective studies in adjuvant radiotherapy for melanoma.[35–40] Recent guidelines from the National Comprehensive Cancer Network support the application of adjuvant radiotherapy, based on lower level evidence.

TRIALS TESTING OTHER ADJUVANT AGENTS
Chemotherapy

Agents like DTIC, bacille Calmette-Guérin (BCG), and levamisole have been tested in the adjuvant setting.[41–44] A few of the trials are summarized in **Table 6**. In summary, chemotherapy with or without combination therapy with other modalities has not shown any improvement in either DFS or OS in any randomized controlled trial to date.

Biochemotherapy

The South West Oncology Group[45] intergroup study S0008 was a phase III adjuvant melanoma study in high-risk, node-positive patients that assessed whether a biochemotherapy (BCT) regimen administered over 9 weeks was more effective than the standard 52-week high-dose IFN (HDI) regimen. The BCT regimen consisted of 3 cycles of cisplatin, vinblastine, and DTIC combined with low doses of IL-2 and IFN-α. At a median follow-up of about 6 years, there was significant improvement in RFS for BCT compared with HDI (median 4.0 years vs 1.9 years), but no improvement in OS and higher grade III/IV toxicity for the BCT group than the HDI group (76% vs 64%). Patients on the HDI arm were more frequently followed during therapy as clinically indicated with IFN-α, whereas patients receiving BCT were seen every 3 months following completion of the 9-week BCT regimen. It is not clear whether this imbalance of early follow-up between the HDI and BCT arms may have affected the RFS outcome. Multiple other agents that have been tested in small nonrandomized trials include vitamin A, megestrol acetate, BCG, *Corynebacterium parvum*, and transfer factor, with no demonstrable benefits.

Immunotherapy with Vaccines

Vaccines in melanoma can be grouped based on the type of antigens incorporated: peptide, ganglioside, and whole cell/cell lysate. Examples of peptide vaccines include vaccination with MART-1/Melan-A, gp100, and tyrosinase peptides that are melanocyte lineage antigens identified by cytotoxic T lymphocytes with the help of HLA-A2 eliciting an antigen-specific cytotoxic T-cell response.

Table 5
Clinical trials testing adjuvant radiation therapy

Name of Trial	Comparison Groups	High-risk Criteria	Dosing RT	RC	Survival/Response
Randomized Controlled Trials					
ANZMTG 1-02/TROG 02.01 Burmeister et al,[34] 2012 n = 217	Observation vs adjuvant RT (2002-2007)	Involvement of parotid ≥1 LN+, or axilla ≥2 LN+, or groin ≥3 LN+, or ECE+, or LN size neck ≥3 cm or axilla/groin ≥4 cm	RT to nodal basin 48 Gy/20 fx	SS HR = 0.56, (95% CI, 0.32–0.98) P = .04	NS
Mayo Clinic Creagan et al,[35] 1978 n = 56	Observation vs adjuvant RT (1972–1977)	Nodal disease with primary on trunk, extremities, or unknown primary	RT 25 Gy/14 fx, then 3–4 wk gap and then 50 Gy over 28 d	—	NS
Retrospective and Prospective Trials					
Queensland Radium Institute, Australia Burmeister et al,[36] 1995 n = 57	1989–1993	Nonspecific nodal disease	Variety of RT schedules	RC 88%	Response rates 84%
Peter MacCallum Institute, Australia Corry et al,[37] 1999 n = 113	1985–95	With/without residual disease after surgery	Adjuvant RT 50/25 Gy or 60/30 Gy	RC 78%	5-y OS 33%
Sydney Melanoma Unit Stevens et al,[38] 2000 n = 174	1989–1998	Stage I–III	30–36 Gy in 5–7 fractions	RC 89%	5-y OS 41%
MD Anderson Ballo et al,[39] 2006 n = 466	1983–2003	Any nodal metastasis treated with LND/chemotherapy	30 Gy in 5 fractions	5-y RC 89%	DFS 42%, DMFS 44%
TROG 96.06 Burmeister et al,[40] 2006 n = 234	Prospective (1989–2001)	Nodal metastasis or soft tissue disease in nodal basin	48 Gy in 20 fractions	5-y RC 91%	5-y PFS 27%, OS 36%
MDACC and Roswell Park Agrawal et al,[32] 2009 n = 615	Observation (106) vs adjuvant RT (509) (1983–2003)	Patients meeting Ballo criteria	30 Gy in 5 fractions	RC: 90% in RT group vs 60% in Obs group (SS)	DSS 30% in Obs vs 51% in RT (SS)

Ballo criteria[31]: For most patients: ECE+, LN greater than or equal to 3 cm, 4+ LN+, recurrent disease.
For cervical patients: ECE+, smaller LNs, fewer LNs, recurrent disease.
For groin patients: 2 of the high-risk features.
For greater than 10 LN+: 2 of the high-risk features, because their risk of systemic disease is high.
Abbreviations: DSS, disease-specific survival; ECE+, extracapsular extension; fx, fractionation; LN+, lymph node metastasis; Obs, observation after surgical resection; RC, regional control; SS, statistically significant.

Table 6 Phase II/III adjuvant studies of chemotherapeutic agents in melanoma					
Study Reference	Number of Patients Eligible for Analysis (Follow-up)	TNM Stage	Treatment Arm	Median Follow-up at Time of Reporting (y)	OS
Veronesi et al,[41] 1982	931	II/III	DTIC BCG DTIC + BCG Obs	5	NS
Lejeune et al,[42] 1988	325	I, IIA, IIB	DTIC Levamisole placebo	4	NS
Fisher et al,[43] 1981	181	II/III	CCNU Obs	3	NS
Koops et al,[44] 1998	632	II/III	Isolated limb perfusion + hyperthermia Obs	6.4	NS

Abbreviation: CCNU, Lomustine.

The MAGE antigens constitute a family of tumor antigens that are expressed in a few cancers, including melanoma, but are not expressed in normal tissues other than testis and placenta. Adjuvant MAGE-A3 protein is being tested in a randomized phase III trial (DERMA) based on promising results from a previous study in advanced melanoma.[46] The Melacine vaccine trial conducted in the United States showed some promise initially, but failed to sustain it. An Australian study using vaccinia viral lysates in high-risk subjects following resection also showed a statistically insignificant increase in RFS.[47] Gangliosides are sialic acid–containing glycosphingolipids that are overexpressed on the surface of melanoma cells. The E1694 trial, which tested GM2 with BCG and with KLH and a QS-21 adjuvant (GMK), as discussed earlier, showed no therapeutic impact for the vaccine.[9]

A phase III trial for resected stage III/IV melanoma compared a polyvalent vaccine known as Canvaxin with BCG vaccination. DFS and OS were worse in the Canvaxin group, likely because of vaccine-induced immunosuppression.[48]

MODALITIES OF THE NEAR FUTURE: UNDER TRIAL
Immunotherapy with Anti–Cytotoxic T-Lymphocyte Antigen 4 Antibodies

Cytotoxic T-lymphocyte antigen 4 (CTLA-4) competes with CD28 for binding B7 on antigen presenting cells and serves as a key inhibitory checkpoint in self-regulating the adaptive immune response. The role of the anti–CTLA-4 monoclonal antibodies was first studied in advanced disease and they were later brought into trials conducted in the adjuvant setting.

Ipilimumab (Medarex Inc/Bristol-Myers Squibb) is a fully humanized immunoglobulin G1 kappa monoclonal antibody that barricades CTLA-4. It has achieved FDA and European regulatory approval for treating advanced melanoma as both first-line and second-line options. The phase III MDX010-20 trial compared ipilimumab alone (3 mg/kg dose), ipilimumab plus a peptide vaccine, and vaccine plus placebo.[49] The trial showed a statistically significant survival benefit for ipilimumab compared with the Gp100 peptide vaccine comparator. The next positive phase III study, CA 184-024, compared ipilimumab (at 10 mg/kg) plus dacarbazine with dacarbazine plus placebo.[50] Adjuvant ipilimumab trials that are underway include the US

Intergroup E1609 trial testing ipilimumab at 3 mg/kg or 10 mg/kg versus HDI and the EORTC 18071 trial investigating ipilimumab at 10 mg/kg against placebo (**Table 7**).

Other Future Concepts

Immunotherapy with anti–programmed death 1 and anti–programmed death L1 agents

Contrary to CTLA-4 blockade, which happens during the initial phase of antigen presentation, programmed death (PD) 1 physiology plays a significant role at the tumor end of the T-cell interaction. The PD-1 receptor is expressed by T cells during long-term antigen exposure and regulates the effector phase of T-cell responses. PD-1 and PD-L1 blockade are subjects of ongoing research and multiple phase I to III trials. In the near future, these agents will be part of trials testing adjuvant therapy.

Targeted therapy with inhibitors of BRAF

Activating mutations have been observed in the BRAF gene of around 40% to 50% of melanomas. Between 80% and 90% are V600E mutations in which glutamic acid has substituted for valine at the V600 locus. BRAF phosphorylates regulatory serine residues on MEK1 and MEK2 and hence mutation of BRAF activates the RAS/RAF/MEK/ERK pathway leading to tumor proliferation. Vemurafenib and dabrafenib have both achieved regulatory approval based on significant phase III trial impact on RFS and OS.[51] Trials are underway testing both vemurafenib (monotherapy) and dabrafenib (in combination with trametinib) as adjuvant therapy in high-risk melanoma.

NEOADJUVANT THERAPY

The term neoadjuvant usually refers to preoperative therapy offered to patients with disease that is difficult to resect surgically, in an attempt to downstage the tumor and improve surgical operability. Given the unique immunogenicity of melanoma, there is greater interest in pursuing immunotherapy in the neoadjuvant setting.

Various chemotherapeutic and biochemotherapeutic regimens have been investigated in phase II studies in the neoadjuvant setting for IIIB/IVA disease. These studies included 3 or more cycles of chemotherapy (dacarbazine, cisplatin, and vinblastine) plus immunomodulators like interleukin (IL)-2 and IFN-α, and objective responses were seen. However, the phase III trials (E3695 and EORTC 18951) that compared them with single-agent chemotherapy showed no significant benefit in either progression-free survival (PFS) or response rate along with significant toxicity.[52,53] Moschos and colleagues[5] tested the effect of HDI in patients with stage IIIB/C disease who underwent biopsy followed by induction HDI (IV 20 MU/m^2 5 days a week for 4 weeks) followed by completion LND and subsequent maintenance HDI (SC 10 MU/m^2 3 days a week for 48 weeks). Among 20 patients studied, 3 had pathologic complete responses (CRs) and 8 had partial responses (PRs) for an objective response rate of 55%. Responders had significantly greater intratumoral (CD3+/CD11+) monocyte-derived dendritic cells and evidence of withdrawal of immune tolerance.[54]

Tarhini and colleagues,[55] studied neoadjuvant ipilimumab in patients with locally and regionally advanced melanoma. Following pretreatment biopsies, induction ipilimumab (IV 10 mg/kg) was given on days 1 and 21 followed by radical regional lymphadenectomy after at least 2 weeks. Two to 4 weeks after surgery, 2 more doses of maintenance ipilimumab (IV 10 mg/kg) were given at 3-week intervals. At 14-month median follow-up, data presented at ASCO 2012 revealed a median PFS of 15.5 months. In addition, significant immunomodulatory findings were reported, such as the downregulation of myeloid-derived suppressor cells in the circulation

Table 7
Ongoing adjuvant trials in high-risk melanoma

Study Reference	No of Patients	TNM Stage	Therapy	Dose and Schedule: Treatment Arm	Primary End Point	ClinicalTrials.gov Identifier
EORTC 18071	950	III (T_{any} N+ except in-transit, M0)	Ipilimumab vs placebo	IV, 10 mg/kg, 4× every 21 d, then starting from week 24 every 12 wk until week 156 or progression, 3 y	RFS	NCT00636168
US Intergroup E1609	1500	III (IIIB, IIIC), IV (M1a, M1b)	Ipilimumab at 10 mg/kg (arm A) or 3 mg/kg (arm C) Vs IFNα (arm B)	IV, 10 mg/kg (A) or 3 mg/kg (C), 4× every 21 d, then starting from week 24 every 12 wk 4× Vs IV 20 MU/m² 5 d a week for 4 wk, then SC 10 MU/m² 3 d a week for 48 wk	RFS and OS	NCT01274338
COMBI-AD	852	III BRAF V600E/K mutation positive	Dabrafenib + trametinib vs placebo	Dabrafenib (150 mg twice daily) and trametinib (2 mg once daily) orally for 12 mo	RFS	NCT01682083
BRIM-8	725	IIC, III BRAF V600 mutation positive by cobas	Vemurafenib vs placebo	Vemurafenib 960 mg orally twice daily for 52 wk	DFS	NCT01667419
DERMA	1349	IIIB or IIIC (tumor expression of MAGE-A3 gene)	GSK 2132231A (D1/3-MAGE-3-His fusion protein) vs placebo	GSK 2132231A IM solution, 13 injections over 27 mo	DFS	NCT00796445

and the tumor microenvironment as well as the induction of tumor-specific T-cell responses and T-cell memory, which were associated with clinical benefit.

SUMMARY

HDI has shown significant reduction in the risk of recurrence and death compared with observation (E1684) and the GMK vaccine (E1694), but it is also associated with significant toxicity and cost. Based on the RFS benefit seen in the EORTC 18991 trial, peg-IFN recently received regulatory approval as adjuvant therapy in node-positive disease. In the most recent and largest meta-analysis of adjuvant IFN-α trials, IFN-α was associated with an 18% risk reduction in recurrence and 11% risk reduction in mortality.[25] Ongoing adjuvant trials are testing ipilimumab CTLA-4 blockade therapy (EORTC 18071 and E1609), BRAF inhibitors (BRIM-8 and COMBI-AD), and MAGE-A3 vaccine (DERMA). Although it has recently been announced that the DERMA trial did not reach its primary end point of RFS, the results of EORTC 18071 are expected in the first quarter of 2014. Research in identifying specific populations that benefit the most from adjuvant systemic therapy is ongoing and is key to identifying therapeutic predictive biomarkers. Adjuvant trials using anti–PD-1 antibody therapy are in the planning phase.

REFERENCES

1. Siegel R, Ma J, Zou Z, et al. Cancer statistics, 2014. CA Cancer J Clin 2014; 64(1):9–29.
2. Balch CM, Gershenwald JE, Soong SJ, et al. Final version of 2009 AJCC melanoma staging and classification. J Clin Oncol 2009;27:6199–206.
3. Sosman JA, Moon J, Tuthill RJ, et al. A phase 2 trial of complete resection for stage IV melanoma: results of Southwest Oncology Group Clinical Trial S9430. Cancer 2011;117:4740-06.
4. Tarhini AA, Gogas H, Kirkwood JM. IFN-alpha in the treatment of melanoma. J Immunol 2012;189:3789–93.
5. Moschos SJ, Edington HD, Land SR, et al. Neoadjuvant treatment of regional stage IIIB melanoma with high-dose interferon alfa-2b induces objective tumor regression in association with modulation of tumor infiltrating host cellular immune responses. J Clin Oncol 2006;24:3164–71.
6. Creagan ET, Dalton RJ, Ahmann DL, et al. Randomized, surgical adjuvant clinical trial of recombinant interferon alfa-2a in selected patients with malignant melanoma. J Clin Oncol 1995;13:2776–83.
7. Kirkwood JM, Strawderman MH, Ernstoff MS, et al. Interferon alfa-2b adjuvant therapy of high-risk resected cutaneous melanoma: the Eastern Cooperative Oncology Group Trial EST 1684. J Clin Oncol 1996;14:7–17.
8. Kirkwood JM, Ibrahim JG, Sondak VK, et al. High- and low-dose interferon alfa-2b in high-risk melanoma: first analysis of intergroup trial E1690/S9111/C9190. J Clin Oncol 2000;18:2444–58.
9. Kirkwood JM, Ibrahim JG, Sosman JA, et al. High-dose interferon alfa-2b significantly prolongs relapse-free and overall survival compared with the GM2-KLH/QS-21 vaccine in patients with resected stage IIB-III melanoma: results of intergroup trial E1694/S9512/C509801. J Clin Oncol 2001;19:2370–80.
10. Kirkwood JM, Ibrahim J, Lawson DH, et al. High-dose interferon alfa-2b does not diminish antibody response to GM2 vaccination in patients with resected melanoma: results of the Multicenter Eastern Cooperative Oncology Group Phase II Trial E2696. J Clin Oncol 2001;19:1430–6.

11. Chao C, Wong SL, Ross MI, et al. Patterns of early recurrence after sentinel lymph node biopsy for melanoma. Am J Surg 2002;184:520–4 [discussion: 5].

12. Chiarion-Sileni V, Guida M, Romanini A, et al. Intensified high-dose intravenous interferon alpha 2b (IFNa2b) for adjuvant treatment of stage III melanoma: a randomized phase III Italian Melanoma Intergroup (IMI) trial [ISRCTN75125874]. J Clin Oncol (ASCO Annual Meeting Abstracts) 2011; 29(Suppl 15):8506.

13. Gogas H, Bafaloukos D, Ioannovich J, et al. Tolerability of adjuvant high-dose interferon alfa-2b: 1 month versus 1 year–a Hellenic Cooperative Oncology Group study. Anticancer Res 2004;24:1947–52.

14. Agarwala SS, Lee SJ, Flaherty LE, et al. Randomized phase III trial of high-dose interferon alfa-2b (HDI) for 4 weeks induction only in patients with intermediate- and high-risk melanoma (intergroup trial E 1697), 2011 ASCO Annual Meeting Abstracts. J Clin Oncol 2011;29:8505.

15. Kleeberg UR, Suciu S, Brocker EB, et al. Final results of the EORTC 18871/DKG 80-1 randomised phase III trial. rIFN-alpha2b versus rIFN-gamma versus ISCADOR M versus observation after surgery in melanoma patients with either high-risk primary (thickness >3 mm) or regional lymph node metastasis. Eur J Cancer 2004;40:390–402.

16. Cascinelli N, Bufalino R, Morabito A, et al. Results of adjuvant interferon study in WHO melanoma programme. Lancet 1994;343:913–4.

17. Hancock BW, Wheatley K, Harris S, et al. Adjuvant interferon in high-risk melanoma: the AIM HIGH Study–United Kingdom Coordinating Committee on Cancer Research randomized study of adjuvant low-dose extended-duration interferon Alfa-2a in high-risk resected malignant melanoma. J Clin Oncol 2004;22:53–61.

18. Cameron DA, Cornbleet MC, Mackie RM, et al. Adjuvant interferon alpha 2b in high risk melanoma - the Scottish study. Br J Cancer 2001;84:1146–9.

19. Hauschild A, Weichenthal M, Rass K, et al. Efficacy of low-dose interferon {alpha}2a 18 versus 60 months of treatment in patients with primary melanoma of >= 1.5 mm tumor thickness: results of a randomized phase III DeCOG trial. J Clin Oncol 2010;28:841–6.

20. Eggermont AM, Suciu S, MacKie R, et al. Post-surgery adjuvant therapy with intermediate doses of interferon alfa 2b versus observation in patients with stage IIb/III melanoma (EORTC 18952): randomised controlled trial. Lancet 2005;366: 1189–96.

21. Eggermont AM, Suciu S, Santinami M, et al. Adjuvant therapy with pegylated interferon alfa-2b versus observation alone in resected stage III melanoma: final results of EORTC 18991, a randomised phase III trial. Lancet 2008; 372:117–26.

22. Grob JJ, Dreno B, de la Salmoniere P, et al. Randomised trial of interferon alpha-2a as adjuvant therapy in resected primary melanoma thicker than 1.5 mm without clinically detectable node metastases. French Cooperative Group on Melanoma. Lancet 1998;351:1905–10.

23. Garbe C, Radny P, Linse R, et al. Adjuvant low-dose interferon {alpha}2a with or without dacarbazine compared with surgery alone: a prospective-randomized phase III DeCOG trial in melanoma patients with regional lymph node metastasis. Ann Oncol 2008;19:1195–201.

24. Pehamberger H, Soyer HP, Steiner A, et al. Adjuvant interferon alfa-2a treatment in resected primary stage II cutaneous melanoma. Austrian Malignant Melanoma Cooperative Group. J Clin Oncol 1998;16:1425–9.

25. Mocellin S, Pasquali S, Rossi CR, et al. Interferon alpha adjuvant therapy in patients with high-risk melanoma: a systematic review and meta-analysis. J Natl Cancer Inst 2010;102:493–501.

26. Eggermont AM, Spatz A, Lazar V, et al. Is ulceration in cutaneous melanoma just a prognostic and predictive factor or is ulcerated melanoma a distinct biologic entity? Curr Opin Oncol 2012;24:137–40.

27. Gogas H, Ioannovich J, Dafni U, et al. Prognostic significance of autoimmunity during treatment of melanoma with interferon. N Engl J Med 2006;354:709–18.

28. Tarhini AA, Stuckert J, Lee S, et al. Prognostic significance of serum S100B protein in high-risk surgically resected melanoma patients participating in Intergroup Trial ECOG 1694. J Clin Oncol 2009;27:38–44.

29. Meyer S, Wild PJ, Vogt T, et al. Methylthioadenosine phosphorylase represents a predictive marker for response to adjuvant interferon therapy in patients with malignant melanoma. Exp Dermatol 2010;19:e251–7.

30. Ballo MT, Ang KK. Radiation therapy for malignant melanoma. Surg Clin North Am 2003;83:323–42.

31. Ballo MT, Bonnen MD, Garden AS, et al. Adjuvant irradiation for cervical lymph node metastases from melanoma. Cancer 2003;97:1789–96.

32. Agrawal S, Kane JM 3rd, Guadagnolo BA, et al. The benefits of adjuvant radiation therapy after therapeutic lymphadenectomy for clinically advanced, high-risk, lymph node-metastatic melanoma. Cancer 2009;115:5836–44.

33. Strojan P, Jancar B, Cemazar M, et al. Melanoma metastases to the neck nodes: role of adjuvant irradiation. Int J Radiat Oncol Biol Phys 2010;77:1039–45.

34. Burmeister BH, Henderson MA, Ainslie J, et al. Adjuvant radiotherapy versus observation alone for patients at risk of lymph-node field relapse after therapeutic lymphadenectomy for melanoma: a randomised trial. Lancet Oncol 2012;13:589–97.

35. Creagan ET, Cupps RE, Ivins JC, et al. Adjuvant radiation therapy for regional nodal metastases from malignant melanoma: a randomized, prospective study. Cancer 1978;42:2206–10.

36. Burmeister BH, Smithers BM, Poulsen M, et al. Radiation therapy for nodal disease in malignant melanoma. World J Surg 1995;19:369–71.

37. Corry J, Smith JG, Bishop M, et al. Nodal radiation therapy for metastatic melanoma. Int J Radiat Oncol Biol Phys 1999;44:1065–9.

38. Stevens G, Thompson JF, Firth I, et al. Locally advanced melanoma: results of postoperative hypofractionated radiation therapy. Cancer 2000;88:88–94.

39. Ballo MT, Ross MI, Cormier JN, et al. Combined-modality therapy for patients with regional nodal metastases from melanoma. Int J Radiat Oncol Biol Phys 2006;64:106–13.

40. Burmeister BH, Mark Smithers B, Burmeister E, et al. A prospective phase II study of adjuvant postoperative radiation therapy following nodal surgery in malignant melanoma-Trans Tasman Radiation Oncology Group (TROG) Study 96.06. Radiother Oncol 2006;81:136–42.

41. Veronesi U, Adamus J, Aubert C, et al. A randomized trial of adjuvant chemotherapy and immunotherapy in cutaneous melanoma. N Engl J Med 1982;307:913–6.

42. Lejeune F, Macher E, Kleeberg U, et al. An assessment of DTIC versus levamisole and placebo in the treatment of high risk stage I patients after removal of a primary melanoma of the skin, a phase III adjuvant study. EORTC protocol 18761. Eur J Cancer Clin Oncol 1988;24:881–90.

43. Fisher RI, Terry WD, Hodes RJ, et al. Adjuvant immunotherapy or chemotherapy for malignant melanoma. Preliminary report of the National Cancer Institute randomized clinical trial. Surg Clin North Am 1981;61:1267–77.

44. Koops HS, Vaglini M, Suciu S, et al. Prophylactic isolated limb perfusion for localized, high-risk limb melanoma: results of a multicenter randomized phase III trial. European Organization for Research and Treatment of Cancer Malignant Melanoma Cooperative Group Protocol 18832, the World Health Organization Melanoma Program Trial 15, and the North American Perfusion Group Southwest Oncology Group-8593. J Clin Oncol 1998;16:2906–12.

45. Flaherty LE, Moon J, Atkins MB, et al. Phase III trial of high-dose interferon alpha-2b versus cisplatin, vinblastine, DTIC plus IL-2 and interferon in patients with high-risk melanoma (SWOG S0008): an intergroup study of CALGB, COG, ECOG, and SWOG. J Clin Oncol (ASCO Annual Meeting) 2012;30(Suppl 15):8504.

46. Kruit W, Suciu S, Dreno B, et al. Active immunization toward the MAGE-A3 antigen in patients with metastatic melanoma: four-year follow-up results from a randomized phase II study (EORTC16032-18031). 2011 ASCO Annual Meeting Abstracts. J Clin Oncol 2011;29(Suppl 15):8535.

47. Hersey P, Coates AS, McCarthy WH, et al. Adjuvant immunotherapy of patients with high-risk melanoma using vaccinia viral lysates of melanoma: results of a randomized trial. J Clin Oncol 2002;20:4181–90.

48. Morton D, Mozzillo N, Thompson JF, et al. An international, randomized, phase III trial of bacillus Calmette-Guerin (BCG) plus allogeneic melanoma vaccine (MCV) or placebo after complete resection of melanoma metastatic to regional or distant sites. 2007 ASCO Annual Meeting Proceedings. J Clin Oncol 2007; 25(18S):8508.

49. Hodi FS, O'Day SJ, McDermott DF, et al. Improved survival with ipilimumab in patients with metastatic melanoma. N Engl J Med 2010;363:711–23.

50. Wolchok JD, Thomas L, Bondarenko IN, et al. Phase III randomized study of ipilimumab (IPI) plus dacarbazine (DTIC) versus DTIC alone as first-line treatment in patients with unresectable stage III or IV melanoma. ASCO Annual Meeting Proceedings. J Clin Oncol 2011;29(Suppl) [abstract: LBA5].

51. Chapman PB, Hauschild A, Robert C, et al. Improved survival with vemurafenib in melanoma with BRAF V600E mutation. N Engl J Med 2011;364:2507–16.

52. Atkins MB, Hsu J, Lee S, et al. Phase III trial comparing concurrent biochemotherapy with cisplatin, vinblastine, dacarbazine, interleukin-2, and interferon alfa-2b with cisplatin, vinblastine, and dacarbazine alone in patients with metastatic malignant melanoma (E3695): a trial coordinated by the Eastern Cooperative Oncology Group. J Clin Oncol 2008;26:5748–54.

53. Keilholz U, Punt CJ, Gore M, et al. Dacarbazine, cisplatin, and interferon-alfa-2b with or without interleukin-2 in metastatic melanoma: a randomized phase III trial (18951) of the European Organisation for Research and Treatment of Cancer Melanoma Group. J Clin Oncol 2005;23:6747–55.

54. Tarhini AA, Pahuja S, Kirkwood JM. Neoadjuvant therapy for high-risk bulky regional melanoma. J Surg Oncol 2011;104:386–90.

55. Tarhini AA, Edington H, Butterfield LH. Neoadjuvant ipilimumab in locally/regionally advanced melanoma: clinical outcome and biomarker analysis. J Clin Oncol 2012;30(Suppl 30) [abstract: 8533].

Targeted Therapies for Cutaneous Melanoma

Damien Kee, MBBS, DMedSc, FRACP[a,b,*], Grant McArthur, MBBS, PhD, FRACP[a,b,c]

KEYWORDS

- Melanoma • Targeted therapy • MAPK signaling • BRAF • MEK • NRAS

KEY POINTS

- The molecular characterization of melanomas for BRAF, NRAS, and KIT mutations is increasingly essential for the optimal selection of targeted therapies and clinical trials in patients with advanced disease.
- In melanomas with BRAF V600 mutations, both RAF-inhibitor and MEK-inhibitor monotherapy improves overall survival. Resistance to both drug classes invariably develops but may be potentially delayed by upfront combination therapy.
- NRAS-mutant disease is more refractory to targeted therapy, although MEK-inhibitor monotherapy appears promising, and combination strategies are under investigation.
- KIT inhibitors are active in melanomas with exon-11 and exon-13 KIT mutations, with several compounds undergoing randomized phase III studies.

INTRODUCTION

Melanoma is the most deadly form of skin cancer, accounting for more than two-thirds of skin cancer–related mortality.[1] Although most patients with localized disease can be cured with complete surgical excision, melanoma is highly malignant, and even small primary tumors have the potential to metastasize.[2] In those who develop disseminated disease, treatment options have been limited. Melanoma has long been proved to be refractory to conventional chemotherapeutics.[3] Dacarbazine has been considered the standard treatment for patients with metastatic melanoma for more than 30 years, yet only 5% to 15% of patients will achieve a response and no overall survival benefit has ever been demonstrated.[4] Comparative trials of dacarbazine with other cytotoxic agents such as temozolomide, fotemustine, or platinum-based regimens, or in combination with biological agents such as interferon-α2b or

[a] Division of Cancer Medicine and Research, Peter MacCallum Cancer Centre, St Andrews Place, East Melbourne, Victoria 3002, Australia; [b] Department of Pathology, University of Melbourne, Grattan Street, Parkville, Victoria 3010, Australia; [c] Department of Medicine, St Vincent Hospital, University of Melbourne, Victoria Parade, Fitzroy, Victoria 3065, Australia
* Corresponding author. Division of Cancer Medicine and Research, Peter MacCallum Cancer Centre, St Andrews Place, East Melbourne, Victoria, Australia.
E-mail address: Damien.Kee@petermac.org

Hematol Oncol Clin N Am 28 (2014) 491–505
http://dx.doi.org/10.1016/j.hoc.2014.02.003
0889-8588/14/$ – see front matter © 2014 Elsevier Inc. All rights reserved.
hemonc.theclinics.com

high-dose interleukin-2, have failed to improve on this benchmark.[4] During this era, the median survival for patients with metastatic melanoma was between 6 and 9 months.[2]

Only more recently have tangible advances in the treatment of metastatic melanoma been realized. Developments in understanding of immune checkpoint regulation and the molecular biology of melanoma have laid the groundwork for 2 distinct treatment approaches that culminated in the successful phase III clinical trials of ipilimumab and vemurafenib in 2011.[5,6] Ipilimumab is an antibody directed against the inhibitory cytotoxic T-lymphocyte associated antigen 4 (CTLA-4) receptor expressed by activated T cells. Disruption of this immune checkpoint mechanism results in an enhanced T-cell–mediated antitumor response. In phase III studies, treatment with ipilimumab was associated with modest response rates and improvements in median overall survival, but a notable 10% improvement in overall survival after 2 and 3 years of follow-up.[6] A subsequent analysis has demonstrated that this plateau in melanoma-related deaths is maintained from 3 years out to beyond 10 years after ipilimumab therapy, suggesting that a proportion of patients will develop truly durable antitumor responses.[7] Risks associated with ipilimumab include a 15% to 20% incidence of clinically significant autoimmunity. Next-generation antibodies targeting the interaction between another negative regulator of T-cell function, programmed cell death 1 (PD-1) receptor and its ligand, appear more specific for T-cell anticancer immunity and may be associated with a higher response rate and less frequent autoimmune effects.[8,9] A more thorough review of immunologic therapies in melanoma is provided elsewhere in this issue.

This article focuses on the second approach: the clinical development of specific targeted therapies in direct response to the recent discoveries characterizing common oncogenic drivers in cutaneous melanoma. In particular, mutations resulting in the constitutive activation of the mitogen-activated protein kinase (MAPK) pathway, a key regulator of normal cellular growth and proliferation, appear to be central to the pathogenesis of most melanomas. Vemurafenib was the first of several agents now proven to target this pathway in cutaneous melanoma.

THE MITOGEN-ACTIVATED PROTEIN KINASE PATHWAY IN CUTANEOUS MELANOMA

Extracellular ligands bind to specific membrane-bound receptor tyrosine kinases (RTKs) to initiate MAPK signaling. Subsequent recruitment and activation of the guanosine triphosphatase (GTPase), RAS, results in a cascade of phosphorylation (activating) events involving the serine/threonine kinases RAF, MEK, and ERK. Active ERK phosphorylates numerous cytoplasmic and nuclear targets regulating processes such as cell proliferation, differentiation, survival, migration, and angiogenesis (**Fig. 1**).[10]

ERK has been demonstrated to be hyperactivated in most melanomas. The most commonly identified abnormality is a mutation in BRAF, with a frequency of 40% to 60%.[11–13] A single valine for glutamine substitution at codon 600 (V600E) accounts for greater than 75% of BRAF mutations,[11] with the resultant protein having a 10-fold greater kinase activity than wild-type BRAF.[14] NRAS mutations occur in about 15% of melanomas and are mutually exclusive to BRAF mutations.[13,15] Other mutations, for instance in KIT (encoding the KIT RTK), have been identified but are far less common.[15] However, the relative frequencies of different genetic mutations appear to cluster with certain clinicopathologic features: whereas BRAF mutations are most common in melanomas arising in skin without evidence of chronic sun damage, in much rarer mucosal or acral melanomas BRAF mutations are uncommon but the frequency of KIT mutations ranges from 10% to greater than 20%.[15–17] These findings allow for more rationalized mutation testing, and have resulted in a shift from the

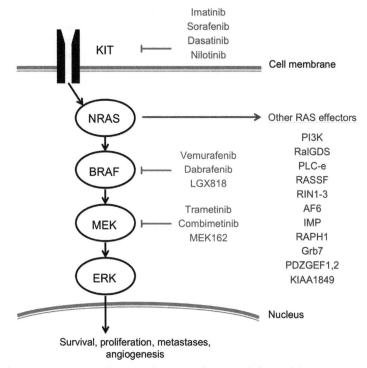

Fig. 1. The mitogen-activated protein kinase pathway and drug inhibitors in melanoma.

traditional histologic classification of melanoma toward a more molecularly based one.[18]

A further point of note is that although MAPK activation seems to be important in melanomagenesis, it is insufficient by itself to result in full malignant transformation. Evidence of this is most clearly found in the demonstration of activating *BRAF* mutations not only across all stages of melanoma progression but also in most benign melanocytic nevi.[19] Other events must also be required, such as a mutation or deletion of the *PTEN* tumor suppressor, which co-occurs in 40% of *BRAF*-mutant melanomas.[20,21] Nevertheless, despite this most melanomas seem to remain dependent on MAPK signaling, making this pathway an excellent therapeutic target.

TARGETING BRAF IN CUTANEOUS MELANOMA
Early RAF-Inhibitor Studies

The earliest attempt to inhibit RAF-mediated MAPK signaling in melanoma was with sorafenib, a broad-spectrum multikinase inhibitor with pan-RAF inhibitory activity.[22] Already in clinical development at the time of the discovery of *BRAF* mutations in melanoma in 2002,[14] it was quickly adapted to be studied in patients with melanoma. Unfortunately, these studies involving sorafenib were disappointing and raised doubts as to the potential of RAF inhibition as a therapeutic strategy. In the initial single-agent phase II studies, sorafenib showed little clinical activity and no survival advantage when compared with historical controls,[23,24] and although a phase I/II clinical trial of sorafenib in combination with carboplatin and paclitaxel showed promising response rates and progression-free survival (PFS) in patients unselected for *BRAF* genotype, no advantage for the addition of sorafenib was demonstrated in the subsequent phase

III study.[25,26] Preclinical experiments had shown that sorafenib could inhibit the MAPK pathway and cellular proliferation in melanoma cell lines with *BRAF* and *NRAS* mutation in vitro; however, only modest pathway inhibition was ever demonstrated in tumor biopsies from treated patients.[27] The failure of sorafenib was therefore likely due to it being unable to achieve sufficient levels of RAF inhibition at maximum tolerated doses that were limited by its off-target multikinase activity. Subsequently, studies involving RAF inhibitors with greater potency and selectivity for mutant BRAF have followed.

Efficacy of the Selective RAF Inhibitors

Vemurafenib was the first highly selective RAF inhibitor to enter clinical trials. This agent was designed prospectively by cocrystallography of the BRAF V600E protein kinase domain and candidate compound structures.[28] In kinase inhibition assays, vemurafenib demonstrated selective inhibition of RAF kinases at nanomolar concentrations and also demonstrated a 3-fold potency against the BRAF V600E versus BRAF wild-type kinase.[29] In fact, in cellular assays where BRAF and CRAF signal as dimers, vemurafenib only inhibits MAPK activation in *BRAF* mutant cells.[30] Surprisingly, in *BRAF* wild-type cells, particularly in the context of activated RAS, RAF inhibitors augmented MAPK signaling, a phenomenon now termed paradoxic MAPK pathway activation.[31,32] Subsequent studies have elucidated a potential mechanism for this behavior whereby the binding of RAF inhibitors to normal CRAF and BRAF dimers induces a conformational change in these complexes that results in increased kinase activity.[31,32] This differential effect of RAF inhibitors on *BRAF* mutant and wild-type cells has since been recognized as a major contributor to the broad therapeutic index and unique toxicity profile of this drug class.

The phase I study of vemurafenib quickly demonstrated marked differences between it and sorafenib.[33] In the initial dose-escalation cohort, a wide therapeutic index was established, with objective tumor regressions observed at doses higher than 240 mg twice daily and dose-limiting toxicities not encountered until doses of 1120 mg twice daily. Responses were limited to patients with *BRAF* V600–mutant melanoma, making this population the exclusive focus of the future phase II and III vemurafenib trials. Within the subsequent expansion cohort, patients treated at the established maximum tolerated dose (MTD) of 960 mg twice daily had an unprecedented response rate of 81% and a median PFS of longer than 7 months (**Table 1**). Paired tumor biopsies showed a strong correlation between tumor response and inhibition of cytoplasmic ERK phosphorylation.[34] Profound inhibition of tumor metabolic activity was also demonstrated on day-15 [18F]fluorodeoxyglucose positron emission tomography (FDG-PET) in all patients treated above the drug threshold of 240 mg twice daily.[35] Similarly impressive results were reported in the phase II study, which involved 132 patients with previously treated melanoma.[36] The confirmed objective response rate was 53%, although most patients obtained some degree of tumor control. The median PFS was 6.8 months, and the median overall survival of 15.9 months far exceeded benchmarks set in previous second-line studies.[37]

Confirmation of improved survival in patients treated with vemurafenib would come with the phase III clinical trial.[5] This study randomly assigned 675 patients with untreated advanced melanoma harboring *BRAF* V600E mutations between either single-agent vemurafenib or dacarbazine. Overall survival was the primary end point, and crossover to vemurafenib was not initially permitted. At the time of the first interim analysis, with a median follow-up of only 3.7 months, the survival outcomes were clearly in favor of patients being treated with vemurafenib. Relative risk of death was reduced by 63% and of tumor progression by 74%. These results led to the early termination of the trial, and dacarbazine-treated patients were allowed to cross over to

Table 1
Main clinical trials of selective RAF inhibitors in metastatic cutaneous melanoma

Study/Treatment Group	BRAF Genotype	Patients (n)	ORR (%)	Median PFS (mo)	Median OS (mo)
Phase I study of vemurafenib: dose escalation and cohort extension in previously treated patients[33]					
Vemurafenib >240 mg bid	V600E	16	69	NR	NR
Vemurafenib 960 mg bid	V600E	32	81	>7.0	NR
Phase II study of vemurafenib in previously treated patients[36]					
Vemurafenib 960 mg bid	V600E	132	53	6.8	15.9
Phase III study of vemurafenib vs dacarbazine in untreated patients[5,38]					
Vemurafenib 960 mg bid	V600E	295	59	6.9	13.3
	V600K	33	45	5.9	14.5
DTIC 1000 mg/m^2 every 21 d	V600E/K	338	8.6	1.6	9.7
Phase I study of dabrafenib: dose escalation and cohort extension in previously treated patients[39]					
Dabrafenib 35–300 mg bid	V600E	27	78	5.5	NR
	V600K	18	39	5.6	NR
Phase II study of dabrafenib in previously treated patients[40]					
Dabrafenib 150 mg bid	V600E	76	60	6.3	13.1
	V600K	16	13	4.5	12.9
Phase III study of dabrafenib vs dacarbazine in untreated patients[41]					
Dabrafenib 150 mg bid	V600E	187	53	5.1	NA
DTIC 1000 mg/m^2 every 21 d	V600E	63	6	2.7	NA

Abbreviations: bid, twice daily; DTIC, dacarbazine; NA, not yet available; NR, not reported; ORR, objective response rate; OS, overall survival; PFS, progression-free survival.

vemurafenib. Later analysis at a median follow-up of 10.5 months showed a median overall survival in vemurafenib-treated patients of 13.6 months, and 9.7 months for patients treated with dacarbazine.[38] Objective response rates were 62.6% versus 9.8% in favor of vemurafenib. Based on these findings, vemurafenib was approved for the treatment of patients with unresectable or metastatic melanoma with *BRAF* V600E mutations by the US Food and Drug Administration in August 2011; and in melanomas with any *BRAF* V600 mutation by the European Medicine Agency in February 2012.

The successes of vemurafenib were not isolated events in the development of highly targeted, mutation-specific therapeutics for melanoma. Clinical trials of other selective RAF inhibitors quickly followed. Chief among these were the trials involving dabrafenib, another inhibitor of RAF kinase with selectivity for mutant BRAF in kinase panel screening. In corresponding phase I, II, and III studies, dabrafenib showed properties similar to those of vemurafenib (see **Table 1**).[39–41] Once again a high therapeutic index was apparent, and investigators had difficulties defining an MTD. Eventually a recommended phase II dose of 150 mg twice daily was brought forward, as beyond this there was little improvement in clinical responses, and near maximal effects were already noted on the pharmacodynamic studies that included tumor biopsies and FDG-PET imaging.[39] At this dose confirmed response rates were consistently higher than 50%, and in the phase III study comparing treatment with dabrafenib versus dacarbazine in patients with untreated *BRAF* V600E–positive melanoma, risk of tumor progression was once again reduced by more than 70%.[41] The median overall survival also favored patients treated with dabrafenib (hazard ratio 0.76, 95% confidence interval 0.48–1.21) but was not statistically significant, with the 36 of 63 (57%) dacarbazine-treated patients crossing over to dabrafenib and potentially obscuring any overall survival benefit obtained with initial treatment. The key differences between the vemurafenib and dabrafenib clinical trials were the intentional inclusion of patients with non–*BRAF* V600E mutations and patients with untreated brain metastases in the phase I and II studies of the latter.

RAF Inhibitors in BRAF Non-V600E Mutant Melanoma

Although most *BRAF*-mutant melanomas are the result of a V600E substitution, approximately 5% to 10% are V600K, 5% V600R or V600D, and a minority involves non-V600 abnormalities. Cellular assays suggest vemurafenib to be active against all 3 of these non-V600E codon 600 *BRAF* mutations,[30] although its clinical trials used a sequencing method that was unable to reliably distinguish between V600E mutations and these variants.[42] However, subsequent Sanger sequencing and pyrosequencing identified 33 patients with V600K mutations from the vemurafenib treatment arm of the phase III study. These patients had a response rate (45%) and survival outcome (see **Table 1**) similar to those with V600E mutations.[38] The phase I and II trials of dabrafenib intentionally enrolled patients with non-V600E mutations and included a total of 67 patients with V600K mutations, including 34 patients with untreated brain metastases.[39,40] Individual trials were not sufficiently powered to detect significant differences between V600K- and V600E-bearing melanomas, and although clear benefits were seen in both, response rates and survival outcomes were slightly inferior in the V600K populations. As the phase III study enrolled only those patients with confirmed V600E mutations, more detailed information is not available. However, like vemurafenib, dabrafenib has similar activity against V600E and V600K mutant BRAF in kinase assays, and on the balance of current evidence it is believed that most patients with codon 600 *BRAF* mutations are likely to benefit from RAF-inhibitor therapy. For patients with noncodon 600 *BRAF* mutations the data are even more limited, although it seems unlikely that these patients benefit. Cell lines expressing BRAF K601E require significantly higher concentrations of vemurafenib to suppress growth that may be difficult to achieve in vivo,[30] and in clinical trials there were no responders among the 3 patients with non-V600 *BRAF* mutations (2 K601E and 1 V600_K601delinsE mutation) treated in the phase I study of dabrafenib.[39]

RAF Inhibitors in Patients with Brain Metastases

Brain metastases are present at diagnosis in up to 20% of patients with metastatic melanoma, and develop in 40% to 45% of patients overall.[43,44] Treatment options have included surgery, stereotactic radiosurgery, or whole brain irradiation. However, the response rate to systemic chemotherapy is less than 10%, and their presence is a poor prognostic feature, signifying a median overall survival of only 4 to 5 months.[45–47]

Because of concerns about the potential for neurotoxicity, dabrafenib was specifically engineered not to cross the blood-brain barrier.[39] Investigators were therefore surprised by evidence of intracranial activity in a small group of patients with brain metastases enrolled in the phase I trial's expansion cohort.[39] These findings resulted in a subsequently designed phase II study that enrolled 172 patients with either untreated or secondarily progressive melanoma brain metastases.[48] In the subset of 139 (81%) patients with V600E mutations, the intracranial response rate was 39.2% in those with untreated brain metastases and 30.8% in those with previously treated brain metastases. Median PFS was just over 16 weeks and the median overall survival just over 31 weeks. Similar to in extracranial disease, slightly less robust results were noted in the 33 patients with *BRAF* V600K mutations. The results suggested superiority to previous systemic agents in patients with intracranial metastases, and confirmed the activity of dabrafenib in this setting.

Based on its physiochemical properties, vemurafenib was also expected to have difficulty crossing the blood-brain barrier,[49] and patients with cerebral disease were specifically excluded from its initial clinical trials. However, a subsequent phase II open-label study in 24 patients with cerebral disease demonstrated similar PFS benefits to patients treated with dabrafenib,[50] and a second larger trial is currently under way to further define its efficacy. The explanation underlying the activity of these RAF inhibitors in central nervous system disease is probably related to the disruption of the normal blood-brain barrier integrity in the presence of melanoma macrometastases.[51] These agents now provide a viable option for the treatment of patients with cerebral disease, and should encourage the inclusion of similar patients in future studies of targeted therapies in melanoma.

RAF-Inhibitor Toxicity

RAF inhibitors as a class have been generally well tolerated. In clinical trials approximately 25% of patients required a dose interruption or modification, and 5% drug cessation.[5,41] Common toxicities include arthralgia, fatigue, headache, and nausea. Particular to vemurafenib is photosensitivity, rare cases of prolonged QT interval, uveitis, and bilateral facial palsies.[5] Febrile reactions are frequent in patients treated with dabrafenib.[41]

Also common to both drugs are prominent cutaneous side effects, which have included rash, hyperkeratosis, and papillomas. However, a particular concern has been the development of either cutaneous squamous cell carcinoma and keratoacanthomas in 20% to 26%[5,33,36] and 6% to 11%[39-41] of patients enrolled in the phase I to III studies of vemurafenib or dabrafenib, respectively. Molecular studies have demonstrated that these squamous cell tumors are caused by the paradoxic activation of the MAPK pathway under the influence of RAF-inhibition.[52] A high percentage of excised lesions have been identified as possessing *RAS* mutations which, combined with the short latency period in their development, have supported a drug interaction with preexisting *RAS* mutations in the skin.[52,53] The combination treatment of a RAF inhibitor and MEK inhibitor attenuates this paradoxic signaling, reducing the incidence of cutaneous tumors.[54] In fact, a reduced incidence of RAF-inhibitor–related rash, hyperkeratosis, and papilloma with BRAF/MEK combination therapy suggests that these are also mediated by paradoxic MAPK pathway activation.[54]

Cases of new nevi and second primary melanomas have also been reported.[55] Genotyping of these lesions have demonstrated them to be consistently *BRAF* wild-type, with one genotyped melanoma so far identified with an *NRAS* mutation. The true incidence (which is probably less than 2%) and significance of these lesions is yet to be determined. There have also been 2 cases of patients developing new second malignancies reported while receiving RAF-inhibitor therapy. Both of these cases were likely related to paradoxic MAPK signaling promoting the growth and expansion of a preexisting, but subclinical, *RAS*-mutant cell population.[56,57] In the context of metastatic melanoma, this low incidence of secondary malignancies is easy to accept. However, caution will be required in the future use of these agents, particularly in the adjuvant setting, or in patients with a history of *RAS*-mutant cancer.

Development of RAF-Inhibitor Resistance

Although most patients will benefit from RAF-inhibitor monotherapy, approximately 10% have primary resistance and half will develop secondary resistance within a median time of 5 to 7 months.[5,41] Postprogression biopsies show reactivation of the MAPK pathway in most patients progressing on vemurafenib.[58] Underlying mechanisms so far identified include secondary mutations in *NRAS*[58,59]; amplification of *BRAF*[60]; expression of BRAF splice variants that form active BRAF dimers[61]; overexpression of the cancer Osaka thyroid (COT) kinase (an alternative MEK activator)[62]; or mutations in MEK itself.[58] In patient biopsies with persistent inhibition of MAPK, the activation of RTKs including PDGFR, IGF1R, FGFR3 and MET, or loss of PTEN expression, can activate the PI3K pathway and confer RAF-inhibitor resistance.[59,63–66] A more detailed review of resistance mechanism to RAF-inhibitor therapy is available elsewhere in this issue; however, it is clear that further strategies will be required to optimize survival in *BRAF*-mutant melanoma.

MEK-Inhibitor Monotherapy and Combination Therapy

As the major substrate of RAF kinase, MEK offers an alternative target for both treatment-naïve *BRAF*-mutant melanoma and for melanomas that develop resistance through the reactivation of the MAPK pathway. In preclinical studies, *BRAF*-mutant cell lines and melanoma xenografts are extremely sensitive to MEK inhibition.[67] However, clinical trials involving early MEK inhibitors were associated with low response rates, presumably as these agents were unable to achieve sufficiently sustained target inhibition.[68–70] Since then, several MEK inhibitors with more favorable pharmacokinetic and pharmacodynamic properties have been developed.[71] Chief among them has been trametinib, which in single-agent studies has consistently shown a greater than 20% confirmed response rate[39,40]; moreover, in a phase III study, trametinib significantly improved both PFS and overall survival when compared with treatment with systemic chemotherapy (**Table 2**).[41] Across its phase I/II studies, trametinib demonstrated a greater breadth of activity than did the selective RAF inhibitors.[39,40] Responses were seen in 3 of 4 noncodon 600 *BRAF*-mutant melanomas, including 2 with K601E and 1 with a L597V mutation; as well as prolonged stable disease in 1 patient with an *NRAS*-mutant disease. Minimal clinical benefit was obtained in the cohort of 40 patients previously treated with RAF inhibitors, suggesting a high cross-selectivity for both RAF-inhibitor and MEK-inhibitor resistance, perhaps involving a switch in dependence to alternative signaling pathways such as the PI3K pathway. Consistent with prior MEK-inhibitor studies, the common and dose-limiting toxicities included diarrhea, acneiform rash, and ocular toxicity including a reversible central serous retinopathy.[39]

It is interesting to consider that whereas the dosing and activity of MEK inhibitors may be limited by toxicities resulting from the direct suppression of MAPK signaling in normal tissues, the toxicities of the selective RAF inhibitors is caused by the paradoxic activation of this pathway within these same cells. It had therefore been speculated that the combination of these 2 drug classes may result in an attenuation of both RAF-inhibitor and MEK-inhibitor specific toxicities while also providing more profound inhibition of the MAPK pathway, and either preventing or delaying the emergence of MAPK-dependent resistance mechanisms in *BRAF*-mutant melanoma cells.

Two subsequent phase I/II studies have demonstrated the feasibility of this approach, safely combining at full dose dabrafenib with trametinib, and vemurafenib with cobimetinib. Published results from the randomized phase II component of the dabrafenib/trametinib combination study further demonstrated that the combined treatment was associated with a significantly higher response rate (76% vs 54%, *P* = .03) and prolonged PFS (9.4 months vs 5.8 months, *P*<.001) when compared with dabrafenib monotherapy.[54] Key dermatologic toxicities such as hyperkeratosis, acneiform rash, squamous cell carcinomas, and keratoacanthomas were also

Table 2
Main clinical trials involving MEK inhibitors in metastatic cutaneous melanoma

Study/Treatment Group	Genotype	Patients (n)	ORR (%)	Median PFS (mo)	Median OS (mo)
Phase I study of trametinib: dose escalation and cohort extension in patients untreated with prior MEKi treatment[39]					
Trametinib, no prior BRAFi	BRAF MT	30	33	5.7	NR
Trametinib, prior BRAFi	BRAF MT	6	1 of 6	NR	NR
Trametinib	BRAF WT	39	10	2.0	NR
Phase II study of trametinib in patients without prior MEKi treatment[40]					
Trametinib, no prior BRAFi	BRAF MT	57	25	4.0	14.2
Trametinib, prior BRAFi	BRAF MT	40	0	1.8	5.8
Phase III study of trametinib vs chemotherapy as second-line therapy in patients untreated by prior RAFi, MEKi, or ipilimumab[41]					
Trametinib 2 mg daily	V600E/K	214	22	4.8	NA
DTIC 1000 mg/m^2 every 21 d or paclitaxel 175 mg/m^2 every 21 d	V600E/K	108	8	1.5	NA
Phase II study of MEK162 in patients without prior MEKi treatment[79]					
MEK162 45 mg bid	NRAS MT	30	20	3.7	NR
MEK162 45 mg bid	BRAF MT	41	20	3.6	NR
Phase I/II study of dabrafenib 150 mg bid in combination with trametinib, extension cohort[54]					
Dab + trametinib 0 mg daily	V600E/K	54	54	5.8	NA
Dab + trametinib 1 mg daily	V600E/K	54	50	9.2	NA
Dab + trametinib 2 mg daily	V600E/K	54	76	9.4	NA

Abbreviations: Dab, dabrafenib; DTIC, dacarbazine; MEKi, MEK inhibitor; MT, mutant; NA, not yet available; NR, not reported; ORR, objective response rate; OS, overall survival; PFS, progression-free survival; RAFi, RAF inhibitor; WT, wild-type.

reduced, although the incidence of pyrexia and chills, and nausea and vomiting, were significantly higher with combination therapy. Coadministration of vemurafenib and cobimetinib has also demonstrated significant efficacy, with the full results currently in press.[72] Regardless, the combination treatment of RAF inhibitors and MEK inhibitors appears promising, and hopefully will further extend the impressive clinical results already achieved in treating *BRAF*-mutant melanoma.

TARGETING NRAS IN CUTANEOUS MELANOMA

NRAS mutations occur in approximately 15% of cutaneous melanomas[13,15] and have been associated with worse patient outcomes.[73,74] Preclinical studies have demonstrated their ability to induce an oncogene-dependent state in melanoma cells, and their potential as a therapeutic target through the use of gene-silencing techniques.[14,75] However, compared with agents that target oncogenic BRAF, the development of clinically effective compounds in cancers harboring *RAS* mutations has been far more challenging. Owing to the structural characteristics of RAS GTPases and high intracellular GTP levels, the direct inhibition of RAS proteins is generally considered as unfeasible.[76] Inhibition of downstream pathways is complicated by the presence of more than 10 identified downstream effectors (see **Fig. 1**), Despite this, however, drug combinations that target multiple pathways have been at the forefront of investigational strategies to combat oncogenic *RAS*.[76–78]

Intriguingly, single-agent MEK inhibitors have demonstrated signs of activity in *NRAS*-mutant melanoma. These agents include: MEK162, which achieved responses in 6 of the 30 (20%) patients tested and stable disease in a further 13 (43%)[79]; pimasertib, with 1 complete response and 3 partial responses seen within a cohort of 17 patients (24% response rate)[80]; and trametinib, where in a phase I study, 2 of 7 patients treated with *NRAS*-mutant melanoma achieved stable disease, with 1 receiving treatment for a total of 48 weeks.[39] It may be that melanomas, having a greater dependence on MAPK signaling, are uncommonly sensitive to MEK-inhibitor monotherapy among *RAS*-mutant cancers. Follow-up randomized studies will look for a survival benefit for either MEK162, or pimasertib, over dacarbazine in patients with untreated *NRAS*-mutant melanoma, with other promising strategies examining the combination of MEK inhibitors with drugs that target the PI3K pathway.

TARGETING KIT-MUTANT MELANOMA

Amplification or mutations in *KIT* are rare in cutaneous melanoma, but are more common in acral or mucosal melanoma subtypes.[15,81] In contrast to *BRAF* or *NRAS*, *KIT* mutations in melanoma tend to be far more diverse, and not all mutations are likely to be necessary drivers of oncogenesis. The clinical experience of KIT inhibitors in patients with cutaneous melanoma is limited. However, in phase II trials of imatinib the presence of known functional mutations, such as those involving *KIT* exons 11 and 13, rather than melanoma subtype, seemed to be the best predictor of treatment response.[17,82,83] Other KIT inhibitors including sorafenib,[84] dasatinib,[85] sunitinib,[86] and nilotinib[87] have also demonstrated responses in *KIT*-mutant melanomas. Each of these inhibitors is active against a spectrum of KIT mutations different to that of imatinib. Moreover, similarly to therapy for gastrointestinal stromal tumors, optimal drug selection and sequencing is likely to be mutation specific.[88]

CURRENT RECOMMENDATIONS

At present, the authors recommend testing tumors from all patients with advanced cutaneous melanoma and who are suitable for active therapy for *BRAF* mutations; and in those who are *BRAF* wild-type, for *NRAS* and *KIT* mutations where suitable clinical trials are available.

In patients with a *BRAF* V600 mutation, either of the approved selective RAF inhibitors vemurafenib or dabrafenib, alone or, in the case of dabrafenib, in combination with MEK inhibitor, are appropriate first-line treatment options. Further trials involving other combinations of RAF and MEK inhibitors are also pending. One central question to be analyzed in clinical trials is whether patients with small-volume or indolent disease should be treated in the first line with targeted therapies, or with ipilimumab or investigational agents targeting PD-1 or PD-1 ligand. These immunologic therapies offer potential long-term survival benefits with the potential for salvage with BRAF-inhibitor therapy in nonresponders. Targeted therapies for other melanoma genotypes remain experimental. MEK inhibitors appear to be the most promising of the targeted therapies in patients with non-V600 *BRAF* and *NRAS*-mutant disease; patients with exon-11 or exon-13 *KIT*-mutant melanomas should consider participating in registration trials involving the various KIT inhibitors.

SUMMARY

Within the last decade, characterization of the main oncogenic drivers in melanoma has paved the way for effective targeted therapies. This development has been most manifest in those agents that target BRAF-mutant disease; however, agents targeting NRAS- and KIT-mutant melanoma are also promising. Future goals will include the optimization of these treatments to address the eventual emergence of resistance; investigation of their extension into the adjuvant setting; and understanding how to best sequence or combine them with novel immunotherapies.

REFERENCES

1. Narayanan DL, Saladi RN, Fox JL. Ultraviolet radiation and skin cancer. Int J Dermatol 2010;49(9):978–86.
2. Balch CM, Gershenwald JE, Soong SJ, et al. Final version of 2009 AJCC melanoma staging and classification. J Clin Oncol 2009;27(36):6199–206.
3. La Porta CA. Drug resistance in melanoma: new perspectives. Curr Med Chem 2007;14(4):387–91.
4. Jilaveanu LB, Aziz SA, Kluger HM. Chemotherapy and biologic therapies for melanoma: do they work? Clin Dermatol 2009;27(6):614–25.
5. Chapman PB, Hauschild A, Robert C, et al. Improved survival with vemurafenib in melanoma with BRAF V600E mutation. N Engl J Med 2011;364(26):2507–16.
6. Robert C, Thomas L, Bondarenko I, et al. Ipilimumab plus dacarbazine for previously untreated metastatic melanoma. N Engl J Med 2011;364(26):2517–26.
7. Schadendorf D, Hodi FS, Robert C, et al. Pooled analysis of long-term survival data from phase II and phase III trials of ipilimumab in metastatic or locally advanced, unresectable melanoma [Abstract 24]. Presented at: European Cancer Congress. Amsterdam, The Netherlands, September 27–October 1, 2013.
8. Brahmer JR, Tykodi SS, Chow LQ, et al. Safety and activity of anti-PD-L1 antibody in patients with advanced cancer. N Engl J Med 2012;366(26):2455–65.
9. Topalian SL, Hodi FS, Brahmer JR, et al. Safety, activity, and immune correlates of anti-PD-1 antibody in cancer. N Engl J Med 2012;366(26):2443–54.
10. Yoon S, Seger R. The extracellular signal-regulated kinase: multiple substrates regulate diverse cellular functions. Growth Factors 2006;24(1):21–44.
11. Greaves WO, Verma S, Patel KP, et al. Frequency and spectrum of BRAF mutations in a retrospective, single-institution study of 1112 cases of melanoma. J Mol Diagn 2013;15(2):220–6.
12. Long GV, Menzies AM, Nagrial AM, et al. Prognostic and clinicopathologic associations of oncogenic BRAF in metastatic melanoma. J Clin Oncol 2011; 29(10):1239–46.
13. Platz A, Egyhazi S, Ringborg U, et al. Human cutaneous melanoma; a review of NRAS and BRAF mutation frequencies in relation to histogenetic subclass and body site. Mol Oncol 2008;1(4):395–405.
14. Davies H, Bignell GR, Cox C, et al. Mutations of the BRAF gene in human cancer. Nature 2002;417(6892):949–54.
15. Curtin JA, Busam K, Pinkel D, et al. Somatic activation of KIT in distinct subtypes of melanoma. J Clin Oncol 2006;24(26):4340–6.
16. Beadling C, Jacobson-Dunlop E, Hodi FS, et al. KIT gene mutations and copy number in melanoma subtypes. Clin Cancer Res 2008;14(21):6821–8.
17. Guo J, Si L, Kong Y, et al. Phase II, open-label, single-arm trial of imatinib mesylate in patients with metastatic melanoma harboring c-Kit mutation or amplification. J Clin Oncol 2011;29(21):2904–9.
18. Romano E, Schwartz GK, Chapman PB, et al. Treatment implications of the emerging molecular classification system for melanoma. Lancet Oncol 2011; 12(9):913–22.

19. Pollock PM, Harper UL, Hansen KS, et al. High frequency of BRAF mutations in nevi. Nat Genet 2003;33(1):19–20.
20. Gast A, Scherer D, Chen B, et al. Somatic alterations in the melanoma genome: a high-resolution array-based comparative genomic hybridization study. Genes Chromosomes Cancer 2010;49(8):733–45.
21. Tsao H, Goel V, Wu H, et al. Genetic interaction between NRAS and BRAF mutations and PTEN/MMAC1 inactivation in melanoma. J Invest Dermatol 2004; 122(2):337–41.
22. Wilhelm SM, Adnane L, Newell P, et al. Preclinical overview of sorafenib, a multikinase inhibitor that targets both Raf and VEGF and PDGF receptor tyrosine kinase signaling. Mol Cancer Ther 2008;7(10):3129–40.
23. Eisen T, Ahmad T, Flaherty KT, et al. Sorafenib in advanced melanoma: a phase II randomised discontinuation trial analysis. Br J Cancer 2006;95(5):581–6.
24. Ott PA, Hamilton A, Min C, et al. A phase II trial of sorafenib in metastatic melanoma with tissue correlates. PLoS One 2010;5(12):e15588.
25. Flaherty KT, Lee SJ, Zhao F, et al. Phase III trial of carboplatin and paclitaxel with or without sorafenib in metastatic melanoma. J Clin Oncol 2013;31(3):373–9.
26. Flaherty KT, Schiller J, Schuchter LM, et al. A phase I trial of the oral, multikinase inhibitor sorafenib in combination with carboplatin and paclitaxel. Clin Cancer Res 2008;14(15):4836–42.
27. Liu L, Cao Y, Chen C, et al. Sorafenib blocks the RAF/MEK/ERK pathway, inhibits tumor angiogenesis, and induces tumor cell apoptosis in hepatocellular carcinoma model PLC/PRF/5. Cancer Res 2006;66(24):11851–8.
28. Tsai J, Lee JT, Wang W, et al. Discovery of a selective inhibitor of oncogenic B-Raf kinase with potent antimelanoma activity. Proc Natl Acad Sci U S A 2008;105(8):3041–6.
29. Joseph EW, Pratilas CA, Poulikakos PI, et al. The RAF inhibitor PLX4032 inhibits ERK signaling and tumor cell proliferation in a V600E BRAF-selective manner. Proc Natl Acad Sci U S A 2010;107(33):14903–8.
30. Yang H, Higgins B, Kolinsky K, et al. RG7204 (PLX4032), a selective BRAFV600E inhibitor, displays potent antitumor activity in preclinical melanoma models. Cancer Res 2010;70(13):5518–27.
31. Hatzivassiliou G, Song K, Yen I, et al. RAF inhibitors prime wild-type RAF to activate the MAPK pathway and enhance growth. Nature 2010;464(7287):431–5.
32. Poulikakos PI, Zhang C, Bollag G, et al. RAF inhibitors transactivate RAF dimers and ERK signalling in cells with wild-type BRAF. Nature 2010;464(7287):427–30.
33. Flaherty KT, Puzanov I, Kim KB, et al. Inhibition of mutated, activated BRAF in metastatic melanoma. N Engl J Med 2010;363(9):809–19.
34. Bollag G, Hirth P, Tsai J, et al. Clinical efficacy of a RAF inhibitor needs broad target blockade in BRAF-mutant melanoma. Nature 2010;467(7315):596–9.
35. McArthur GA, Puzanov I, Amaravadi R, et al. Marked, homogeneous, and early [18F]fluorodeoxyglucose-positron emission tomography responses to vemurafenib in BRAF-mutant advanced melanoma. J Clin Oncol 2012;30(14):1628–34.
36. Sosman JA, Kim KB, Schuchter L, et al. Survival in BRAF V600-mutant advanced melanoma treated with vemurafenib. N Engl J Med 2012;366(8): 707–14.
37. Korn EL, Liu PY, Lee SJ, et al. Meta-analysis of phase II cooperative group trials in metastatic stage IV melanoma to determine progression-free and overall survival benchmarks for future phase II trials. J Clin Oncol 2008;26(4):527–34.
38. McArthur GA, Chapman PB, Robert C, et al. Safety and efficacy of vemurafenib in BRAFV600E and BRAFV600K mutation-positive melanoma (BRIM-3): extended

follow-up of a phase 3, randomised, open-label study. Lancet Oncol 2014;15(3): 323–32.

39. Falchook GS, Long GV, Kurzrock R, et al. Dabrafenib in patients with melanoma, untreated brain metastases, and other solid tumours: a phase 1 dose-escalation trial. Lancet 2012;379(9829):1893–901.

40. Ascierto PA, Minor D, Ribas A, et al. Phase II trial (BREAK-2) of the BRAF inhibitor dabrafenib (GSK2118436) in patients with metastatic melanoma. J Clin Oncol 2013;31(26):3205–11.

41. Hauschild A, Grob JJ, Demidov LV, et al. Dabrafenib in BRAF-mutated metastatic melanoma: a multicentre, open-label, phase 3 randomised controlled trial. Lancet 2012;380(9839):358–65.

42. Anderson S, Bloom KJ, Vallera DU, et al. Multisite analytic performance studies of a real-time polymerase chain reaction assay for the detection of BRAF V600E mutations in formalin-fixed, paraffin-embedded tissue specimens of malignant melanoma. Arch Pathol Lab Med 2012;136(11):1385–91.

43. Davies MA, Liu P, McIntyre S, et al. Prognostic factors for survival in melanoma patients with brain metastases. Cancer 2011;117(8):1687–96.

44. Fife KM, Colman MH, Stevens GN, et al. Determinants of outcome in melanoma patients with cerebral metastases. J Clin Oncol 2004;22(7):1293–300.

45. Agarwala SS, Kirkwood JM, Gore M, et al. Temozolomide for the treatment of brain metastases associated with metastatic melanoma: a phase II study. J Clin Oncol 2004;22(11):2101–7.

46. Margolin K, Ernstoff MS, Hamid O, et al. Ipilimumab in patients with melanoma and brain metastases: an open-label, phase 2 trial. Lancet Oncol 2012;13(5): 459–65.

47. Mornex F, Thomas L, Mohr P, et al. A prospective randomized multicentre phase III trial of fotemustine plus whole brain irradiation versus fotemustine alone in cerebral metastases of malignant melanoma. Melanoma Res 2003;13(1):97–103.

48. Long GV, Trefzer U, Davies MA, et al. Dabrafenib in patients with Val600Glu or Val600Lys BRAF-mutant melanoma metastatic to the brain (BREAK-MB): a multicentre, open-label, phase 2 trial. Lancet Oncol 2012;13(11):1087–95.

49. Buckmelter AJ, Ren L, Laird ER, et al. The discovery of furo[2,3-c]pyridine-based indanone oximes as potent and selective B-Raf inhibitors. Bioorg Med Chem Lett 2011;21(4):1248–52.

50. Dummer R, Goldinger SM, Turtschi CP, et al. Vemurafenib in patients with BRAF mutation-positive melanoma with symptomatic brain metastases: final results of an open-label pilot study. Eur J Cancer 2014;50(3):611–21.

51. Gerstner ER, Fine RL. Increased permeability of the blood-brain barrier to chemotherapy in metastatic brain tumors: establishing a treatment paradigm. J Clin Oncol 2007;25(16):2306–12.

52. Su F, Viros A, Milagre C, et al. RAS mutations in cutaneous squamous-cell carcinomas in patients treated with BRAF inhibitors. N Engl J Med 2012;366(3): 207–15.

53. Oberholzer PA, Kee D, Dziunycz P, et al. RAS mutations are associated with the development of cutaneous squamous cell tumors in patients treated with RAF inhibitors. J Clin Oncol 2012;30(3):316–21.

54. Flaherty KT, Infante JR, Daud A, et al. Combined BRAF and MEK inhibition in melanoma with BRAF V600 mutations. N Engl J Med 2012;367(18):1694–703.

55. Zimmer L, Hillen U, Livingstone E, et al. Atypical melanocytic proliferations and new primary melanomas in patients with advanced melanoma undergoing selective BRAF inhibition. J Clin Oncol 2012;30(19):2375–83.

56. Callahan MK, Rampal R, Harding JJ, et al. Progression of RAS-mutant leukemia during RAF inhibitor treatment. N Engl J Med 2012;367(24):2316–21.
57. Andrews M, Behren A, Chiohn F, et al. BRAF inhibitor-driven tumor proliferation in a KRAS-mutated colon carcinoma is not overcome by MEK1/2 inhibition. J Clin Oncol 2013;31(35):e448–51.
58. Trunzer K, Pavlick AC, Schuchter L, et al. Pharmacodynamic effects and mechanisms of resistance to vemurafenib in patients with metastatic melanoma. J Clin Oncol 2013;31(14):1767–74.
59. Nazarian R, Shi H, Wang Q, et al. Melanomas acquire resistance to B-RAF(V600E) inhibition by RTK or N-RAS upregulation. Nature 2010;468(7326):973–7.
60. Shi H, Moriceau G, Kong X, et al. Melanoma whole-exome sequencing identifies (V600E)B-RAF amplification-mediated acquired B-RAF inhibitor resistance. Nat Commun 2012;3:724.
61. Poulikakos PI, Persaud Y, Janakiraman M, et al. RAF inhibitor resistance is mediated by dimerization of aberrantly spliced BRAF(V600E). Nature 2011;480(7377):387–90.
62. Johannessen CM, Boehm JS, Kim SY, et al. COT drives resistance to RAF inhibition through MAP kinase pathway reactivation. Nature 2010;468(7326):968–72.
63. Straussman R, Morikawa T, Shee K, et al. Tumour micro-environment elicits innate resistance to RAF inhibitors through HGF secretion. Nature 2012;487(7408):500–4.
64. Villanueva J, Vultur A, Lee JT, et al. Acquired resistance to BRAF inhibitors mediated by a RAF kinase switch in melanoma can be overcome by cotargeting MEK and IGF-1R/PI3K. Cancer Cell 2010;18(6):683–95.
65. Wilson TR, Fridlyand J, Yan Y, et al. Widespread potential for growth-factor-driven resistance to anticancer kinase inhibitors. Nature 2012;487(7408):505–9.
66. Yadav V, Zhang X, Liu J, et al. Reactivation of mitogen-activated protein kinase (MAPK) pathway by FGF receptor 3 (FGFR3)/Ras mediates resistance to vemurafenib in human B-RAF V600E mutant melanoma. J Biol Chem 2012;287(33):28087–98.
67. Solit DB, Garraway LA, Pratilas CA, et al. BRAF mutation predicts sensitivity to MEK inhibition. Nature 2006;439(7074):358–62.
68. Rinehart J, Adjei AA, Lorusso PM, et al. Multicenter phase II study of the oral MEK inhibitor, CI-1040, in patients with advanced non-small-cell lung, breast, colon, and pancreatic cancer. J Clin Oncol 2004;22(22):4456–62.
69. LoRusso PM, Krishnamurthi SS, Rinehart JJ, et al. Phase I pharmacokinetic and pharmacodynamic study of the oral MAPK/ERK kinase inhibitor PD-0325901 in patients with advanced cancers. Clin Cancer Res 2010;16(6):1924–37.
70. Kirkwood JM, Bastholt L, Robert C, et al. Phase II, open-label, randomized trial of the MEK1/2 inhibitor selumetinib as monotherapy versus temozolomide in patients with advanced melanoma. Clin Cancer Res 2012;18(2):555–67.
71. Gilmartin AG, Bleam MR, Groy A, et al. GSK1120212 (JTP-74057) is an inhibitor of MEK activity and activation with favorable pharmacokinetic properties for sustained in vivo pathway inhibition. Clin Cancer Res 2011;17(5):989–1000.
72. McArthur G, Gonzalez R, Pavlick A, et al. Vemurafenib (VEM) and MEK inhibitor, cobimetinib (GDC-0973), in advanced BRAFV600-mutated melanoma (BRIM7): dose-escalation and expansion results of a phase IB study [Abstract 3703]. Paper presented at: European Cancer Congress. Amsterdam, The Netherlands. September 27–October 1, 2013. Available at: http://eccamsterdam2013.ecco-org.eu/Scientific-Programme/Abstract-search.aspx?abstractid=7015.

73. Devitt B, Liu W, Salemi R, et al. Clinical outcome and pathological features associated with NRAS mutation in cutaneous melanoma. Pigment Cell Melanoma Res 2011;24(4):666–72.

74. Jakob JA, Bassett RL Jr, Ng CS, et al. NRAS mutation status is an independent prognostic factor in metastatic melanoma. Cancer 2012;118(16):4014–23.

75. Eskandarpour M, Kiaii S, Zhu C, et al. Suppression of oncogenic NRAS by RNA interference induces apoptosis of human melanoma cells. Int J Cancer 2005; 115(1):65–73.

76. Gysin S, Salt M, Young A, et al. Therapeutic strategies for targeting ras proteins. Genes Cancer 2011;2(3):359–72.

77. Kelleher FC, McArthur GA. Targeting NRAS in melanoma. Cancer J 2012;18(2): 132–6.

78. Kwong LN, Costello JC, Liu H, et al. Oncogenic NRAS signaling differentially regulates survival and proliferation in melanoma. Nat Med 2012;18(10):1503–10.

79. Ascierto PA, Schadendorf D, Berking C, et al. MEK162 for patients with advanced melanoma harbouring NRAS or Val600 BRAF mutations: a non-randomised, open-label phase 2 study. Lancet Oncol 2013;14(3):249–56.

80. Delord JP, Houédé N, Awada A, et al. Pimasertib (MSC1936369B/AS703026), a selective oral MEK1/2 inhibitor, shows clinical activity in melanoma. Eur J Cancer 2012;48(Suppl):190.

81. Curtin JA, Fridlyand J, Kageshita T, et al. Distinct sets of genetic alterations in melanoma. N Engl J Med 2005;353(20):2135–47.

82. Carvajal RD, Antonescu CR, Wolchok JD, et al. KIT as a therapeutic target in metastatic melanoma. JAMA 2011;305(22):2327–34.

83. Hodi FS, Corless CL, Giobbie-Hurder A, et al. Imatinib for melanomas harboring mutationally activated or amplified KIT arising on mucosal, acral, and chronically sun-damaged skin. J Clin Oncol 2013;31(26):3182–90.

84. Quintas-Cardama A, Lazar AJ, Woodman SE, et al. Complete response of stage IV anal mucosal melanoma expressing KIT Val560Asp to the multikinase inhibitor sorafenib. Nat Clin Pract Oncol 2008;5(12):737–40.

85. Woodman SE, Trent JC, Stemke-Hale K, et al. Activity of dasatinib against L576P KIT mutant melanoma: molecular, cellular, and clinical correlates. Mol Cancer Ther 2009;8(8):2079–85.

86. Minor DR, Kashani-Sabet M, Garrido M, et al. Sunitinib therapy for melanoma patients with KIT mutations. Clin Cancer Res 2012;18(5):1457–63.

87. Cho JH, Kim KM, Kwon M, et al. Nilotinib in patients with metastatic melanoma harboring KIT gene aberration. Invest New Drugs 2012;30(5):2008–14.

88. Kee D, Zalcberg JR. Current and emerging strategies for the management of imatinib-refractory advanced gastrointestinal stromal tumors. Ther Adv Med Oncol 2012;4(5):255–70.

Treatments for Noncutaneous Melanoma

Danny N. Khalil, MD, PhD[a], Richard D. Carvajal, MD[b],*

KEYWORDS

- Uveal melanoma • Ocular melanoma • Mucosal melanoma • Anorectal melanoma
- Vulvovaginal melanoma

KEY POINTS

- Molecular characterization of uncommon subsets of melanoma has revealed that mucosal and ocular melanomas are distinct disease subtypes with unique biologic features that have a direct bearing on treatment.
- Surgery, if feasible, offers the best chance for cure in localized ocular and mucosal melanoma. However, in select patients with ocular melanoma, plaque therapy can substitute for enucleation, with similar outcomes.
- Although systemic treatment of advanced disease has historically been guided by the experience with cutaneous melanoma, targeted treatments addressing the unique genetics of ocular and cutaneous melanomas are showing significant promise.

INTRODUCTION
Biology and Epidemiology

Recent advances in the understanding of melanoma have allowed clinicians to move away from a classification system organized according to histologic differences toward a genetics-based system that has important therapeutic and prognostic implications.[1] One consequence of this is that clinicians are now better equipped to understand and exploit the unique characteristics of melanomas that do not arise from the skin.

The number of cases of skin melanoma in the United States in 2013 was estimated to be 76,690.[2] Among melanomas, 5% to 10% are noncutaneous. Such malignancies can be broadly separated into those arising from the eye and those arising from the mucosal surfaces of the body.

Funding Sources and Conflicts of Interest: No relevant funding or conflicts of interest to report.
[a] Department of Medicine, Memorial Sloan-Kettering Cancer Center, 1275 York Avenue, New York, NY 10065, USA; [b] Developmental Therapeutics, Department of Medicine, Memorial Sloan-Kettering Cancer Center, 300 East 66th Street, No. 1071, New York, NY 10065, USA
* Corresponding author.
E-mail address: carvajar@mskcc.org

Hematol Oncol Clin N Am 28 (2014) 507–521
http://dx.doi.org/10.1016/j.hoc.2014.02.006
0889-8588/14/$ – see front matter © 2014 Elsevier Inc. All rights reserved.

Mucosal melanoma

Approximately 55% of mucosal melanomas (MMs) arise from the head and neck while 24% and 18% arise from the anorectal and vulvovaginal regions, respectively. Melanomas arising from the urinary tract, cervix, esophagus, and gallbladder constitute the remaining 3%.[3]

The epidemiology of MM differs significantly from that of cutaneous melanoma.[3] The median age at diagnosis for MM is 67 years, approximately 1 decade later than for cutaneous disease. Because of the mucosal area associated with the female genital tract, women are approximately 80% more likely than men to be diagnosed with MM, whereas cutaneous melanoma has a slight male predominance. The incidence of MM has remained stable, whereas cutaneous melanomas are being diagnosed with increasing frequency[3]; moreover, unlike the association between exposure to ultraviolet light and fair skin with cutaneous melanoma, there is no well-established risk factor or race predilection for MM.

Prognostically MM is also unique. Irrespective of stage, the 5-year overall survival of MM is 25%, in stark contrast to the 80% survival at 5 years for cutaneous melanoma. Suggested explanations for poor outcomes with mucosal disease include the challenge of diagnosing MM early in its evolution, and the rich lymphovascular supply at mucosal surfaces. Among the subtypes, vulvovaginal disease has the bleakest prognosis, with only 11.4% surviving at 5 years.[3] 19.8% of patients with anorectal MM and 31.7% of patients with head and neck MM are alive at 5 years.[3] There is no universal staging system for MM, as prognosticators remain elusive. Depending on subtype, nodal involvement and size greater than 3 cm appear to correlate with prognosis in retrospective analyses; prospective validation, however, is lacking.[4,5]

Approximately half of all melanomas harbor mutations in BRAF, and only 28% are wild-type for BRAF, NRAS, and KIT. Among MMs, however, 55% are wild-type for these oncogenes. One-quarter of MMs harbor mutations in KIT, 12% have mutations in NRAS, and the remaining 9% contain BRAF mutations.[1,6] The therapeutic implications of these findings are discussed later in this article.

Ocular melanoma

Approximately 95% of ocular melanomas arise from the uvea, including the iris, the ciliary body, and the choroid. Less than 5% arise from the conjunctiva, and less than 1% arise from the eyelid or the orbit. Five percent of all melanomas are ocular, yet most primary ocular cancers in adults are melanomas. Uveal melanoma accounts for 70% of all malignancies arising from the eye.[7]

Approximately 1500 cases of ocular melanoma are diagnosed in the United States annually,[8–10] and cases occur 30% more frequently in men than in women. Independent risk factors for uveal melanoma are light eye or skin color,[11] nevi of the skin or iris,[12] and possibly exposure to ultraviolet light, including occupational exposures (eg, welding).[13]

Although only 1% of patients harbor distant disease at presentation,[14] approximately half of all patients with ocular melanoma succumb to metastatic disease. The precise site of origin has important prognostic implications. Melanomas arising from the iris have a 10-year survival rate of 95%, whereas ciliochoroidal tumors have a 77% survival rate at 10 years after diagnosis. Tumor size, tumor pigmentation, iris color, and degree of local invasion correlate with poor outcomes.[15]

Like MMs, ocular melanomas have unique genetic features that correspond to a distinct biology. GNAQ and GNA11, genes encoding the α subunits of G proteins, are mutated in more than 80% of uveal melanomas, whereas such mutations are present in only 4% of melanomas generally. Such mutations are thought to drive tumor growth by activating downstream growth pathways including the mitogen-activated protein kinase (MAPK) pathway.[16–18] Mutations in the deubiquitinating gene BAP1, and in codon 625 of splicing factor 3B (SF3B) have also been implicated in the pathogenesis and progression of uveal melanoma.[19,20]

CLINICAL MANAGEMENT OF LOCOREGIONAL DISEASE
Evaluation and Workup

Staging mucosal melanoma
In part owing to the rarity of the disease, staging systems that have been proposed to date, including the American Joint Committee on Cancer (AJCC) staging system for cutaneous melanoma, have failed to reliably separate MM into distinct prognostic categories across subtypes. The Ballantyne staging system,[21] presented in 1970 as a way of staging MMs of the head and neck, has subsequently been used to stage MMs more broadly. This system divides cases into those with clinically localized disease (Stage 1), those with regional lymph node involvement (Stage 2), and those with distant metastases (Stage 3). Its ease of use and straightforward descriptive nature have allowed it to gain acceptance for anorectal and vulvovaginal disease in addition to head and neck MM. However, given that most patients with MM present with localized disease, and that positive lymph nodes are of indeterminate significance, even for MM of the head and neck the practical value of this system is limited.

A more useful method for staging MM takes into account the unique prognostic and therapeutic implications of the site from which the disease stems. A recently proposed staging system from the AJCC specifically for MMs of the head and neck has been shown to predict prognosis.[22] To account for the poor prognosis in even the most limited disease, the lowest possible stage is III and patients can be diagnosed with stage IV disease by local invasion alone, without nodal or distant spread. The key distinction between disease of stages IVA, IVB, and IVC is resectability.

With regard to anorectal disease, the Ballantyne staging system has been shown to correlate with prognosis in a retrospective series.[23] Proposed schema to stage vulvovaginal melanoma,[24–28] whether adaptations from systems devised for the skin or systems that are specific to the female genital tract, have been unable to consistently predict prognosis. The 2002 modified AJCC system for staging cutaneous melanoma, however, has been shown to predict recurrence-free survival for vulvar melanoma.[29,30] While much work remains to be done to better understand how best to stage MM, particularly when it arises from the vagina or anorectum, a suggested approach to selecting a staging system that takes into account subtype and avoids unnecessary complexity is presented in **Table 1**.

Table 1	
Suggested staging systems for mucosal melanoma by subtype	
Subtype	**Suggested Staging Method**
Head and neck	AJCC head and neck system for mucosal melanoma
Anorectal	Ballantyne staging system
Vulvar	AJCC cutaneous melanoma staging system
Vaginal	Ballantyne staging system
Cervical	FIGO staging system[31]
Urethral	Levine system for urethral carcinoma[32]

Abbreviations: AJCC, American Joint Committee on Cancer; FIGO, Fédération Internationale de Gynécologie et d'Obstétrique.

Staging ocular melanoma

Three prognostic systems have a place in uveal melanoma, based on anatomy, cyto-genetics, and gene expression profiling, respectively. The 2010 version of the AJCC staging system for uveal melanoma has been demonstrated to accurately predict prognosis by taking into account tumor size and invasion.[33] Cytogenetically, mono-somy of the third chromosome has been correlated with a poor prognosis,[34] particu-larly when found in the setting of alterations in chromosome 8.[35] Finally, a commercially available 15-gene expression profile array[36] has demonstrated excellent prognostic power in a validation cohort.[37,38]

Treating Locoregional Mucosal Melanoma

Surgery

Although cure rates for localized disease remain dismal, both surgery and radiation are potentially definitive modalities, with surgery typically offering the best chance for cure. However, the use of surgery is frequently limited by the multifocal nature of tu-mors' growth and the fact that local recurrence rates are generally greater than 50%.[39] For most localized tumors, anatomic constraints ultimately determine whether surgery is feasible.

For MM of the sinuses or nasal cavity without nodal involvement, wide surgical resec-tion without lymph node dissection with consideration of postoperative radiation ther-apy to the primary site is advocated. This approach may entail craniofacial resection for tumors involving the cribriform plate, orbital exenteration for orbital involvement, and radical nasal exenteration for diffuse mucosal disease.[40] An endoscopic approach may reduce morbidity and improve functional outcomes.[41] Some consider forgoing radiation for limited tumors that do not involve deep soft tissues, cartilage, bone, or skin.

If regional lymph nodes are involved but the tumor does not involve the brain, masti-cator space, skull base, dura, carotid artery, cranial nerves IX through XII, or the pre-vertebral space, the lesion is still considered potentially resectable. In this case a wide surgical resection with neck dissection and postoperative radiation to the primary site and the neck is advocated, based on reports of improvement in local control.[42,43] For MM of the oral cavity, oropharynx, larynx, or hypopharynx, even if regional lymph node involvement is not suspected, neck dissection is advocated if the primary lesion in-volves deep soft tissues, cartilage, bone, or skin.[44] More advanced disease can be treated with either radiation or systemic therapy (see later discussion).

Historically, anorectal MMs were managed with abdominopelvic resections, whereas vulvovaginal MMs were treated with anterior pelvic exenteration. Despite the aggressive nature of this surgery and the high associated morbidity, local and distant recurrence rates remained high. For this reason it was hypothesized that wide local excisions may offer similar outcomes without the need for more radical surgery. Although retrospective data suggest that this more restrained approach may increase the rate of local recurrence, it does not appear to confer a worse overall survival,[4,5,23,30,45–48] possibly because of the high rate of distant metastasis that frequently determines survival.

The role for lymph node dissection in this setting remains undetermined and, as dis-cussed earlier, nodal status is not an established prognosticator for anorectal or vul-vovaginal MM. Furthermore, the presence of distant metastases in the absence of nodal involvement is a well-documented phenomenon.[29,47,49]

Radiotherapy

Whereas historical in vitro data suggest that melanoma cells are able to survive sub-lethal doses of ionizing radiation, more recent data have called these results into question.[50] In fact, some have even reported local control rates for MM as high as 85% with definitive radiotherapy.[51,52]

A logical extrapolation from these data is that adjuvant radiation can be used to improve local disease control after surgery, and indeed this has been reported.[42,53,54] Nevertheless, radiation is yet to show improved overall survival when used after surgery, in part because of the high rate of distant recurrence. This situation may change in light of the fact that optimal dosing schedules, particularly with regard to anorectal and vulvovaginal disease, are still being determined.

Adjuvant chemotherapy

The high rate of recurrence after definitive treatment of primary MM has stimulated great interest in the role of adjuvant systemic treatment. Unfortunately, there has been a paucity of clinical data to guide treatment in this domain. In the only randomized study of adjuvant treatment for MM to demonstrate a survival advantage, Lian and colleagues[55] have shown improved outcomes with a regimen of cisplatin and temozolomide. In this study of 189 patients, those who were randomized to adjuvant temozolomide with cisplatin had an improved overall survival (median 48.7 months) when compared with those who were randomized to surgery alone (21.2 months) or adjuvant treatment with interferon (40.4 months). These results, however, should be interpreted with caution given that melanomas arising in Chinese populations are genetically distinct from those arising in Western patients.[56,57] Furthermore, it is difficult to reconcile an improved overall survival with the use of chemotherapy in the adjuvant setting when no such benefit has been demonstrated in the metastatic setting. Nevertheless, this study clearly establishes a role for adjuvant chemotherapy in the treatment of resectable MM.

Treating Locoregional Ocular Melanoma

Every effort should be made to optimize the chance for cure of ocular melanoma with first-line treatment, as local recurrence confers an increased risk for metastatic disease.[58,59] Current approaches to the use of radiotherapy offer outcomes comparable with those of enucleation while sparing the eye, provided that radiotherapy can be initiated promptly after diagnosis.[60] Radiotherapy for ocular melanoma can be divided into 2 categories: brachytherapy, which includes several radioactive plaques containing various radioisotopes, and external beam radiation, which includes charged-particle radiation and photon-based stereotactic radiotherapy.

Radiotherapy: brachytherapy

Radioactive plaques that have been used to treat ocular melanoma include iodine-125 (^{125}I), cobalt-60, iridium-192, palladium-103, and ruthenium 106–rhodium 106. ^{125}I is often favored, as its off-target effects can be easily shielded while maintaining good tissue penetration. Although higher rates of local recurrence have been reported with plaque therapy in comparison with particle radiation,[15,58,61–66] identifying optimal candidates for brachytherapy may offset this effect. For example, ruthenium plaque therapy has been reported to yield a 2% 5-year recurrence rate for patients with small tumors distal from the optic disc.

Radiation retinopathy is a common adverse effect associated with plaque therapy, reported to occur in 6% of patients at 1 year and 50% of patients at 5 years. Proximity to the optic disc and fovea, in addition to high radiation dose, correlates with the risk of retinopathy. Other side effects of plaque therapy include cataracts, glaucoma, vitreous hemorrhage, and scleral necrosis.[67]

Radiotherapy: external beam radiation

Photon-based external beam stereotactic radiation therapy is an alternative to radio-active plaque therapy. Treatment with this modality is generally administered at a dose of 50 to 70 Gy as 5 daily fractions. Local control at 10 years is approximately 93% for choroidal disease.[68]

Charged particles used to irradiate uveal melanoma include protons, carbon ions, and helium ions. This technique is favored for medium to large choroidal tumors, particularly when they occur near the fovea or optic disc, as this approach provides a sharp decrease in radiation dose outside of the targeted area.[59,62,69,70]

A single-institution study of more than 2000 patients treated with proton therapy reported a local control rate of 95% at 15 years of follow-up, with eye preservation in 84% of patients.[15] Risk factors for visual loss in this experience included tumor location near the optic disc or macula, large tumor size, poor vision at baseline, retinal detachment, and diabetes. A meta-analysis that included 8809 patients showed a significantly lower rate of local recurrence among those who received charged-particle therapy compared with those who received ^{125}I brachytherapy.

Surgery

Given the success of radiotherapy in controlling localized ocular melanoma while sparing the involved eye, surgery has generally been reserved for cases whereby radiation is not feasible because of large tumor size or extrascleral extension, for example. In 2006, the Collaborative Ocular Melanoma Study Group reported the results of a large randomized study in which patients with choroidal melanoma received either ^{125}I brachytherapy or enucleation.[71] At 12 years' follow-up, there was no statistically significant survival benefit for patients randomized to enucleation.

Although enucleation remains the most commonly performed surgery for the treatment of localized ocular melanoma, local resection (eg, with the use of scleral lamellar dissection) continues to be performed for a small subset of patients with ocular melanoma.[72] This procedure has been associated with retinal detachment and vitreous hemorrhage, as well as higher rates of recurrence in comparison with radiotherapy or enucleation.[73,74] For this reason, such procedures should be performed at high-volume centers, and possibly followed by adjuvant brachytherapy[75,76] or external beam radiation.[77]

Other approaches

Transpupillary thermotherapy (TTT) is a modality whereby electromagnetic radiation is delivered via an infrared laser to cause tumor necrosis. Complications include vision loss secondary to either maculopathy or retinopathy. Given the superior efficacy of radiotherapy, the use of TTT as definitive treatment for ocular melanoma is not favored; moreover, given its side-effect profile, its use in combination with brachytherapy to improve local control remains questionable.[78–82]

Photocoagulation involves the delivery of thermal energy to the tumor with the goal of directly lysing melanoma cells and rendering the local vasculature inadequate to sustain the malignancy. Its use had previously been limited to the treatment of small choroidal melanomas; however, owing to its unfavorable side-effect profile including vascular occlusion of the retina, vitreous hemorrhage, and retinal detachment, its use is now limited to a subset of disease that recurs after proton therapy.[83]

Photodynamic therapy using photosensitizing chemicals injected directly into the tumor has also been used. Photosensitive compounds including porfimer and hematoporphyrin, which are activated by light at specific wavelengths, are administered to generate free radicals that damage endothelial cells and induce vascular occlusion to cause tumor necrosis.[84,85] Results with this method have been discouraging. In one small series, 62% of patients with locoregional disease had recurrent disease within 5 years.[86]

Adjuvant chemotherapy

To date, no adjuvant treatment has demonstrated a survival advantage for patients with ocular melanoma. A trial with maintenance interferon-α2a given over a 2-year period after either enucleation or proton radiation in 121 patients with increased-risk uveal melanoma failed to demonstrate an improvement in overall survival when compared with matched historical controls.[87]

Surveillance

Few objective data exist to guide surveillance after definitive treatment of localized ocular melanoma. However, given that up to 50% of such patients will develop metastatic disease, surveillance is reasonable. Repeat imaging done every 3 to 12 months with particular attention to the liver is reasonable. As magnetic resonance imaging (MRI) is the most sensitive imaging modality for identifying hepatic metastasis, the authors generally use MRI of the abdomen and pelvis together with computed tomography of the chest. Basic blood work including liver function tests may be done on a similar schedule.

The interval of testing can be tailored to risk of recurrence as determined by gene-expression profile,[37,88] the size of the primary tumor, and histologic findings (eg, degree of plasma-cell infiltration, presence of vasculogenic mimicry). Recent data suggest that inactivating mutations in BAP-1 may also portend a high risk of recurrence,[19,89] whereas mutations in codon 625 of the splicing factor SF3B1 may confer a more favorable prognosis.[20]

CLINICAL MANAGEMENT OF ADVANCED DISEASE
Local Modalities for the Treatment of Systemic Disease

Surgery

Metastasectomy has been used in the treatment of metastatic uveal melanoma. In a relatively large case series of patients with metastatic uveal melanoma, 24 were treated surgically. All but 2 of these patients had a single metastasis, generally outside of the liver. Five-year survival for those treated surgically was 39%, compared with 0% for those who were not.

Liver-directed therapy

For patients with hepatic metastases from uveal melanoma, liver-directed therapy has shown activity in select patients. Chemoembolization is one such technique that has been associated with some objective responses. In a single-institution, retrospective study, chemoembolization with cisplatin-based regimens demonstrated a response rate of 36%, compared with a response rate of less than 1% with systemic chemotherapy.[90]

Hepatic artery infusion has also been studied. In a trial of patients with ocular melanoma and liver metastases, patients were randomized to either hepatic artery infusion with melphalan or to best alternative therapy. This study resulted in improved hepatic progression-free survival for those who received liver-directed therapy, but no significant difference in overall survival.[91] Fotemustine, an alkylating agent, has also been studied for use as a hepatic artery infusion. Based on an early clinical study showing objective responses to this approach,[92] a phase III study comparing intrahepatic with intravenous fotemustine for the treatment of uveal melanoma with liver metastases is currently under way (NCT00110123).

Local modalities for the treatment of metastatic MM are less developed than those used for metastatic ocular melanoma, and as such are generally limited to use in the context of a clinical trial.

Systemic Therapy

Despite the unique biology of ocular and MM, the rarity of these 2 disease entities has meant that in most cases the approach to systemic treatment is largely guided by the experience with cutaneous melanoma.

Before 2011, dacarbazine and high-dose interleukin-2 were the only 2 medical treatments approved in the United States for metastatic cutaneous melanoma. Neither had demonstrated improved overall survival for skin melanoma.

In March of 2011, a fully human monoclonal antibody, ipilimumab, designed to block the inhibitory T-cell receptor CTLA-4 (cytotoxic T-lymphocyte antigen 4) was approved by the Food and Drug Administration based on phase III data showing an overall survival benefit in pretreated patients with advanced cutaneous melanoma.[93] In a single-institution series of 20 patients with advanced uveal melanoma, most of whom had received prior treatment, 25% had clinical benefit, defined as stable disease or objective response, at 24 weeks,[94] which is comparable with the experience with advanced cutaneous disease. In a multicenter, retrospective series of 33 patients with metastatic or unresectable MM treated with ipilimumab, the median overall survival was 6.4 months, with a poorer overall response rate than that associated with cutaneous melanoma.[95]

The next agent to be approved for the treatment of advanced melanoma was vemurafenib, a small-molecule inhibitor of the serine/threonine kinase B-Raf. In a randomized phase III trial of untreated patients with metastatic cutaneous melanomas harboring *BRAF* V600E mutations, patients who received vemurafenib achieved a 6-month overall survival of 84%, compared with 64% in patients treated with dacarbazine.[96] The following caveats, however, should be kept in mind: Such *BRAF* mutations are significantly more common in cutaneous melanoma than they are in noncutaneous melanomas. Furthermore, vemurafenib has been associated with the growth of non–BRAF-driven malignancies.[97,98] Nevertheless, although the role of BRAF inhibition has not been studied in ocular melanoma and MM to the extent that it has been in cutaneous melanoma, it would not be unreasonable to use this approach in the minority of patients with noncutaneous melanomas whose tumors are found to have actionable BRAF mutations.

Dabrafenib, a second BRAF inhibitor, was subsequently approved based on phase III data from 250 patients harboring BRAF V600E–positive melanoma who were randomized to receive either the targeted agent or dacarbazine. Median progression-free survival was 5.1 months in patients receiving dabrafenib and 2.7 months in those receiving dacarbazine. A third targeted agent approved for melanoma patients with activating BRAF mutations is the protein kinase inhibitor trametinib. This agent targets the MAPK pathway protein MEK, which is downstream of BRAF. In a phase III study of 322 patients with BRAF V600E or V600K positive metastatic melanoma who were randomized to either trametinib or chemotherapy, overall survival at 6 months was 81% in the trametinib arm in comparison with 67% in the chemotherapy arm.[99]

Another target of small-molecule inhibition in melanoma, particularly MM, is the receptor tyrosine kinase KIT, an oncogene mutated in approximately 25% of MMs.[100] The tyrosine kinase inhibitor imatinib has shown objective responses in both cutaneous melanomas and MMs with KIT mutations,[100] with mutations in exons 11 and 13 appearing to predict clinical response.[101–103]

Table 2
Published series on specific agents in ocular and mucosal melanoma

Drug	Ocular	Mucosal
Dacarbazine/ temozolomide	Bedikian et al[105]	Yi et al[106]
Interleukin-2	—	Kim et al[107]; Harting and Kim[108]; Moreno et al[42]
Ipilimumab	Danielli et al[109]; Khattak et al[110]; Luke et al[111]; Maio et al[112]	Postow et al[95]; Del Vecchio et al[113]
Trametinib	Falchook et al[114]	—
Vemurafenib	—	—
Dabrafenib	—	—
Imatinib	Fiorentini et al[115]	Carvajal et al[100]; Guo et al[101]; Hodi et al[116]

With regard to uveal melanoma, inhibition of MEK is emerging as a highly promising option. The MAPK pathway is activated downstream of GNAQ and GNA11, mutations of which occur in 70% to 85% of patients with uveal melanoma.[104] At the 2013 annual meeting of the American Society for Clinical Oncology, phase II data were presented showing improved progression-free survival in patients treated with the MEK inhibitor selumetinib in comparison with those receiving temozolomide (15.9 vs 7 weeks). This study was the first to show efficacy for any systemic agent in the treatment of uveal melanoma.[104] Based on these results, it would not be unreasonable to consider a MEK inhibitor, such as trametinib, for the treatment of GNAQ/GNA11-mutant metastatic ocular melanoma as part of a study protocol. Given that the phosphoinositide-3-kinase (PI3K) pathway is also downstream of GNAQ and GNA11, dual MAPK and PI3K pathway inhibition are currently being investigated. **Table 2** lists published case series investigating the role of various systemic agents in the treatment of ocular melanoma and MM.

The decision of whether to use immunotherapy rather than targeted therapy depends largely on the extent of disease in the patient at the time of treatment. Although immunotherapy tends to offer a higher rate of durable responses, the response is often delayed, and this modality may therefore not be appropriate for a patient who is experiencing significant morbidity secondary to the disease burden.

REFERENCES

1. Curtin JA, Fridlyand J, Kageshita T, et al. Distinct sets of genetic alterations in melanoma. N Engl J Med 2005;353(20):2135–47.
2. Siegel R, Naishadham D, Jemal A. Cancer statistics, 2013. CA Cancer J Clin 2013;63(1):11–30.
3. Chang AE, Karnell LH, Menck HR. The American College of Surgeons Commission on Cancer and the American Cancer Society. The National Cancer Data Base report on cutaneous and noncutaneous melanoma: a summary of 84,836 cases from the past decade. Cancer 1998;83(8):1664–78.
4. Weinstock MA. Malignant melanoma of the vulva and vagina in the United States: patterns of incidence and population-based estimates of survival. Am J Obstet Gynecol 1994;171(5):1225–30.

5. Ragnarsson-Olding BK, Kanter-Lewensohn LR, Lagerlöf B, et al. Malignant melanoma of the vulva in a nationwide, 25-year study of 219 Swedish females. Cancer 1999;86(7):1273–84.

6. Postow MA, Harding J, Wolchok JD. Targeting immune checkpoints: releasing the restraints on anti-tumor immunity for patients with melanoma. Cancer J 2012;18(2):153–9.

7. Strickland D, Lee JA. Melanomas of eye: stability of rates. Am J Epidemiol 1981; 113(6):700–2.

8. Singh AD, Topham A. Incidence of uveal melanoma in the United States: 1973-1997. Ophthalmology 2003;110(5):956–61.

9. Singh AD, Bergman L, Seregard S. Uveal malignant melanoma: epidemiologic aspects. In: Essentials of ophthalmic oncology. 2009. p. 78.

10. Rietschel P, Panageas KS, Hanlon C, et al. Variates of survival in metastatic uveal melanoma. J Clin Oncol 2005;23(31):8076–80.

11. Weis E, Shah CP, Lajous M, et al. The association between host susceptibility factors and uveal melanoma: a meta-analysis. Arch Ophthalmol 2006;124(1):54.

12. Weis E, Shah CP, Lajous M, et al. The association of cutaneous and iris nevi with uveal melanoma: a meta-analysis. Ophthalmology 2009;116(3):536–43.e2.

13. Shah CP, Weis E, Lajous M, et al. Intermittent and chronic ultraviolet light exposure and uveal melanoma: a meta-analysis. Ophthalmology 2005;112(9):1599–607.

14. Diener-West M, Reynolds S, Agugliaro D, et al. Development of metastatic disease after enrollment in the COMS trials for treatment of choroidal melanoma: Collaborative Ocular Melanoma Study Group report no. 26. Arch Ophthalmol 2005;123(12):1639–43.

15. Gragoudas E, Li W, Goitein M, et al. Evidence-based estimates of outcome in patients irradiated for intraocular melanoma. Arch Ophthalmol 2002;120(12): 1665.

16. Van Raamsdonk CD, Griewank KG, Crosby MB, et al. Mutations in GNA11 in uveal melanoma. N Engl J Med 2010;363(23):2191–9.

17. Van Raamsdonk CD, Bezrookove V, Green G, et al. Frequent somatic mutations of GNAQ in uveal melanoma and blue naevi. Nature 2008;457(7229):599–602.

18. Onken MD, Worley LA, Long MD, et al. Oncogenic mutations in GNAQ occur early in uveal melanoma. Invest Ophthalmol Vis Sci 2008;49(12):5230–4.

19. Harbour JW, Onken MD, Roberson ED, et al. Frequent mutation of BAP1 in metastasizing uveal melanomas. Science 2010;330(6009):1410–3.

20. Harbour JW, Roberson ED, Anbunathan H, et al. Recurrent mutations at codon 625 of the splicing factor SF3B1 in uveal melanoma. Nat Genet 2013;45(2): 133–5.

21. Ballantyne AJ. Malignant melanoma of the skin of the head and neck: an analysis of 405 cases. Am J Surg 1970;120(4):425–31.

22. Shuman AG, Light E, Olsen SH, et al. Mucosal melanoma of the head and neck: predictors of prognosis. Arch Otolaryngol Head Neck Surg 2011;137(4):331.

23. Iddings DM, Fleisig AJ, Chen SL, et al. Practice patterns and outcomes for anorectal melanoma in the USA, reviewing three decades of treatment: is more extensive surgical resection beneficial in all patients? Ann Surg Oncol 2010;17(1):40–4.

24. Breslow A. Thickness, cross-sectional areas and depth of invasion in the prognosis of cutaneous melanoma. Ann Surg 1970;172(5):902.

25. Clark WH, From L, Bernardino EA, et al. The histogenesis and biologic behavior of primary human malignant melanomas of the skin. Cancer Res 1969;29(3): 705–27.

26. Chung AF, Woodruff JM, Lewis JL Jr. Malignant melanoma of the vulva: a report of 44 cases. Obstet Gynecol 1975;45(6):638–46.
27. Benedet JL, Pecorelli S, Ngan HY, et al. Staging classifications and clinical practice guidelines for gynaecological cancers. Int J Gynaecol Obstet 2000;70: 207–312.
28. Balch CM, Gershenwald JE, Soong S, et al. Final version of 2009 AJCC melanoma staging and classification. J Clin Oncol 2009;27(36):6199–206.
29. Phillips GL, Bundy BN, Okagaki T, et al. Malignant melanoma of the vulva treated by radical hemivulvectomy. A prospective study of the Gynecologic Oncology Group. Cancer 1994;73(10):2626–32.
30. Moxley KM, Fader A, Rose P, et al. Malignant melanoma of the vulva: an extension of cutaneous melanoma? Gynecol Oncol 2011;122(3):612–7.
31. Pecorelli S, Zigliani L, Odicino F. Revised FIGO staging for carcinoma of the cervix. Int J Gynaecol Obstet 2009;105(2):107–8.
32. Levine RL. Urethral cancer. Cancer 1980;45(Suppl 7):1965.
33. Shields CL, Kaliki S, Furuta M, et al. American Joint Committee on Cancer classification of posterior uveal melanoma (tumor size category) predicts prognosis in 7731 patients. Ophthalmology 2013;120:2066–71.
34. Bronkhorst IH, Maat W, Jordanova ES, et al. Effect of heterogeneous distribution of monosomy 3 on prognosis in uveal melanoma. Arch Pathol Lab Med 2011; 135(8):1042–7.
35. Thomas S, Pütter C, Weber S, et al. Prognostic significance of chromosome 3 alterations determined by microsatellite analysis in uveal melanoma: a long-term follow-up study. Br J Cancer 2012;106(6):1171–6.
36. Harbour JW, Chen R. The decisionDx-UM gene expression profile test provides risk stratification and individualized patient care in uveal melanoma. PLoS Curr 2012;5.
37. Onken MD, Worley LA, Char DH, et al. Collaborative Ocular Oncology Group report number 1: prospective validation of a multi-gene prognostic assay in uveal melanoma. Ophthalmology 2012;119(8):1596–603.
38. Harbour JW. A prognostic test to predict the risk of metastasis in uveal melanoma based on a 15-gene expression profile. Molecular diagnostics for melanoma. Methods Mol Biol 2014;1102:427–40.
39. Lee SP, Shimizu KT, Tran LM, et al. Mucosal melanoma of the head and neck: the impact of local control on survival. Laryngoscope 1994;104(2):121–6.
40. Carvajal RD, Spencer SA, Lydiatt W. Mucosal melanoma: a clinically and biologically unique disease entity. J Natl Compr Canc Netw 2012;10(3):345–56.
41. Hanna E, DeMonte F, Ibrahim S, et al. Endoscopic resection of sinonasal cancers with and without craniotomy: oncologic results. Arch Otolaryngol Head Neck Surg 2009;135(12):1219.
42. Moreno MA, Roberts DB, Kupferman ME, et al. Mucosal melanoma of the nose and paranasal sinuses, a contemporary experience from the MD Anderson Cancer Center. Cancer 2010;116(9):2215–23.
43. Temam S, Mamelle G, Marandas P, et al. Postoperative radiotherapy for primary mucosal melanoma of the head and neck. Cancer 2005;103(2):313–9.
44. NCCN clinical practice guidelines in oncology—national. 2005. October 8, 2013. Available at: http://www.nccn.org/professionals/physician_gls/.
45. Brady MS, Kavolius EP, Quan SH. Anorectal melanoma. Dis Colon Rectum 1995; 38(2):146–51.
46. Pessaux P, Pocard M, Elias D, et al. Surgical management of primary anorectal melanoma. Br J Surg 2004;91(9):1183–7.

47. Yeh JJ, Shia J, Hwu WJ, et al. The role of abdominoperineal resection as surgical therapy for anorectal melanoma. Ann Surg 2006;244(6):1012.

48. Suwandinata FS, Bohle R, Omwandho C, et al. Management of vulvar melanoma and review of the literature. Eur J Gynaecol Oncol 2007;28(3):220–4.

49. Sugiyama VE, Chan JK, Shin JY, et al. Vulvar melanoma: a multivariable analysis of 644 patients. Obstet Gynecol 2007;110(2 Pt 1):296–301.

50. Stevens G, McKay MJ. Dispelling the myths surrounding radiotherapy for treatment of cutaneous melanoma. Lancet Oncol 2006;7(7):575–83.

51. Gilligan D, Slevin NJ. Radical radiotherapy for 28 cases of mucosal melanoma in the nasal cavity and sinuses. Br J Radiol 1991;64(768):1147–50.

52. Yanagi T, Mizoe J, Hasegawa A, et al. Mucosal malignant melanoma of the head and neck treated by carbon ion radiotherapy. Int J Radiat Oncol Biol Phys 2009; 74(1):15–20.

53. Krengli M, Masini L, Kaanders JH, et al. Radiotherapy in the treatment of mucosal melanoma of the upper aerodigestive tract: analysis of 74 cases. A Rare Cancer Network study. Int J Radiat Oncol Biol Phys 2006;65(3):751–9.

54. Ballo MT, Gershenwald JE, Zagars GK, et al. Sphincter-sparing local excision and adjuvant radiation for anal-rectal melanoma. J Clin Oncol 2002;20(23): 4555–8.

55. Lian B, Si L, Cui C, et al. Phase II randomized trial comparing high-dose IFN-α2b with temozolomide plus cisplatin as systemic adjuvant therapy for resected mucosal melanoma. Clin Cancer Res 2013;19(16):4488–98.

56. Zhou QM, Li W, Zhang X, et al. The mutation profiles of common oncogenes involved in melanoma in southern china. J Invest Dermatol 2012;132(7):1935–7.

57. Kong Y, Si L, Zhu Y, et al. Large-scale analysis of KIT aberrations in Chinese patients with melanoma. Clin Cancer Res 2011;17(7):1684–91.

58. Egger E, Zografos L, Schalenbourg A, et al. Eye retention after proton beam radiotherapy for uveal melanoma. Int J Radiat Oncol Biol Phys 2003;55(4): 867–80.

59. Egan KM, Ryan LM, Gragoudas ES. Survival implications of enucleation after definitive radiotherapy for choroidal melanoma: an example of regression on time-dependent covariates. Arch Ophthalmol 1998;116(3):366.

60. Straatsma BR, DienerWest M, Caldwell R, et al. Mortality after deferral of treatment or no treatment for choroidal melanoma. Am J Ophthalmol 2003;136(1): 47–54.

61. Damato B, Kacperek A, Chopra M, et al. Proton beam radiotherapy of choroidal melanoma: the Liverpool-Clatterbridge experience. Int J Radiat Oncol Biol Phys 2005;62(5):1405–11.

62. Char DH, Quivey JM, Castro JR, et al. Helium ions versus iodine 125 brachytherapy in the management of uveal melanoma. A prospective, randomized, dynamically balanced trial. Ophthalmology 1993;100(10):1547.

63. Jensen AW, Petersen IA, Kline RW, et al. Radiation complications and tumor control after 125 I plaque brachytherapy for ocular melanoma. Int J Radiat Oncol Biol Phys 2005;63(1):101–8.

64. Char DH, Kroll S, Phillips TL, et al. Late radiation failures after iodine 125 brachytherapy for uveal melanoma compared with charged-particle (proton or helium ion) therapy. Ophthalmology 2002;109(10):1850–4.

65. Jampol LM, Moy CS, Murray TG, et al. The COMS randomized trial of iodine 125 brachytherapy for choroidal melanoma: IV. Local treatment failure and enucleation in the first 5 years after brachytherapy. COMS report no. 19. Ophthalmology 2002;109(12):2197–206.

66. Gündüz K, Shields CL, Shields JA, et al. Radiation complications and tumor control after plaque radiotherapy of choroidal melanoma with macular involvement. Am J Ophthalmol 1999;127(5):579–89.
67. Kaliki S, Shields CL, Rojanaporn D, et al. Scleral necrosis after plaque radiotherapy of uveal melanoma: a case-control study. Ophthalmology 2013;120: 1004–11.
68. Dunavoelgyi R, Dieckmann K, Gleiss A, et al. Local tumor control, visual acuity, and survival after hypofractionated stereotactic photon radiotherapy of choroidal melanoma in 212 patients treated between 1997 and 2007. Int J Radiat Oncol Biol Phys 2011;81(1):199–205.
69. Tsuji H, Ishikawa H, Yanagi T, et al. Carbon-ion radiotherapy for locally advanced or unfavorably located choroidal melanoma: a Phase I/II dose-escalation study. Int J Radiat Oncol Biol Phys 2007;67(3):857–62.
70. Caujolle JP, Mammar H, Chamorey E, et al. Proton beam radiotherapy for uveal melanomas at nice teaching hospital: 16 years' experience. Int J Radiat Oncol Biol Phys 2010;78(1):98–103.
71. Collaborative Ocular Melanoma Study Group. The COMS randomized trial of iodine 125 brachytherapy for choroidal melanoma: V. Twelve-year mortality rates and prognostic factors: COMS report No. 28. Arch Ophthalmol 2006;124(12): 1684–93.
72. Foulds WS. Results of local excision of uveal tumors. In: Lommatzsch PK, et al, editors. Intraocular tumors. Springer Verlag; 1983. p. 374–7.
73. Damato B. The role of eyewall resection in uveal melanoma management. Int Ophthalmol Clin 2006;46(1):81–93.
74. Bechrakis NE, Petousis V, Willerding G, et al. Ten-year results of transscleral resection of large uveal melanomas: local tumour control and metastatic rate. Br J Ophthalmol 2010;94(4):460–6.
75. Bechrakis NE, Bornfeld N, Zöller I, et al. Iodine 125 plaque brachytherapy versus transscleral tumor resection in the treatment of large uveal melanomas. Ophthalmology 2002;109(10):1855–61.
76. Kivelä T, Puusaari I, Damato B. Transscleral resection versus iodine brachytherapy for choroidal malignant melanomas 6 millimeters or more in thickness: a matched case-control study. Ophthalmology 2003;110(11):2235–44.
77. Char DH, Miller T, Crawford JB. Uveal tumour resection. Br J Ophthalmol 2001; 85(10):1213–9.
78. Oosterhuis JA, Journee-de Korver HG, Kakebeeke-Kemme HM, et al. Transpupillary thermotherapy in choroidal melanomas. Arch Ophthalmol 1995;113(3):315.
79. Oosterhuis JA, Journée-de Korver HG, Keunen JE. Transpupillary thermotherapy: results in 50 patients with choroidal melanoma. Arch Ophthalmol 1998; 116(2):157.
80. Bartlema YM, Oosterhuis J, Journee-De Korver J, et al. Combined plaque radiotherapy and transpupillary thermotherapy in choroidal melanoma: 5 years' experience. Br J Ophthalmol 2003;87(11):1370–3.
81. Shields CL, Cater J, Shields JA, et al. Combined plaque radiotherapy and transpupillary thermotherapy for choroidal melanoma: tumor control and treatment complications in 270 consecutive patients. Arch Ophthalmol 2002;120(7):933.
82. Kreusel KM, Bechrakis N, Riese J, et al. Combined brachytherapy and transpupillary thermotherapy for large choroidal melanoma: tumor regression and early complications. Graefes Arch Clin Exp Ophthalmol 2006;244(12):1575–80.
83. Gragoudas ES. Current approaches in the management of uveal melanomas. Int Ophthalmol Clin 1992;32(2):129–38.

84. Favilla I, Barry WR, Gosbell A, et al. Phototherapy of posterior uveal melanomas. Br J Ophthalmol 1991;75(12):718–21.

85. Bruce RA. Evaluation of hematoporphyrin photoradiation therapy to treat choroidal melanomas. Lasers Surg Med 1984;4(1):59–64.

86. Favilla I, Favilla M, Gosbell A, et al. Photodynamic therapy: a 5-year study of its effectiveness in the treatment of posterior uveal melanoma, and evaluation of haematoporphyrin uptake and photocytotoxicity of melanoma cells in tissue culture. Melanoma Res 1995;5(5):355–64.

87. Lane AM, Egan KM, Harmon D, et al. Adjuvant interferon therapy for patients with uveal melanoma at high risk of metastasis. Ophthalmology 2009;116(11):2206–12.

88. Onken MD, Worley LA, Ehlers JP, et al. Gene expression profiling in uveal melanoma reveals two molecular classes and predicts metastatic death. Cancer Res 2004;64(20):7205–9.

89. Matatall KA, Agapova OA, Onken MD, et al. BAP1 deficiency causes loss of melanocytic cell identity in uveal melanoma. BMC Cancer 2013;13(1):1–12.

90. Bedikian AY, Legha SS, Mavligit G, et al. Treatment of uveal melanoma metastatic to the liver. A review of the MD Anderson Cancer Center experience and prognostic factors. Cancer 1995;76(9):1665–70.

91. Pingpank JF, Hughes M, Faries M, et al. A phase III random assignment trial comparing percutaneous hepatic perfusion with melphalan (PHP-mel) to standard of care for patients with hepatic metastases from metastatic ocular or cutaneous melanoma. J Clin Oncol 2010;28(Suppl 18):LBA8512.

92. Leyvraz S, Spataro V, Bauer J, et al. Treatment of ocular melanoma metastatic to the liver by hepatic arterial chemotherapy. J Clin Oncol 1997;15(7):2589–95.

93. Hodi FS, O'Day SJ, McDermott DF, et al. Improved survival with ipilimumab in patients with metastatic melanoma. N Engl J Med 2010;363(8):711–23.

94. Khan SA, Callahan M, Postow MA, et al. Ipilimumab in the treatment of uveal melanoma: the Memorial Sloan-Kettering Cancer Center experience. J Clin Oncol 2012;20.

95. Postow MA, Luke JJ, Bluth MJ, et al. Ipilimumab for patients with advanced mucosal melanoma. Oncologist 2013;18:726–32.

96. Chapman PB, Hauschild A, Robert C, et al. Improved survival with vemurafenib in melanoma with BRAF V600E mutation. N Engl J Med 2011;364(26):2507–16.

97. Callahan MK, Rampal R, Harding JJ, et al. Progression of RAS-mutant leukemia during RAF inhibitor treatment. N Engl J Med 2012;367(24):2316–21.

98. Lacouture ME, Duvic M, Hauschild A, et al. Analysis of dermatologic events in vemurafenib-treated patients with melanoma. Oncologist 2013;18:314–22.

99. Flaherty KT, Robert C, Hersey P, et al. Improved survival with MEK inhibition in BRAF-mutated melanoma. N Engl J Med 2012;367(2):107–14.

100. Carvajal RD, Antonescu CR, Wolchok JD, et al. KIT as a therapeutic target in metastatic melanoma. JAMA 2011;305(22):2327.

101. Guo J, Si L, Kong Y, et al. Phase II, open-label, single-arm trial of imatinib mesylate in patients with metastatic melanoma harboring c-Kit mutation or amplification. J Clin Oncol 2011;29(21):2904–9.

102. Fisher DE, Barnhill R, Hodi F, et al. Melanoma from bench to bedside: meeting report from the 6th international melanoma congress. Pigment Cell Melanoma Res 2010;23(1):14–26.

103. Hodi FS, Friedlander P, Corless CL, et al. Major response to imatinib mesylate in KIT-mutated melanoma. J Clin Oncol 2008;26(12):2046–51.

104. Carvajal RD, Sosman J, Quevedo F, et al. Phase II study of selumetinib (sel) versus temozolomide (TMZ) in gnaq/Gna11 (Gq/11) mutant (mut) uveal melanoma (UM). J Clin Oncol 2013;31.
105. Bedikian AY, Papadopoulos N, Plager C, et al. Phase II evaluation of temozolomide in metastatic choroidal melanoma. Melanoma Res 2003;13(3):303–6.
106. Yi JH, Yi SY, Lee HR, et al. Dacarbazine-based chemotherapy as first-line treatment in noncutaneous metastatic melanoma: multicenter, retrospective analysis in Asia. Melanoma Res 2011;21(3):223–7.
107. Kim KB, Sanguino AM, Hodges C, et al. Biochemotherapy in patients with metastatic anorectal mucosal melanoma. Cancer 2004;100(7):1478–83.
108. Harting MS, Kim KB. Biochemotherapy in patients with advanced vulvovaginal mucosal melanoma. Melanoma Res 2004;14(6):517–20.
109. Danielli R, Ridolfi R, ChiarionSileni V, et al. Ipilimumab in pretreated patients with metastatic uveal melanoma: safety and clinical efficacy. Cancer Immunol Immunother 2012;61(1):41–8.
110. Khattak MA, Fisher R, Hughes P, et al. Ipilimumab activity in advanced uveal melanoma. Melanoma Res 2013;23(1):79–81.
111. Luke JJ, Callahan MK, Postow MA, et al. Clinical activity of ipilimumab for metastatic uveal melanoma. Cancer 2013;119(20):3687–95.
112. Maio M, Danielli R, ChiarionSileni V, et al. Efficacy and safety of ipilimumab in patients with pre-treated, uveal melanoma. Ann Oncol 2013;24(11):2911–5.
113. Del Vecchio M, Di Guardo L, Ascierto PA, et al. Efficacy and safety of ipilimumab 3mg/kg in patients with pretreated, metastatic, mucosal melanoma. Eur J Cancer 2014;50:121–7.
114. Falchook GS, Lewis KD, Infante JR, et al. Activity of the oral MEK inhibitor trametinib in patients with advanced melanoma: a phase 1 dose-escalation trial. Lancet Oncol 2012;13:782–9.
115. Fiorentini G, Rossi S, Lanzanova G, et al. Tyrosine kinase inhibitor imatinib mesylate as anticancer agent for advanced ocular melanoma expressing immunohistochemical C-KIT (CD 117): preliminary results of a compassionate use clinical trial. J Exp Clin Cancer Res 2003;22(4):17–20.
116. Hodi FS, Corless CL, GiobbieHurder A, et al. Imatinib for melanomas harboring mutationally activated or amplified kit arising on mucosal, acral, and chronically sun-damaged skin. J Clin Oncol 2013;31:3182–90.

Targeted Therapy Resistance Mechanisms and Therapeutic Implications in Melanoma

Guo Chen, PhD, Michael A. Davies, MD, PhD*

KEYWORDS

- BRAF^{V600} • Melanoma • Drug resistance • MAPK • PI3K/AKT
- Tumor heterogeneity • Combination therapy

KEY POINTS

- The clinical benefit of BRAF and MEK inhibitors is limited by both de novo and acquired resistance mechanisms.
- The presence of molecular changes that cause reactivation of the MAPK pathway is the most common feature of tumors that have progressed on BRAF-inhibitor therapy.
- Activation of the PI3K/AKT pathway is commonly seen concurrently with reactivation of MAPK pathway signaling in BRAF inhibitor–resistant tumors.
- Resistance may be mediated by genetic and epigenetic events, and there is growing evidence of intrapatient and intratumoral heterogeneity of resistance mechanisms.
- Inhibiting multiple pathways simultaneously may be required to overcome resistance to MAPK pathway inhibitors.

INTRODUCTION

The era of personalized therapy in melanoma launched with the identification of recurrent *BRAF^{V600}* mutations in more than 50% of melanomas.[1] Valine-600 is a key residue in the activation segment of the kinase domain of the BRAF protein, and mutation of this residue to glutamate (V600E) increases the protein's catalytic activity by 500 fold or more.[2] Expression of the BRAF^{V600} oncoprotein constitutively activates the mitogen-activated protein kinase (MAPK) signaling pathway, thereby promoting proliferation and survival.[3] Although initial clinical trials with nonselective BRAF inhibitors (ie, sorafenib) yielded disappointing results,[4] 2 different small molecules (vemurafenib

Department of Melanoma Medical Oncology, The University of Texas MD Anderson Cancer Center, 1515 Holcombe Boulevard, Unit 904, Houston, TX 77030, USA
* Corresponding author.
E-mail address: mdavies@mdanderson.org

Hematol Oncol Clin N Am 28 (2014) 523–536
http://dx.doi.org/10.1016/j.hoc.2014.03.001
0889-8588/14/$ – see front matter © 2014 Elsevier Inc. All rights reserved.

and dabrafenib) that selectively inhibit the V600-mutant form of BRAF demonstrated unprecedented single-agent activity in early-phase clinical trials.[5,6] Both agents went on to demonstrate significant improvements in objective response rates (ORR) (~50%) and progression-free survival (PFS) (median 5–6 months) in phase III randomized clinical trials versus chemotherapy, leading to their regulatory approval by the US Food and Drug Administration (FDA) for $BRAF^{V600}$-positive metastatic melanoma.[7,8]

The rapid progress from the identification of this driver mutation to FDA-approved therapies stands as a prime example of the potential benefit of translational research and personalized cancer therapy. However, although the development of the BRAFi was a breakthrough in this highly aggressive disease, the benefit of these agents in patients is critically limited by resistance. Multiple clinical studies have demonstrated that even in patients with the same activating BRAF mutation, the degree of tumor shrinkage achieved can be markedly heterogeneous, with approximately 10% of patients failing to achieve any reduction in tumor burden.[7,8] These observations reflect the presence of de novo, or preexisting, resistance mechanisms that limit the efficacy of the BRAFi. Although most patients achieve some degree of tumor shrinkage, approximately 90% demonstrate disease progression within 12 months of starting treatment. This renewed growth is due to the acquisition of molecular changes that mediate resistance (ie, acquired resistance).

Numerous studies have been undertaken to identify the predictors and mechanisms of resistance to mutant-selective BRAFi. These studies have identified alterations in several key signaling molecules and pathways that mediate resistance, and have presented new therapeutic targets for combinatorial strategies for melanomas with $BRAF^{V600}$ mutations (**Table 1**). Furthermore, these studies have generated numerous insights that will inform and facilitate the development of new treatments for other candidate targets in this disease.

REACTIVATION OF THE MAPK SIGNALING PATHWAY IN RESISTANCE

In normal cells, the MAPK pathway functions to transduce growth signal from receptors at the cell surface to transcriptional machinery in the nucleus, and it accomplishes this task through RAS guanosine triphosphatases (GTPases) and the serine/threonine kinases RAF, mitogen-activated protein kinase kinase (MEK), and extracellular signal receptor kinase (ERK) (**Fig. 1**). The MAPK pathway is constitutively activated by $BRAF^{V600}$ mutant proteins.[2,3] In a clinical trial with vemurafenib, only patients whose tumors demonstrated more than 80% inhibition of the MAPK pathway achieved a clinical response.[9] This finding suggested that marked inhibition of the MAPK pathway is critical to the clinical efficacy of the BRAFi. This hypothesis is supported by analyses showing that 70% to 90% of tumors with acquired resistance are characterized by reactivation of downstream effectors of this pathway.[10,11] Of note, all melanomas with acquired resistance that have been analyzed have retained the same $BRAF^{V600}$ mutation that was present before treatment. However, several other molecular changes that reactivate the pathway have been identified (**Fig. 2**).

Somatic mutations in the NRAS gene that affect residues G12, G13, or Q61 lock the NRAS protein in the active, guanosine triphosphate (GTP)-bound state, resulting in constitutive activation of the MAPK pathway. Activating NRAS mutations are detected in approximately 20% of treatment-naïve melanomas. NRAS mutations are generally mutually exclusive with $BRAF^{V600}$ mutations, and mutant NRAS appears to predominantly use CRAF to activate MEK and ERK.[12] In contrast to treatment-naïve tumors, $BRAF^{V600}$ tumors with acquired resistance to BRAFi have NRAS mutations in 18% to 23% of cases.[10,11,13] In preclinical studies, treatment with MEK inhibitors was

Table 1
BRAFi resistance mechanisms

Pathway	Type of Aberration	Aberration	Type of Resistance	Prevalence in Resistant Tumors (%)	References
MAPK	Genetic	Activating mutations in NRAS	Acquired	18–23	10,11,13,14
	Genetic	Activating mutations in KRAS	Acquired	7	11
	Genetic	BRAF amplification	Acquired	9–19	11,13,16
	Genetic	Activating mutations in MAP2K1	Acquired	4–7	11,13,20
	Genetic	Activating mutations in MAP2K2	De novo and acquired	9	13,51
	Genetic	Loss-of-function mutations in NF1	De novo and acquired	2	13,21,22
	Epigenetic	BRAF splicing	Acquired	14–31	11,17
PI3K/AKT	Genetic or epigenetic	Inactivating mutation, deletion, or loss of expression in PTEN	De novo and acquired	~9	10,11,13,26
	Genetic	Activating mutations in PIK3CA or PIK3CG	Acquired	4–6	11,13
	Genetic	Inactivating mutations in PIK3R2	Acquired	2	11
	Genetic	Activating mutations in AKT1 or AKT3	Acquired	4	11
Others	Epigenetic	RTK overexpression or activation	Acquired	Not available	14,31–35
	Genetic	CDKN2A copy loss	De novo and acquired	7	11
	Genetic	MITF amplification	Acquired	2	13

able to suppress the growth and survival of BRAFi-resistant cells expressing mutant NRAS,[14] suggesting that reactivation of the MAPK pathway, not other pathways implicated in RAS signaling, was the key mediator of resistance. In addition to NRAS, mutations in KRAS, another gene encoding a member of the RAS family of proteins, have been detected in 7% of BRAFi-resistant tumors.[11]

Although secondary mutations in BRAF have not been linked with BRAFi resistance, other alterations to the $BRAF^{V600}$ allele have been implicated, such as amplification and aberrant splicing. The only study that has systematically examined both the DNA and the RNA from BRAFi-resistant melanomas found that amplification (~18%) and erroneous splicing of $BRAF^{V600}$ (~14%) exist in a mutually exclusive fashion in 32% of tumors with acquired resistance,[11] suggesting $BRAF^{V600}$ alteration as the leading cause of BRAFi resistance. In addition, increased $BRAF^{V600}$ expression attributable to epigenetic mechanisms has also been shown to mediate BRAFi resistance in patient-derived xenografts.[15] BRAFi resistance mediated by amplification of the $BRAF^{V600}$ allele can be countered by elevating the dose of BRAFi or combining the

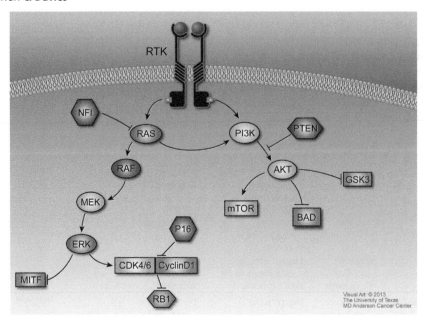

Fig. 1. Core signaling pathways mediating resistance to BRAFi. The MAPK signaling pathway (RAS, RAF, MEK, and ERK) and the PI3K/AKT signaling pathway are the 2 core pathways mediating BRAFi resistance. Mammalian target of rapamycin (mTOR), Bcl-2-associated death promoter (BAD), and glycogen synthase kinase 3 (GSK3) are key signaling molecules phosphorylated by AKT.

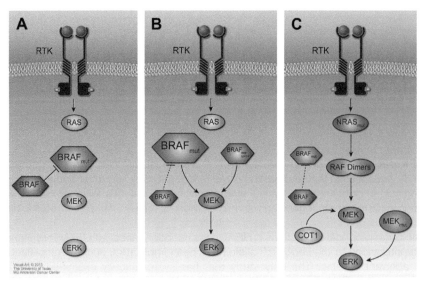

Fig. 2. Aberrations in the MAPK signaling pathway that cause BRAFi resistance. (A) BRAF^{V600} is inhibited by BRAFi, causing MAPK pathway inactivation in tumors responding to BRAFi. (B) Amplification or alternative splicing of *BRAF^{V600}* reactivates the MAPK pathway in a subset of tumors resistant to BRAFi. (C) In addition, the MAPK pathway may be reactivated by mutations in NRAS or MEK in BRAFi-resistant tumors. (*From* Bucheit AD, Davies MA. Emerging insights into resistance to BRAF inhibitors in melanoma. Biochem Pharmacol 2014;87:383; with permission.)

BRAFi with a MEK inhibitor (MEKi),[16] and dosing BRAFi intermittently seems to prevent the emergence of resistant clones overexpressing BRAF^{V600} through epigenetic mechanisms.[15] By contrast, alternative splicing results in the expression of truncated BRAF^{V600} proteins that lack the N-terminal RAS-binding domain but retain the kinase domain.[17] The shortened BRAF^{V600} proteins form homodimers that are resistant to BRAFi, and the resistance cannot be overcome by increasing the concentration of the BRAFi.[17] However, such cells remain dependent on activation of the MAPK pathway, as they are sensitive to MEK and/or ERK inhibition.

Possible gain-of-function mutations in genes encoding MEK1 and MEK2 (*MAP2K1* and *MAP2K2*) have been identified in 8% of BRAFi-naïve melanomas.[18] Whereas some mutations in MEK1 and MEK2 have been identified in pretreatment tumor biopsies of patients and may not confer BRAFi resistance (eg, MEK1^{I111S}, MEK1^{P124S}, MEK1^{P124L}),[10,13,19] others have been detected only in samples with acquired resistance. Mutations associated with resistance include MEK1^{K57N}, MEK1^{Q56P}, MEK1^{V60E}, MEK1^{C121S}, MEK1^{G128V}, MEK1^{E203K}, MEK2^{V35M}, MEK2^{L46F}, MEK2^{C125S}, and MEK2^{N126D}.[10,11,13,20] The incidence of activating mutations in MEK1 and MEK2 in tumors with acquired resistance is 7% to 16%.[11,13] Activating mutations of MEK1/2 may also bestow resistance to allosteric MEK inhibitors, but cells expressing such mutations remain sensitive to ERK inhibition.[13]

Neurofibromin 1 (NF1) negatively regulates RAS activity by promoting the hydrolysis of RAS-bound GTP to guanosine diphosphate. In addition to gene copy loss and loss-of-function mutations, NF1 function may be lost in melanoma because of excessive proteasomal degradation.[21] Depletion of *NF1* elevated HRAS, KRAS, and CRAF activities in *BRAF^{V600E}* melanoma cells, which restored ERK reactivation in the presence of BRAFi.[21,22] NF1-null cells were resistant to not only BRAFi monotherapy but also the combined inhibition of BRAF^{V600} and MEK1/2.[22] However, NF1 loss did not alter the sensitivity to an ERK inhibitor.[22] *NF1* nonsense mutations ($\sim$2%, *NF1^{R2450*}*) and putative splice site mutations (*NF1^{T135C}*, *NF1^{G4023A}*, and *NF1^{C3018T}*) were identified in tumors from patients who had either a short PFS or experienced a relapse after initial response, suggesting that loss of NF1 function may be associated with both de novo and acquired BRAFi resistance.[13,22]

THE PI3K/AKT PATHWAY IN RESISTANCE TO BRAF AND MEK INHIBITORS

The phosphatidylinositide-3-kinase (PI3K)/AKT pathway can also mediate resistance to MAPK-pathway inhibitors. The PI3K/AKT pathway functions in parallel to the MAPK pathway to promote cell growth and suppress programmed cell death (see **Fig. 1**). Aberrant activation of the pathway in BRAFi-resistant tumors can be caused by activation of receptor tyrosine kinases (RTKs), activating mutations of PI3K/AKT pathway components, and inactivation of the phosphatase and tensin homologue (PTEN) lipid phosphatase (**Fig. 3**).[23] Of note, although analyses of resistant cells have occasionally found isolated aberrations in this pathway, such alterations are frequently detected with concurrent alterations in the MAPK pathway.[11]

The PI3K lipid kinase family members catalyze the phosphorylation of the 3′ hydroxyl group on the inositol ring of phosphatidylinositols in the cell membrane.[24] Two PI3K products located at the plasma membrane, phosphatidylinositol-(3,4)-bisphosphate (PIP$_2$) and phosphatidylinositol-(3,4,5)-triphosphate (PIP$_3$), are important signaling intermediaries required for AKT kinase activation. PI3Ks consist of 2 subunits: a regulatory unit encoded by *PIK3R1*, *PIK3R2*, *PIK3R3*, *PIK3R4*, or *PIK3R5*, and a catalytic unit encoded by *PIK3CA*, *PIK3CB*, *PIK3CD*, or *PIK3CG*.[24] Mutations in *PIK3R2* ($\sim$2%, *PIK3R2^{N561D}*), *PIK3CA* ($\sim$4%, *PIK3CA^{D350G}*, *PIK3CA^{E545G}*, and *PIK3CA^{H1047R}*), and

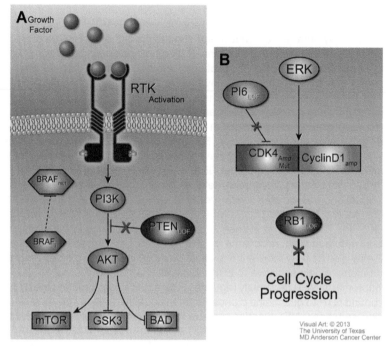

Fig. 3. Resistant mechanisms independent of MAPK reactivation. (*A*) RTK activation, mutations in PI3K or AKT, or loss-of-function aberrations in PTEN, may mediate BRAFi resistance through PI3K/AKT pathway activation. (*B*) In addition, copy number gains in CCND1 or loss-of-function aberrations in CDKN2A may cause BRAFi resistance by deregulating the G1/S cell-cycle checkpoint. (*From* Bucheit AD, Davies MA. Emerging insights into resistance to BRAF inhibitors in melanoma. Biochem Pharmacol 2014;87:384; with permission.)

PIK3CG (~2%, *PIK3CG^{V983E}*) have been found in melanomas that have progressed on BRAFi but not the matched treatment-naïve tumors.[11] PIK3R2^{N561D}, PIK3CA^{D350G}, and PIK3CA^{E545G} mutations increase AKT phosphorylation and decrease sensitivity to vemurafenib in vitro, suggesting that these mutations may drive BRAFi resistance in refractory tumors.[11]

AKT is a group of serine/threonine kinases (AKT1, AKT2, and AKT3) that phosphorylate a variety of proteins with critical roles in cell proliferation and survival. Detection of activating mutations in AKT1 (AKT1^{Q79K}) and AKT3 (AKT3^{E17K}) in approximately 4% of progressing melanomas after BRAFi treatment associates these mutations with acquired resistance.[11] *AKT1^{Q79K}* and *AKT3^{E17K}* mutations activate AKT both in vivo and in vitro, and cells expressing mutant AKT tolerated vemurafenib at higher doses than those expressing the wild-type AKT, establishing a causal link between activating AKT mutations and BRAFi resistance.[11]

PTEN is a phosphatase that acts to remove the 3′ phosphate from the inositol ring of PIP$_2$ and PIP$_3$, thus attenuating PI3K signaling. Up to 30% of cutaneous melanomas have loss of PTEN expression, which can be caused by chromosomal deletions and loss-of-function mutations, or epigenetically by DNA methylation and/or microRNA-regulated gene expression.[25] Examination of pretreatment biopsies showed reduced PTEN expression (*P* = .04) in tumors that did not respond to BRAFi,[10] and another group found a 43% decrease (*P* = .06) in PFS among patients whose tumors harbored

PTEN deletion/mutation,[26] suggesting that loss of PTEN function may be associated with de novo resistance to BRAFi. This result is consistent with several preclinical studies that demonstrated that PTEN loss is associated with diminished cell death in *BRAF^V600E* melanoma cells treated with BRAFi.[27–29] In the 2 recent studies where patient-matched tumor biopsies before and after BRAFi treatment underwent whole-exome sequencing, deletions or inactivating mutations (*PTEN^fs40* and *PTEN^M134del*) of *PTEN* were found in 9% to 11% of tumors with acquired resistance.[11,13] *PTEN* loss/mutation activated AKT and decreased sensitivity to BRAFi in *BRAF^V600E* melanoma cells, and both effects were reversed after wild-type PTEN function was restored.[11] Overall, molecular aberrations that activate the PI3K/AKT pathway were found in 22% of melanomas with acquired resistance to BRAFi, with 82% of these tumors harboring aberrations that concurrently activate the MAPK signaling pathway.[11]

OTHER MECHANISMS THAT MAY MEDIATE BRAFI RESISTANCE
Activation of Receptor Tyrosine Kinases

RTKs are transmembrane cell surface proteins that function as receptors for extracellular growth signals and initiators of various intracellular signaling pathways.[30] Aberrant RTK activation has been established as a prevalent mechanism in the mediation of melanoma resistance to BRAFi. Several signaling pathways downstream from RTK have been associated with BRAFi resistance, such as the MAPK pathway, the PI3K/AKT pathway, and the SRC family kinase/signal transducer and activator of transcription (SFK/STAT) pathway.[14,31–35] So far 5 RTKs (insulin-like growth factor 1 receptor [IGF1R], platelet-derived growth factor receptor [PDGFR], MET, epidermal growth factor receptor [EGFR], and ERBB3) have been implicated in mediating resistance to BRAFi through various mechanisms, including protein overexpression for PDGFR, IGF1R, and ERBB3, relief of negative regulation for IGF1R (through reduced expression of IGFBP3) and EGFR (through reduced expression of SPRY2 or dephosphorylation of MIG6), and production by stroma of cognate growth factor for MET.[14,31–35] Targeting RTK signaling at the receptor level can abolish RTK-mediated BRAFi resistance,[31,32,34] and inhibiting signaling pathways downstream from RTKs may also be a viable strategy. Targeting of the MAPK pathway,[32] the PI3K/AKT pathway,[31] and the SFK/STAT pathway[35] have all shown efficacy in reversing RTK-mediated resistance to BRAFi.

Cell-Cycle Regulators

D-type cyclin-dependent activation of cyclin-dependent kinase (CDK4) promotes cell-cycle progression through the G1/S checkpoint, and aberrant activation of CDK4 leads to uncontrolled cell proliferation.[36] Whereas cyclin D1 (CCND1) activates CDK4, p16^INK4A (CDKN2A) inhibits CDK4 activity.[36] Germline mutations that inactivate CDKN2A or disrupt the CDKN2A binding site on CDK4 predispose the carriers to melanoma, indicating that aberrant activation of CDK4 plays a key role in melanomagenesis. In sporadic melanoma, amplification of *CCND1* and *CDK4* occurs more frequently in tumors without activating *BRAF* or *NRAS* mutations,[37] suggesting that regulation of G1/S transition may be a critical downstream event of MAPK signaling in melanoma. Experiments in BRAF^V600E melanoma cell lines have shown that although *CDK4* mutations had no effect on responses to dabrafenib, *CCND1* amplification conferred resistance.[38] Furthermore, loss of retinoblastoma 1 (RB1), a negative regulator of cell-cycle progression that is phosphorylated and inactivated by CDK4, has been shown to mediate BRAFi resistance in *BRAF^V600E*/PTEN-null melanoma cells.[29] These results suggest that dysregulated cell cycle regulators may bestow BRAFi resistance. Supporting this proposition, copy number gains in *CCND1* and copy number losses in *CDKN2A* were significantly associated with shortened PFS in patients with melanoma who were treated with dabrafenib (see **Fig. 3**).[26] Moreover, *CDKN2A* copy loss has been identified as a new event in tumors progressing on BRAFi, implicating this pathway in acquired resistance.[11]

Amplification of Microphthalmia-Associated Transcription Factor

Microphthalmia-associated transcription factor (MITF) is a transcription factor exclusively expressed in the melanocyte lineage. As a promoter for cell survival, *MITF* is amplified in 15% of metastatic melanomas.[39] MITF appears to be regulated by the MAPK pathway, although the direction of this regulation is controversial.[40,41] In addition, MITF may be regulated at the transcription level by the G-protein–coupled receptor/adenylyl cyclase/protein kinase A/cyclic adenosine monophosphate response element binding protein (GPCR/ADCY/PKA/CREB) pathway.[41] A role for MITF in mediating BRAFi resistance has recently been uncovered, which involves the redirection of cellular metabolism toward oxidative phosphorylation via MITF-induced upregulation of peroxisome proliferator–activated receptor γ coactivator 1α (PGC1α), a master regulator of mitochondrial function.[40] In line with these observations, constitutive expression of MITF desensitized cells to BRAFi in $BRAF^{V600E}$ melanoma cells.[13] Furthermore, *MITF* amplification was found in 1 of 45 (2%) melanomas with acquired resistance to BRAFi.[13] Cells overexpressing MITF are resistant to BRAFi, MEKi, BRAFi + MEKi, and ERKi,[13] but these cells may be sensitive to histone deacetylase inhibitor (HDACi).[41]

Potential Novel Resistance Mechanisms

Exome sequencing of clinical samples has identified new mutations in BRAFi-resistant lesions in RAC1 ($RAC1^{P29S}$), a small GTPase; HOXD8 ($HOXD8^{W252*}$), a member of the homeobox transcription factor family; and PHLPP1 ($PHLPP1^{K596E}$), a phosphatase that inactivates AKT, S6K, and, possibly, ERK. While $RAC1^{P29S}$ and $HOXD8^{W252*}$ are associated with de novo resistance and $PHLPP1^{K596E}$ is implicated in acquired resistance, whether these mutants genuinely induce BRAFi resistance awaits experimental confirmation.[11,13] Despite exhaustive characterization using both exome sequencing and RNA sequencing (RNAseq), resistance mechanisms in 26% to 40% of tumors that progressed on BRAFi or BRAFi + MEKi were unknown,[11,42] suggesting that aberrations at the posttranscriptional level may also play a role in BRAFi resistance.

HETEROGENEITY AND RESISTANCE MECHANISMS

Caused by genomic instability, tumors continuously give rise to molecularly distinct subclones during the course of disease progression. Different genetic aberrations are harbored not only by homologous metastatic lesions derived from the same primary tumor (intrapatient heterogeneity) but also by different regions of a single tumor (intratumoral heterogeneity).[43] Intratumoral heterogeneity was first described in patients receiving BRAFi when only part of a refractory tumor was found to have acquired the $NRAS^{G13V}$ mutation.[44] A second case was reported later when $NRAS^{Q61K}$ was found in one region of a tumor with ERK hyperactivation.[10] The scope and prevalence of intrapatient heterogeneity were assessed in a recent study in which multiple BRAFi-resistant tumors from the same patients (N = 16) were subjected to whole-exome sequencing and RNAseq.[11] Strikingly, 5 different resistance mechanisms were identified in 9 BRAFi-resistant clones from a single patient. Overall, intrapatient divergence in BRAFi resistance mechanisms was identified in 13 of 16 patients (81%). Such diversity carries profound therapeutic implications, as 8 of 44 patients (18%) in the same study showed activation of both MAPK and PI3K/AKT pathways in their progressive lesion(s).[11]

THERAPEUTIC STRATEGIES TO OVERCOME BRAFI RESISTANCE

Reactivation of the MAPK pathway appears to be the most common feature and cause of BRAFi resistance. Molecular changes that can reactivate the pathway have been detected in more than 50% of progressing tumors in several reports.[10,11] One strategy to further suppress MAPK signaling is to combine mutant BRAF inhibition with MEK1/2 blockade. In initial preclinical studies, this strategy ablated the residual ERK phosphorylation that is seen with BRAFi alone and prevented the emergence of resistant clones.[45] Trametinib is a selective MEK1/2 inhibitor that has received FDA approval for the treatment of $BRAF^{V600E}$ or $BRAF^{V600K}$ mutation–positive metastatic melanoma as a single agent (ORR = 22%, PFS = 4.8 months for trametinib vs ORR = 8%, PFS = 1.5 months for chemotherapy).[46] The combination of dabrafenib and trametinib was tested in clinical trials and showed superior PFS (10.5 months) and ORR (76%) over single-agent dabrafenib (PFS = 5.6 months and ORR = 54%) in patients with $BRAF^{V600}$ mutations that had not been previously exposed to BRAFi therapy.[47] Despite these promising results, and the evidence that reactivation of MEK is a consequence of many of the aberrations that reactivate MAPK pathway signaling in resistant samples, the combination of dabrafenib and trametinib achieved a response rate of only 15% and a median PFS of only 3.6 months in patients whose disease had progressed on previous BRAFi therapy.[48] Similar results have been reported with the combination of vemurafenib (BRAFi) and cobimetinib (MEKi) in BRAFi-resistant disease.[49] No data have been reported correlating the resistance mechanisms that were present in the patients whose disease did respond to these combinations, which could identify patients for whom the regimen is sufficient. There are also only limited data about the molecular characteristics of tumors that progressed after BRAFi + MEKi combination therapy. Recently, the results of whole-exome sequencing analysis and RNAseq of pretreatment and progressing tumors from 5 previously BRAFi-naïve patients whose disease responded to dabrafenib + trametinib were reported.[20] Surprisingly, 3 of the 5 resistant tumors showed aberrations that have also been observed in tumors progressing on BRAFi monotherapy: 1 with $MEK2^{Q60P}$ mutation, 1 with $BRAF^{V600E}$ alternative splicing, and 1 with $BRAF^{V600E}$ amplification. Although $MEK2^{Q60P}$ is predicted to cause resistance to combined BRAF and MEK1/2 inhibition,[50,51] preclinical studies suggested that tumors with amplification or alternative splicing of $BRAF$ would be sensitive to MEK inhibition.[16,17] However, no data were presented indicating whether activation of the MAPK pathway was suppressed in the patient samples. No clear resistance mechanisms were identified in the other 2 progressing tumors, although many new molecular changes were identified in each.[20]

The finding that 3 of 5 tumors with resistance to BRAFi + MEKi may have reactivated MAPK signaling suggests that further inhibition of this pathway may help overcome such resistance. One way to improve inhibition of the MAPK pathway may be to escalate the doses of BRAFi and MEKi in combination regimens. For example, in the phase I study of dabrafenib and trametinib, patients tolerated combined treatment with the single-agent maximum tolerated dose of each agent quite well, with a marked reduction in cutaneous toxic effects in comparison with what is observed with each agent alone.[47] Thus, it is possible that one or both of the agents would be tolerated at higher doses when used in combination. As described previously, preclinical studies supported the idea that resistance mediated by BRAF^{V600E} amplification could be overcome by increasing the dose of the BRAFi.[16] Similarly, increasing the dose of the MEKi may help to overcome resistance mechanisms that require MEK reactivation, such as BRAF splicing and NRAS mutations. Alternatively, better clinical activity might be achieved by targeting ERK. Inhibiting ERK using a small-molecule inhibitor or WW domain peptide that disrupts ERK binding to signaling scaffold IQGAP1 inhibited the proliferation of BRAFi-resistant cells in preclinical settings.[13,20,52–54] In these experiments, ERK inhibition overcame resistance to both BRAFi monotherapy and BRAFi + MEKi combinatorial therapy, and also overcame multiple resistance mechanisms such as activating RAS mutations, BRAF amplification, activating MEK1/2 mutations, and RTK upregulation.[13,20,52,53] Whether these promising preclinical results with ERK-inhibiting therapies can be translated into clinical settings awaits further investigation. It also remains unclear if ERK inhibitors will be most beneficial when used alone, or whether they should be combined with a BRAF and/or MEK inhibitor.

Multiple agents that target components of the PI3K/AKT pathway are currently undergoing clinical testing. Combining PI3K/AKT inhibition with either BRAF inhibition or dual BRAF/MEK inhibition overcomes resistance to BRAFi mediated by RTK activation,[31] activating AKT1 mutations[55] or concurrent BRAF^{V600E} amplification/MEK2^{Q60P} mutation in preclinical settings.[51] Clinical trials are now ongoing or planned that combine PI3K/AKT pathway inhibitors with BRAF and/or MEK inhibitors in metastatic melanoma and other diseases. However, it is unclear which of the many small-molecule inhibitors against different targets in the PI3K/AKT pathway (eg, inhibitors of panPI3K, specific isoforms of PI3K, AKT, mammalian target of rapamycin [mTOR], or dual PI3K/mTOR) will confer the most therapeutic benefit with acceptable toxicity. A notable limitation in evaluating the various agents and doses in patients is the lack of a standardized biomarker that correlates with not only pathway inhibition but also clinical benefit.

A subset of melanomas resistant to BRAFi harbor copy number aberrations in CCND1 or CDKN2A,[11,26] suggesting that these tumors may be sensitive to CDK4 inhibition. Palbociclib (PD0332991) is a potent CDK4/6 inhibitor that has shown low toxicity and promising anticancer activity in a phase II clinical trial in ER$^+$/HER2$^-$ breast cancer.[56] Palbociclib induced cell-cycle arrest in melanoma cells that had lost CDKN2A function.[57] Whether palbociclib can overcome BRAFi resistance mediated by dysregulated cell-cycle regulation pathway awaits further investigation.

MITF amplification mediates BRAFi resistance in 2% of resistant melanomas. MITF expression is suppressed by vorinostat (SAHA),[41,58] an HDACi that has been approved for treating cutaneous T-cell lymphoma. Combining vorinostat with BRAFi inhibited growth of BRAFi-resistant melanoma cells overexpressing MITF, but the growth-inhibitory effect was not specific to MITF suppression.[41] These results suggest that vorinostat may reverse BRAFi resistance driven by MITF amplification.

Besides the tremendous emphasis placed on developing rational combinations of targeted therapies based on the molecular characteristics of resistance, it is also possible that combinations with other types of therapies may be clinically beneficial. Analyses in cell lines and clinical specimens have demonstrated that inhibition of the MAPK pathway increases antigen presentation on the surface of melanoma cells, and recognition and infiltration of tumors by T cells.[59–61] Studies have demonstrated that the mutant-selective BRAFi do not affect T-cell function or viability,[59,62] although this may be a concern with MEK inhibitors. Based on preclinical synergy studies,[63] multiple clinical trials have been initiated to determine the safety and efficacy of combining BRAFi with immunotherapies. Although a clinical trial testing the combination of vemurafenib and ipilimumab (an antibody blocking immunosuppressive molecule CTLA4) was stopped early because of unexpected hepatotoxicity, it is hoped that combinations of other BRAFi (eg, dabrafenib and LGX818) and immunotherapies (eg, antibodies against programmed cell death [PD-1] and PD-1 ligand, adoptive T-cell therapy) will circumvent this toxicity. Pretreatment and/or on-treatment biomarkers that correlate with clinical benefit will facilitate the clinical application of this strategy.

SUMMARY

The treatment of melanoma has been revolutionized by an improved understanding of the molecular basis and drivers of this disease, particularly tumors with $BRAF^{V600E}$ mutations. The successful development of multiple active targeted therapies for patients with $BRAF^{V600}$ melanoma demonstrates the promise of dedicated analysis and translation of molecular biology for cancer treatment. However, this experience has also revealed several challenges that must be addressed in the development of therapeutic strategies for other molecular targets. The frequent co-occurrence of activating *BRAF* and *NRAS* mutations in progressing tumors after BRAFi therapy, in comparison with the virtual mutual exclusion of these events in untreated tumors, underscores the critical need to perform dedicated molecular analysis of resistance. This example specifically demonstrates how therapies can change the molecular biology of this disease, and the need to free such analyses from the constraints of prior findings and assumptions. The evolving understanding of the prevalence of the heterogeneity of resistance, including that between patients, within individual patients, and even within individual tumors, is also an important insight as new agents are developed and evaluated. Similar to the experience in other cancers, such as childhood leukemia, this heterogeneity likely necessitates the use of combinatorial approaches that are capable of overcoming multiple resistance mechanisms to maximize clinical benefit. The treatment of patients with metastatic melanoma is in an important transformative era in which multiple treatment modalities are now available for testing and combination.

REFERENCES

1. Davies H, Bignell GR, Cox C, et al. Mutations of the BRAF gene in human cancer. Nature 2002;417:949–54.
2. Wan PT, Garnett MJ, Roe SM, et al. Mechanism of activation of the RAF-ERK signaling pathway by oncogenic mutations of B-RAF. Cell 2004;116:855–67.
3. Karasarides M, Chiloeches A, Hayward R, et al. B-RAF is a therapeutic target in melanoma. Oncogene 2004;23:6292–8.
4. Eisen T, Ahmad T, Flaherty KT, et al. Sorafenib in advanced melanoma: a phase II randomised discontinuation trial analysis. Br J Cancer 2006;95:581–6.
5. Flaherty KT, Puzanov I, Kim KB, et al. Inhibition of mutated, activated BRAF in metastatic melanoma. N Engl J Med 2010;363:809–19.
6. Falchook GS, Long GV, Kurzrock R, et al. Dabrafenib in patients with melanoma, untreated brain metastases, and other solid tumours: a phase 1 dose-escalation trial. Lancet 2012;379:1893–901.
7. Chapman PB, Hauschild A, Robert C, et al. Improved survival with vemurafenib in melanoma with BRAF V600E mutation. N Engl J Med 2011;364:2507–16.
8. Hauschild A, Grob JJ, Demidov LV, et al. Dabrafenib in BRAF-mutated metastatic melanoma: a multicentre, open-label, phase 3 randomised controlled trial. Lancet 2012;380:358–65.

9. Bollag G, Hirth P, Tsai J, et al. Clinical efficacy of a RAF inhibitor needs broad target blockade in BRAF-mutant melanoma. Nature 2010;467:596–9.

10. Trunzer K, Pavlick AC, Schuchter L, et al. Pharmacodynamic effects and mechanisms of resistance to vemurafenib in patients with metastatic melanoma. J Clin Oncol 2013;31:1767–74.

11. Shi H, Hugo W, Kong X, et al. Acquired resistance and clonal evolution in melanoma during BRAF inhibitor therapy. Cancer Discov 2014;4:80–93.

12. Dumaz N, Hayward R, Martin J, et al. In melanoma, RAS mutations are accompanied by switching signaling from BRAF to CRAF and disrupted cyclic AMP signaling. Cancer Res 2006;66:9483–91.

13. Van Allen EM, Wagle N, Sucker A, et al. The genetic landscape of clinical resistance to RAF inhibition in metastatic melanoma. Cancer Discov 2014;4:94–109.

14. Nazarian R, Shi H, Wang Q, et al. Melanomas acquire resistance to B-RAF(V600E) inhibition by RTK or N-RAS upregulation. Nature 2010;468:973–7.

15. Das Thakur M, Salangsang F, Landman AS, et al. Modelling vemurafenib resistance in melanoma reveals a strategy to forestall drug resistance. Nature 2013; 494:251–5.

16. Shi H, Moriceau G, Kong X, et al. Melanoma whole-exome sequencing identifies (V600E)B-RAF amplification-mediated acquired B-RAF inhibitor resistance. Nat Commun 2012;3:724.

17. Poulikakos PI, Persaud Y, Janakiraman M, et al. RAF inhibitor resistance is mediated by dimerization of aberrantly spliced BRAF(V600E). Nature 2011;480: 387–90.

18. Nikolaev SI, Rimoldi D, Iseli C, et al. Exome sequencing identifies recurrent somatic MAP2K1 and MAP2K2 mutations in melanoma. Nat Genet 2012;44:133–9.

19. Shi H, Moriceau G, Kong X, et al. Preexisting MEK1 exon 3 mutations in V600E/KBRAF melanomas do not confer resistance to BRAFi. Cancer Discov 2012;2: 414–24.

20. Wagle N, Emery C, Berger MF, et al. Dissecting therapeutic resistance to RAF inhibition in melanoma by tumor genomic profiling. J Clin Oncol 2011;29: 3085–96.

21. Maertens O, Johnson B, Hollstein P, et al. Elucidating distinct roles for NF1 in melanomagenesis. Cancer Discov 2013;3:338–49.

22. Whittaker SR, Theurillat JP, Van Allen E, et al. A genome-scale RNA interference screen implicates NF1 loss in resistance to RAF inhibition. Cancer Discov 2013; 3:350–62.

23. Kwong LN, Davies MA. Targeted therapy for melanoma: rational combinatorial approaches. Oncogene 2014;33:1–9.

24. Fruman DA, Meyers RE, Cantley LC. Phosphoinositide kinases. Annu Rev Biochem 1998;67:481–507.

25. Davies MA. The role of the PI3K-AKT pathway in melanoma. Cancer J 2012;18: 142–7.

26. Nathanson KL, Martin AM, Wubbenhorst B, et al. Tumor genetic analyses of patients with metastatic melanoma treated with the BRAF inhibitor dabrafenib (GSK2118436). Clin Cancer Res 2013;19:4868–78.

27. Paraiso KH, Xiang Y, Rebecca VW, et al. PTEN loss confers BRAF inhibitor resistance to melanoma cells through the suppression of BIM expression. Cancer Res 2011;71:2750–60.

28. Deng W, Gopal YN, Scott A, et al. Role and therapeutic potential of PI3K-mTOR signaling in de novo resistance to BRAF inhibition. Pigment Cell Melanoma Res 2012;25:248–58.

29. Xing F, Persaud Y, Pratilas CA, et al. Concurrent loss of the PTEN and RB1 tumor suppressors attenuates RAF dependence in melanomas harboring (V600E) BRAF. Oncogene 2012;31:446–57.

30. Schlessinger J. Cell signaling by receptor tyrosine kinases. Cell 2000;103: 211–25.

31. Villanueva J, Vultur A, Lee JT, et al. Acquired resistance to BRAF inhibitors mediated by a RAF kinase switch in melanoma can be overcome by cotargeting MEK and IGF-1R/PI3K. Cancer Cell 2010;18:683–95.

32. Lito P, Pratilas CA, Joseph EW, et al. Relief of profound feedback inhibition of mitogenic signaling by RAF inhibitors attenuates their activity in BRAFV600E melanomas. Cancer Cell 2012;22:668–82.

33. Straussman R, Morikawa T, Shee K, et al. Tumour micro-environment elicits innate resistance to RAF inhibitors through HGF secretion. Nature 2012;487: 500–4.

34. Abel EV, Basile KJ, Kugel CH 3rd, et al. Melanoma adapts to RAF/MEK inhibitors through FOXD3-mediated upregulation of ERBB3. J Clin Invest 2013;123: 2155–68.

35. Girotti MR, Pedersen M, Sanchez-Laorden B, et al. Inhibiting EGF receptor or SRC family kinase signaling overcomes BRAF inhibitor resistance in melanoma. Cancer Discov 2013;3:158–67.

36. Hunter T, Pines J. Cyclins and cancer. II: cyclin D and CDK inhibitors come of age. Cell 1994;79:573–82.

37. Curtin JA, Fridlyand J, Kageshita T, et al. Distinct sets of genetic alterations in melanoma. N Engl J Med 2005;353:2135–47.

38. Smalley KS, Lioni M, Dalla Palma M, et al. Increased cyclin D1 expression can mediate BRAF inhibitor resistance in BRAF V600E-mutated melanomas. Mol Cancer Ther 2008;7:2876–83.

39. Garraway LA, Widlund HR, Rubin MA, et al. Integrative genomic analyses identify MITF as a lineage survival oncogene amplified in malignant melanoma. Nature 2005;436:117–22.

40. Haq R, Shoag J, Andreu-Perez P, et al. Oncogenic BRAF regulates oxidative metabolism via PGC1alpha and MITF. Cancer Cell 2013;23:302–15.

41. Johannessen CM, Johnson LA, Piccioni F, et al. A melanocyte lineage program confers resistance to MAP kinase pathway inhibition. Nature 2013;504:138–42.

42. Wagle N, Van Allen EM, Treacy DJ, et al. MAP kinase pathway alterations in BRAF-mutant melanoma patients with acquired resistance to combined RAF/MEK Inhibition. Cancer Discov 2014;4:61–8.

43. Burrell RA, McGranahan N, Bartek J, et al. The causes and consequences of genetic heterogeneity in cancer evolution. Nature 2013;501:338–45.

44. Wilmott JS, Tembe V, Howle JR, et al. Intratumoral molecular heterogeneity in a BRAF-mutant, BRAF inhibitor-resistant melanoma: a case illustrating the challenges for personalized medicine. Mol Cancer Ther 2012;11:2704–8.

45. Paraiso KH, Fedorenko IV, Cantini LP, et al. Recovery of phospho-ERK activity allows melanoma cells to escape from BRAF inhibitor therapy. Br J Cancer 2010;102:1724–30.

46. Flaherty KT, Robert C, Hersey P, et al. Improved survival with MEK inhibition in BRAF-mutated melanoma. N Engl J Med 2012;367:107–14.

47. Flaherty KT, Infante JR, Daud A, et al. Combined BRAF and MEK inhibition in melanoma with BRAF V600 mutations. N Engl J Med 2012;367:1694–703.

48. Sosman JA, Daud A, Weber JS, et al. BRAF inhibitor (BRAFi) dabrafenib in combination with the MEK1/2 inhibitor (MEKi) trametinib in BRAFi-naive and

BRAFi-resistant patients (pts) with BRAF mutation-positive metastatic melanoma (MM) [abstract 9005]. In: Abstracts of 2013 American Society of Clinical Oncology Annual Meeting. Chicago: J Clin Oncol 2013;31:9005.

49. Menzies AM, Long GV. New combinations and immunotherapies for melanoma: latest evidence and clinical utility. Ther Adv Med Oncol 2013;5:278–85.

50. Emery CM, Vijayendran KG, Zipser MC, et al. MEK1 mutations confer resistance to MEK and B-RAF inhibition. Proc Natl Acad Sci U S A 2009;106:20411–6.

51. Villanueva J, Infante JR, Krepler C, et al. Concurrent MEK2 mutation and BRAF amplification confer resistance to BRAF and MEK inhibitors in melanoma. Cell Rep 2013;4:1090–9.

52. Morris EJ, Jha S, Restaino CR, et al. Discovery of a novel ERK inhibitor with activity in models of acquired resistance to BRAF and MEK inhibitors. Cancer Discov 2013;3:742–50.

53. Jameson KL, Mazur PK, Zehnder AM, et al. IQGAP1 scaffold-kinase interaction blockade selectively targets RAS-MAP kinase-driven tumors. Nat Med 2013;19: 626–30.

54. Carlino MS, Todd JR, Gowrishankar K, et al. Differential activity of MEK and ERK inhibitors in BRAF inhibitor resistant melanoma. Mol Oncol 2014. [Epub ahead of print].

55. Shi H, Hong A, Kong X, et al. A novel AKT1 mutant amplifies an adaptive melanoma response to BRAF inhibition. Cancer Discov 2014;4:69–79.

56. Finn RS, Crown JP, Lang I, et al. Results of a randomized phase 2 study of PD 0332991, a cyclin-dependent kinase (CDK) 4/6 inhibitor, in combination with letrozole vs letrozole alone for first-line treatment of ER+/HER2- advanced breast cancer (BC) [Abstract nr S1–6]. In: Abstracts of the 35th Annual Cancer Therapy & Research Center at UT Health Science Center San Antonio -American Association for Cancer Research Breast Cancer Symposium. San Antonio: Ann Oncol 2012;23:ii43–5.

57. Young RJ, Waldeck K, Martin C, et al. Loss of CDKN2A Expression is a frequent event in primary invasive melanoma and correlates with Sensitivity to the CDK4/6 inhibitor PD0332991 in melanoma cell lines. Pigment Cell Melanoma Res 2014. [Epub ahead of print]. http://dx.doi.org/10.1111/pcmr.12228.

58. Yokoyama S, Feige E, Poling LL, et al. Pharmacologic suppression of MITF expression via HDAC inhibitors in the melanocyte lineage. Pigment Cell Melanoma Res 2008;21:457–63.

59. Boni A, Cogdill AP, Dang P, et al. Selective BRAFV600E inhibition enhances T-cell recognition of melanoma without affecting lymphocyte function. Cancer Res 2010;70:5213–9.

60. Wilmott JS, Long GV, Howle JR, et al. Selective BRAF inhibitors induce marked T-cell infiltration into human metastatic melanoma. Clin Cancer Res 2012;18: 1386–94.

61. Frederick DT, Piris A, Cogdill AP, et al. BRAF inhibition is associated with enhanced melanoma antigen expression and a more favorable tumor microenvironment in patients with metastatic melanoma. Clin Cancer Res 2013;19: 1225–31.

62. Hong DS, Vence L, Falchook G, et al. BRAF(V600) inhibitor GSK2118436 targeted inhibition of mutant BRAF in cancer patients does not impair overall immune competency. Clin Cancer Res 2012;18:2326–35.

63. Liu C, Peng W, Xu C, et al. BRAF inhibition increases tumor infiltration by T cells and enhances the antitumor activity of adoptive immunotherapy in mice. Clin Cancer Res 2013;19:393–403.

Introduction to the Role of the Immune System in Melanoma

Kim Margolin, MD

KEYWORDS

- Melanoma • Immune system • Acute and chronic inflammation • Molecular biology
- Microenvironment • Radiation • Metastasis

KEY POINTS

- Inflammation and immune reactions, particularly involving the innate immune system, are important elements in melanomagenesis.
- Host and tumor characteristics of an immunologic nature determine the fate of melanoma, from the oncogenesis of the primary tumor to the characteristics of the draining lymph node to the microenvironment of melanoma in sites of metastasis.
- Therapeutic strategies need to exploit the existing features of the host-tumor immunologic interactions as well as alter selected feature of the tumor and/or immune system to improve treatment outcomes.
- The amount of heterogeneity among tumors and the host's immune reactions to them provide the basis for recognizing that all forms of therapy require careful patient selection to provide the best therapeutic index at all stages of malignancy.

BACKGROUND
Inflammation and Immunosurveillance in Melanomagenesis

Common knowledge holds that cutaneous melanoma is caused by harmful ultraviolet (UV) radiation, largely from intermittent scorching sunburns, particularly in childhood, an observation based on epidemiologic associations. The contribution of intentional exposure to erythema-inducing doses of UV wavelengths from tanning beds has been the focus of efforts to alter sun behaviors and enact legislation against access, particularly by minors, to tanning salons. It is also commonly thought that cancer immunosurveillance plays a large role in preventing or reducing the risk of invasive cancers, and there are plentiful examples in the literature for a strong association between immunosuppression or immunodeficiency and the occurrence of malignancy. However, despite a large and growing role for immunomodulatory therapies in advanced stages, melanoma is not one of the neoplasms occurring at significantly increased frequency among patients with compromised immunity. It is likely that the precise type

Medical Oncology, Seattle Cancer Care Alliance, University of Washington, 825 Eastlake Avenue E, Seattle, WA 98109, USA
E-mail address: kmargoli@seattlecca.org

Hematol Oncol Clin N Am 28 (2014) 537–558
http://dx.doi.org/10.1016/j.hoc.2014.02.005
0889-8588/14/$ – see front matter © 2014 Elsevier Inc. All rights reserved.

and severity of immunodeficiency required to promote melanomagenesis or emergence of invasive, overt disease from a precursor or indolent disease occur only rarely.

Inflammation plays an important role in melanomagenesis, and inflammation is also a critical component of the liaisons between innate and adaptive immune responses, both of which have been shown to play roles in controlling tumors and protecting against new malignancy. Starting with the earliest stages of melanomagenesis, inflammation induced by UV light is associated with enhanced blood flow, vascular permeability, and damage to subcellular structures resulting from reactive oxygen species. In the earliest example of a tumor microenvironment reactive to oncogenic environmental factors, both the melanocytes and keratinocytes are induced by UV light to produce inflammatory substances that cooperate to prepare for tumor promotion and an immunosuppressive milieu and eventually the elaboration of growth factors that further support tumor growth, invasion, and metastasis.

Immunosuppression induced by UV light contributes to melanomagenesis via the reduction in the number of Langerhans cells; decreased antigen presentation; and elaboration of type 2 cytokines and other substances with suppressive effects, such as interleukin (IL)-4, IL-10, and prostaglandin-E2. UV light also stimulates the production of growth factors with tumor-promoting effects such as alpha-melanocyte–stimulating factor and platelet-activating factor. Neuropilin-1, a member of the vascular endothelial growth factor (VEGF) receptor family, contributes to the protumoral effects of a subset of regulatory T cells in melanoma, and its effects seem to be mediated by transforming growth factor beta (TGF-β) and to be synergistic with those of VEGF.[1–3]

The role of chronic inflammation in melanomagenesis is less clear, although it has been suggested that solar elastosis, a consequence of prolonged rather than acute UV skin damage, may be protective and confer a more favorable prognosis in melanoma[4]; however, this observation may also be explained by some other favorable feature(s) of melanoma arising as a result of chronic UV damage rather than as a direct result of the solar elastosis. A promising therapeutic target is related to the phenomenon of T-cell immune exhaustion, caused in part by the interactions between ligands on the tumor cell as well as on other inflammatory cells, the programmed-death (PD)-1/PD-ligand (PD-L1) interaction, which is detailed later in this article and elsewhere in this issue by Naidoo and colleagues.[5] Established melanoma is likely to represent successful tumor evolution through the 3 stages of immunoediting described by Schreiber and colleagues,[6] beginning with elimination, evolving to equilibrium, and eventually resulting in escape. Also of likely immunotherapeutic importance are recent observations that the common molecular driver of melanoma and some other tumors, BRAF v600[E], confers alterations in melanocytes resulting in an immunosuppressive microenvironment that can be overcome by inhibitors of the enhanced mitogen-associated protein kinase (MAPK) pathway signaling (**Fig. 1**).[7–13] Whether other, less commonly occurring oncogenic drivers are similarly immunosuppressive remains to be shown, and the growing number of molecularly targeted inhibitors need to be carefully tested for their impact on cells of the immune system (both in the circulation and in the tumor microenvironment), because their on-target and off-target effects may be varied and unpredictable. Because molecularly and immunologically targeted therapies and the opportunities for combinatorial strategies are increasing rapidly, it is necessary to examine each component carefully in order to design regimens with the optimal therapeutic index.

Prognostic Value of Studying the Immune Tumor Microenvironment

The importance of immune-mediated events in the response of malignancy to traditional cytotoxic therapies, including chemotherapies and radiation, has recently undergone a resurgence of interest, with evidence that most antitumor therapies

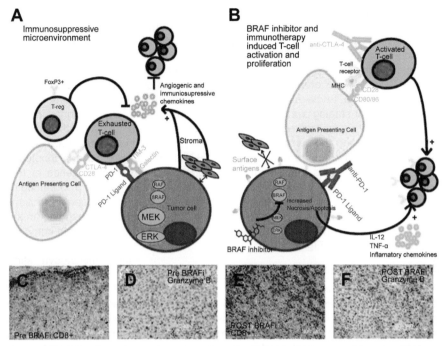

Fig. 1. Inhibition of constitutively activated mutant BRAF in melanoma driven by this onco-gene has a favorable effect on immunotherapy. (*A*) The tumor microenvironment features immunosuppressive chemokines from tumor and stromal cells. (*B*) BRAF inhibition may reduce these chemokines and the resulting recruited monocytes as well as inducing necrosis and increasing tumor antigen expression. (*C*) Pretreatment biopsy showing a low density of CD8+ lymphocytes. (*D*) Pretreatment biopsy showing a low density of granzyme B+ lympho-cytes. (*E*) Post–BRAF inhibitor biopsy showing a high density of CD8+ lymphocytes. (*F*) Post–BRAF inhibitor biopsy showing a high density of granzyme B+ lymphocytes. (*From* Wilmott JS, Scolyer RA, Long GV, et al. Combined targeted therapy and immunotherapy in the treatment of advanced melanoma. Oncoimmunology 2012;1:998; with permission.)

work at least in part through immune control and do not work in the absence of im-mune effectors. Examples of immunogenic chemotherapy have recently been studied by investigators at the Institut Gustav-Roussy (IGR), who analyzed the immunomodu-latory effects of many different cytotoxic and targeted anticancer agents. Because there were substantial differences in the effects and mechanisms of different agents on responses, which included both innate and adaptive immune systems, it is not possible to distinguish those drugs that work predominantly through a contribution to immunogenic cancer cell death. Furthermore, the importance of schedule and cell targets (immune effectors, tumor cells, vascular endothelium, and stromal cells) responding to various anticancer drugs needs to be taken into account in designing regimens to exploit these findings.[14] The transcription factor signal transducer of acti-vated T cells-3 (STAT3) may be of particular importance in mediating the expression of a broad spectrum of immunosuppressive, inflammatory, and proangiogenic factors that contribute to the growth and survival of tumor cells and the immunosuppressive state of the peritumoral milieu, and efforts to suppress its activity in combinatorial anti-tumor strategies have been encouraging.[15,16]

A series of additional studies from the IGR have provided the foundations for a systematic approach to the definition of immune system–tumor interactions with important implications for prognostic and predictive considerations in the further design of strategies to answer biological questions and to optimize clinical trials. These principles are best illustrated by **Fig. 2**. This model describes the immunoscore, a method for quantitating the CD8 effector and memory cells in different locations of the immune tumor microenvironment, which has a strong independent prognostic value (and allows a dichotomization of relapse-free and overall survival) in colorectal cancer and seems to be superior to earlier systems such as the tumor-node-metastasis (TNM) staging systems commonly used for solid tumor prognostication. The immunoscore was derived from a more complex system, termed the immune contexture, including the same T-cell subsets as the immunoscore but also taking into account the orientation, density, organizational characteristics, and functional characteristics of T cells in the tumor microenvironment.[17] The relevance of this approach to the melanoma immune tumor microenvironment and the importance of other nontumor cells such as stromal, vascular, and other cells of immune and inflammatory lineages remains to be elucidated and is also likely to differ depending on the primary location/biology, sites of metastatic disease, driver mutations, and immunogenetics of the patient (**Fig. 3**).

Inflammatory and Immune Gene Signatures in the Biology of Melanoma

Extensive studies of melanoma gene expression have supported the concept that it may be possible to recognize a dichotomy of biological behaviors characterized by patterns of gene expression reflecting differences in the immunologic interactions among tumor cells, stroma, and infiltrating immune and inflammatory cells. In an attempt to elucidate why some melanoma metastases seem to be heavily infiltrated by CD8 (potentially cytotoxic) T cells but nevertheless grow and eventually kill the patient, whereas other lethal melanomas do not feature an immune cell infiltrate, investigators at the University of Chicago described 2 distinct patterns of gene expression, one termed inflamed gene signature and the other noninflamed.[18] In addition to elegantly working out the cellular and molecular biology of the associated cell-cell interactions through gamma-interferon, intracellular sensing of tumor DNA, and

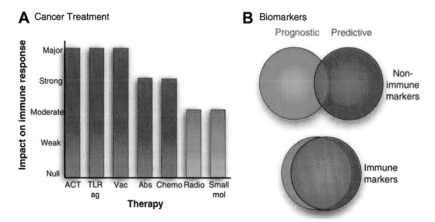

Fig. 2. (*A*) The impact of cancer treatments on the host immune system, and (*B*) the likely differences between immune-based and non–immune-based biomarkers with prognostic and/or predictive value for various cancer treatments. (*From* Angell H, Galon J. From the immune contexture to the Immunoscore: the role of prognostic and predictive immune markers in cancer. Curr Opin Immunol 2013;25:264; with permission.)

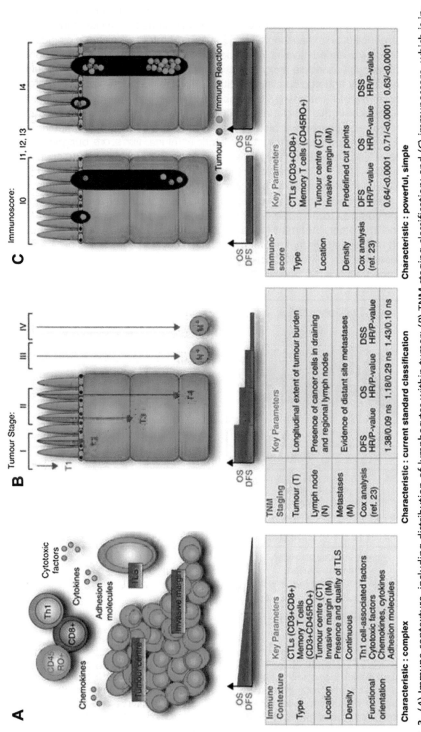

Fig. 3. (A) Immune contexture, including distribution of lymphocytes within tumor; (B) TNM staging classification; and (C) immunoscore, which is in-dependent of tumor burden. (*From* Angell H, Galon J. From the immune contexture to the Immunoscore: the role of prognostic and predictive immune markers in cancer. Curr Opin Immunol 2013;25:262; with permission.)

chemokines that mediate T-cell homing to tumor, these investigators proposed that the biology underlying melanoma growth despite an inflamed gene signature depends on the emergence of an exhaustion phenotype (thus identifying an immunologic target for which therapy is already available [antibodies to PD-1 or PD-L1]) or other suppressive mediators such as indole dioxygenase, for which therapeutic small molecule inhibitors are already undergoing clinical testing (**Fig. 4**).[19,20]

Additional forms of T-cell anergy, tolerance, or immunologic ignorance of tumor also exist (detailed later in this article) and may be possible to overcome therapeutically using other immune checkpoint blockers, such as anti–cytotoxic T lymphocyte antigen-4 (CTLA-4), immunostimulatory/homeostatic cytokines like IL-15, or agonistic antibodies mimicking the action of the natural ligands for costimulatory receptors (OX40, CD137, and CD40L).[21,22] Pleiotropic factors like TGF-β, IL-10, and the transcriptional regulator STAT3 and its downstream targets are also likely to play important supporting roles in cancer immunotherapy strategies, but their functions and targeting are currently too complex to incorporate into therapeutic strategies. Stimulation of antigen presentation and other important functions mediating crosstalk between cells traditionally part of the innate immune system and those considered responsible for adaptive responses include a wide variety of dendritic cell (DC) signaling agonists derived from pathogen-associated molecular pattern molecules like bacterial cell wall

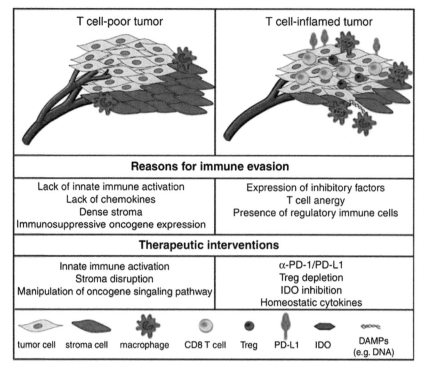

Fig. 4. A model for T cell–noninflamed (*left*) versus T cell–inflamed (*right*) tumor microenvironments. Left panel shows failed innate immune activation, dense stroma as a physical barrier, and possible immunosuppressive oncogene pathways. Right panel shows possible inhibition by PD-1/PD-L1 axis, indole dioxygenase (IDO), T-cell anergy, and T$_{reg}$ suppression. DAMPs, damage associated molecular patterns. (*From* Gajewski TF, Woo SR, Zha Y, et al. Cancer immunotherapy strategies based on overcoming barriers within the tumor microenvironment. Curr Opin Immunol 2013;25:269; with permission.)

components or nucleic acid fragments, or damage-associated molecular pattern molecules like double-stranded RNA that bind to specialized receptors on or within DCs.[23] Other agents, including the interferons (IFN), both type I (IFN-α and IFN-β) and type II or immune (IFN-γ), can enhance major histocompatibility complex (MHC) (human leukocyte antigen [HLA]) molecule expression on tumor cells and increase the expression and presentation by class I and II MHC molecules of immunogenic peptide epitopes derived from tumor antigens, in part by altering the ratio of different types of proteasomes responsible for antigen processing.[24,25] IFN-α also enhances the responsiveness of cytotoxic CD8 T cells to homeostatic cytokines such as IL-15 and IL-7, as well as to recall antigens.[25] Many elements of the immune tumor microenvironment influence the processing and transport of antigens within the tumor cell to their final site of presentation in the epitope-binding site of the HLA molecule to the peptide-recognition portion of the T-cell receptor. The expression of some of the genes involved in these tightly regulated pathways, as well as the intracellular transport of tumor antigen–derived peptides, can be modulated therapeutically by drugs that are already in the clinic or in development. These drugs include demethylating agents like 5-aza-2-deoxycytidine[26] and investigational heat-shock protein inhibitors that can alter intracellular patterns of antigen transport.[27]

Role of the Immune System in Dissemination of Melanoma to the Nodes and Distant Organs

Among the critical unresolved questions regarding the biology of melanoma is the control of dissemination to regional lymph nodes and the role played by cells and molecules of the immune system. It is increasingly evident that lymph nodes are not merely passive recipients of melanoma cells as they traverse the local lymphatics but that important intercellular interactions and intracellular events also control this phenomenon, which is likely set in motion before the appearance of melanoma cells in the node. Homing to the nodes is controlled in part by the expression of interacting pairs of chemokines and their receptors, and other intercellular interactions are mediated by adhesion molecules that allow melanoma cells to interact with endothelial cells.[28] Important interactions with the vasculature are also mediated by inflammatory cytokines, VEGFs, and other vasoactive molecules.[29] Lymph nodes may play a more active role in the dissemination of melanoma cells, via the elaboration of chemokine 1 (CCL1) by the lymphatic endothelial cells, which binds to chemokine receptor 8 (CCR8) on tumor cells, inducing chemotaxis to the node and controlling the transmigration of tumor cells from the subcapsular sinus to the cortex of the node.[30]

Recent studies have shown that premetastatic lymph nodes from patients with melanoma have alterations in their T-cell receptor function as shown by the expression of the zeta subunit of the CD3 signaling molecule.[31] Established nodal metastases also feature cellular infiltrates characteristic of chronic inflammation, including regulatory T cells (T_{reg}), myeloid-derived suppressor cells, tolerogenic DCs, and tumor-associated macrophages (TAM), which produce suppressive small molecules and other factors that mediate immunosuppression.[32,33] Further studies of melanoma-positive sentinel lymph nodes revealed that those from patients with either additional positive nodes at completion of lymph node dissection or from patients who relapse within 5 years differed significantly in their numbers of CD30+ lymphocytes from those who experienced neither unfavorable outcome. The CD30+ cell population consisted of a heterogeneous distribution of cells with phenotypic markers of suppression or exhaustion and that were also found in the peripheral blood of patients with advanced melanoma.[34] A potential role for activated natural killer (NK) cells in nodal immunosurveillance and adjuvant therapy is supported by the recent report of a unique population of

NK cells in melanoma-containing lymph nodes that can be stimulated to high lytic activity by IL-12 or IL-15.[35] The immunophenotypic and functional characteristics of melanoma-draining lymph node cells provides a rich foundation for both prognostic and predictive factors in the design of adjuvant trials for resected melanoma that complements the information increasingly available from the molecular and immunologic features of the primary tumor.

Immunosurveillance Against Primary and Relapsing Melanoma

It has long been thought that some form of immunosurveillance provides protection from cancer and that among the reasons for most cancers' predilection for older individuals is the gradual erosion of immune competence with advancing age. Recent observations on the impact of known molecular drivers and other modulators of melanoma biology have provided some understanding of different categories of melanoma, a disease that also has a lower median age and affects even children, adolescents, and young adults. It is likely that the role of immunosurveillance and the potential for immunotherapy strategies differ substantially among these different classes of melanoma that take into account not only patient age but also other tumor-host interactions and tumor-intrinsic factors such as their molecular drivers, which also change over time (melanoma has a high rate of acquisition of new mutations). Thus, despite the recent successes resulting from new immunotherapies for advanced melanoma (in particular, immune checkpoint blockade with antibodies as well as therapeutic infusions of expanded autologous cytotoxic T lymphocytes), the control of melanoma at every point along the continuum from melanomagenesis to proliferation and metastasis of advanced tumors requires specific alignment of cellular and molecular determinants of the interactions among these cells (including stroma and vasculature, which are also affected by the complex immunogenetic background of human patients). Thus, although the principles of immunosurveillance and immunotherapy for melanoma share many elements with other tumor types, there remain important differences that make it necessary to design investigational strategies based on the precise requirements for melanoma, and even for different types of melanoma (eg, uveal vs mucosal vs cutaneous). However, it may be possible to find methods to render melanomas more immunogenic using some of the interventions discussed in this article (eg, epigenetic modification of tumor, and radiotherapy and intralesional injection of immunomodulatory molecules) and thus cause it to behave more like those tumors that are known to depend more heavily on the immunosuppressed host, such as Merkel cell carcinoma, or that are virally induced, such as cervical cancer or cancers resulting from both viral and chronic inflammatory contributions (hepatitis B-associated and C-associated hepatocellular cancer).

Despite the presence of identified driver oncogenic mutations in at least 70% of cutaneous melanomas (and likely a high percentage of the others, yet to be identified), these mutations alone are not sufficient to confer the fully malignant phenotype, suggesting that additional modifying factors are required[36]; however, the role and the precise parameters of the host immune response in preventing or modifying melanomagenesis and subsequent melanoma behavior remains ill defined. To date, there is little evidence that the incidence of melanoma or the likelihood of an unfavorable outcome (earlier relapse, shorter survival) of previously diagnosed melanoma is substantially higher in patients who are overtly immunosuppressed, such as those with B-cell malignancies, solid organ transplant, or hematopoietic cell transplant.[37] It is likely that successful efforts to control and possibly even prevent melanoma using strategies that exploit the immune system will depend not only on the identification of the factors involved in tumor-host interactions but also in large part on tumor-specific immunogenic mutations that confer tumor cell onco-gene addiction.[38]

Immunosuppression, Tolerance Mechanisms, and Chronic Inflammation Induced by Melanoma

Although melanoma is not among the malignancies arising in the setting of chronic inflammation, its establishment is associated with the development of a local inflammatory microenvironment that initiates and maintains the suppressive or Th2 pattern of molecular and cellular components critical to its highly invasive and metastatic behavior. Many of these cells and molecules have been addressed earlier, and more detailed descriptions are beyond the scope of this article, but some of the important biological determinants and therapeutic targets include selected chemokines and their receptors (particularly CCL5 or regulated on activation, normal T cell expressed and secreted [RANTES], CCL11 or eotaxin, and CX chemokine 10 (CXCL10) or interferon gamma-induced protein 10 [IP-10]); VEGF; TGF-β; tumor necrosis factor alpha (TNF-α); and the cytokines IL-1, IL-6, and IL-8, all of which exert pleiotropic inflammatory effects on the surrounding cellular milieu. It is likely that the melanoma microenvironment exploits the inflammation amplifier, a circuit of cytokines, chemokines, neurotransmitters, growth factors/receptors, stromal elements, transcription factors, and inflammatory cells that work in concert to potentiate a state of local inflammation and tumor promotion and maintenance (**Fig. 5**).[39]

The immune tumor microenvironment has become the focus of intense scrutiny, because it has recently been shown to hold many of the secrets of tumor cell resistance to or escape from controlling mechanisms, which include but are not limited to those resulting from immune effector mechanisms. Although the current state of the field derived in large part from the study of phenotype and function of effectors and other inflammatory cells in the peripheral circulation, it is now clear that only by carefully dissecting and interrogating the tumor microenvironment can the precise impact of cell-cell and associated interactions be understood (as well as the role of cell populations that migrate in and out of sites of antigen presentation, including tumor). Further, these elements must be studied in several dimensions: histologic organization, quantitation of cell types, functional assays including serial analyses over time and in response to interventions, and sophisticated studies of the layers of omics reflecting genetics and gene expression in the various cell types comprising the tumor microenvironment. The results to date of such studies and the relative characteristics of the tumor immune contexture and the immunoscore are detailed earlier in this article (**Fig. 6**).

These observations have also provided corroboration of the immunoediting model of tumor–immune system interactions that features 3 broad phases: elimination of the tumor, equilibrium with the tumor, and escape by the tumor from immune control. These phases correspond with the experimental observations that more immunogenic tumors grow poorly in immunocompetent hosts and require host immunosuppression to grow well, whereas nonimmunogenic tumors grow well in immunocompetent hosts; a situation that is most closely related to human patients with melanoma (**Fig. 7**).[6]

Experimental evidence for these phases is also consistent with the concept of 3 mechanisms that explain the failure of T-cell immune reactions to control cancer. The first 2 are likely the related results of antigen presented without adequate costimulation and consist of (1) self-tolerance (which can include the immunologic ignorance, whereby antigenic signals are delivered in a concentration or orientation insufficient to activate T cells but can be enhanced by higher concentration or exogenous

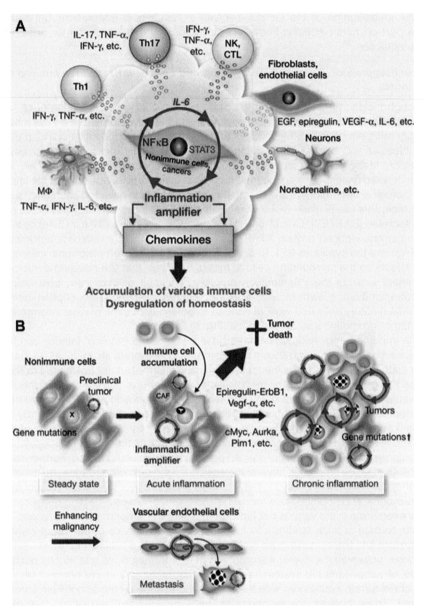

Fig. 5. The so-called inflammation amplifier, featuring tumor and stromal cell secretion of cytokines, chemokines, and growth factors that recruit immunosuppressive leukocytes that, in turn, secrete additional factors with tumor-promoting and/or immunosuppressive effects. (*A*) Pathways mediated by transcription factors NF-κB and STAT3. (*B*) Tumor cells are usually eliminated during acute inflammation, whereas the expression of inflammation amplifier–related genes by tumors, inflammatory cells, and endothelial cells during chronic inflammation might induce survival and/or new mutations to increase tumor cell aggressiveness. (*From* Atsumi T, Singh R, Sabharwal L, et al. Inflammation amplifier, a new paradigm in cancer biology. Cancer Res 2014;74(1):10; with permission.)

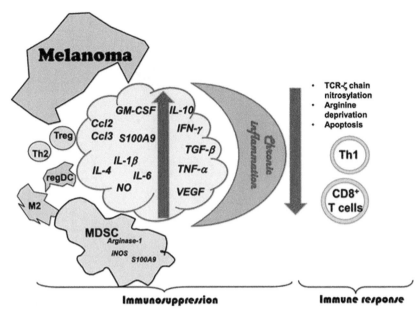

Fig. 6. Inflammatory and immunosuppressive relationships in the melanoma microenvironment, including the elements of chronic inflammation detailed in **Fig. 5** and showing the inflammatory mediators (cytokines, chemokines, and growth factors) secreted by the tumor and stroma cells. These mediators induce recruitment to tumor and activation of immunosuppressive leukocytes. Immunosuppressive activity of myeloid-derived suppressor cell (MDSC) includes inducible nitric oxide synthase and arginase-1, which contribute to inhibiting antitumor responses mediated by effector CD4 (Th1) and CD8 T cells via the induction of T cell receptor zeta chain downregulation, arginine deprivation, and apoptosis. (*From* Umansky V, Sevko A. Overcoming immunosuppression in the melanoma microenvironment induced by chronic inflammation. Cancer Immunol Immunother 2012;61:276; with permission.)

inflammatory signals; a unique state of T-cell differentiation with a tolerance-specific gene program); and (2) anergy, defined as the inability to produce IL-2 or proliferate to antigen delivered under optimal conditions. The third phenomenon, which has been the focus of considerable investigation and some notable therapeutic successes over the last several years, is termed exhaustion, and refers to the state of immunologic inaction resulting from the downmodulatory response of T cells to chronic antigenic stimulation (**Fig. 8**).

All of the factors associated with the immunosuppressed characteristics of the tumor microenvironment, including MDSC, T_{reg}, IL-10, TGF-β, IDO, tumor-associated macrophage, and the low-pH/high–reactive oxygen species local chemical milieu are associated with the expression by tumor-infiltrating T cells of exhaustion markers such as PD receptor-1 and T-cell immunoglobulin and mucin domain-3 (TIM-3).[40] Although maneuvers such as therapeutic lymphodepletion using chemotherapy can lead to the expansion of antigen-specific T cells and reverse tolerance, this approach alone is usually insufficient to induce tumor regression. However, many of the elements of the tumor immune microenvironment listed earlier are now amenable to therapeutic targeting with antibodies or small molecules and are currently under active investigation for melanoma and other malignancies, with encouraging results that are covered in detail elsewhere in this issue.

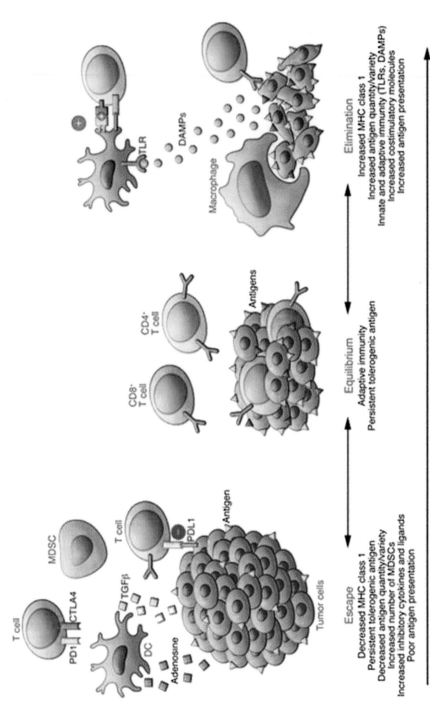

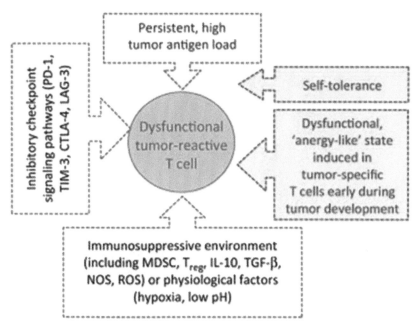

Fig. 8. Factors mediating exhaustion in tumor-induced T-cell dysfunction share phenotypic and functional characteristics with those of chronic viral infections, including expression of PD-1, LAG-3, 2B4, TIM-2, and CTLA-4. Also, TIL can be heterogeneous in their states of dysfunction, which are mediated by cell-intrinsic programs such as a tolerance program imprinted in self/tumor antigen-specific T cells or in tumor-specific T cells that encounter tumor antigen early during a premalignant noninflammatory phase of tumor development. (*From* Schietinger A, Greenberg PD. Tolerance and exhaustion: defining mechanisms of T cell dysfunction. Trends Immunol 2014;35:52; with permission.)

CLINICAL STATUS OF IMMUNOTHERAPY FOR MELANOMA: BRIEF OVERVIEW
Cancer Vaccines, Adoptive T-cell Therapies, and Antigen-specific Escape from Effector T-cell Response

Melanoma is one of the first malignancies to have been therapeutically targeted with immunomodulation, based in part on observations in animal models, occasional human anecdotes of tumors regressing in response to an inflammatory event, and on the well-documented refractoriness of melanoma to cytotoxic chemotherapy. Cancer vaccines based on tumor cells (autologous or allogeneic) and their crude products such as lysates or cells chemically altered to enhance their immunogenicity have been disappointing and have given way to more defined vaccine strategies based on a wide

◄─────────────────────────────────────

Fig. 7. The cancer immunoediting hypothesis, in which the tumor–immune system balance shifts among the states of equilibrium or coexistence to elimination (occurring early in tumor development, when highly antigenic clones are recognized and eradicated by innate and/or adaptive immune cell responses) or to escape (in which many of the unfavorable or suppressive tumor–immune system interactions shown earlier provide a net advantage to the tumor). CTLA4, cytotoxic T lymphocyte antigen 4; TLR, Toll-like receptor. (*From* Kalbasi A, June CH, Haas N, et al. Radiation and immunotherapy: a synergistic combination. J Clin Invest 2013;123:2757; with permission.)

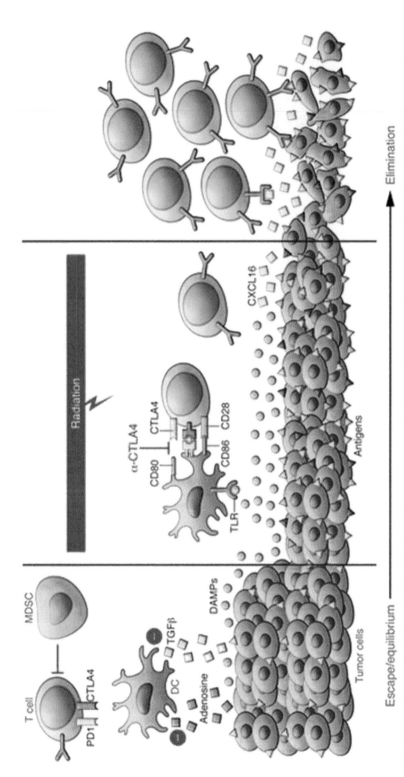

Fig. 9. The role of radiation in inducing effective antitumor responses includes enhancement of antigen expression, release of proinflammatory chemokines that recruit immune effector cells, other proteins that promote antigen cross-presentation by DCs, and the induction of apoptosis-mediating receptor expression on tumor cells. (*From* Kalbasi A, June CH, Haas N, et al. Radiation and immunotherapy: a synergistic combination. J Clin Invest 2013;123:2759; with permission.)

variety of antigens derived from melanoma-specific differentiation antigens such as tyrosinase, gp100, and MELAN-A/MART-1; cancer-testis antigens without specificity for melanoma but with restriction to embryonal tissues and germ cells as well as malignant cells in adults (eg, NY-ESO-1 and MAGE-A3 in melanoma); and other molecules with potential for immunogenicity based on mutation in tumor and/or different patterns of expression between malignant cells and normal tissue, such as survivin and telomerase.[41–46] In addition to the need to overcome the highly immunosuppressive tumor milieu detailed earlier, the remaining challenges of vaccine development include the identification of optimal antigenic peptides for class I and II MHC–binding and T-cell receptor engagement, selecting the best targets and agonists for costimulation, designing the most potent antigen-presentation strategies, monitoring the immune and clinical responses to immunotherapy, and maintaining these responses once achieved. Animal models of immunotherapy against experimental tumors, often showing a critical window for optimal intervention, have poorly represented human spontaneous cancers, particularly melanoma with its high rate of mutations and the low immunogenicity of the antigens identified to date in human patients with advanced disease and even those with fully resected melanoma at high risk of recurrence.

The most promising forms of adoptive T-cell therapy derive from the expansion of tumor-infiltrating lymphocytes (TIL) cultivated in T-cell growth factors and administered to patients pretreated with lymphodepleting chemotherapy and/or radiotherapy to increase the availability of homeostatic cytokines (IL-7, IL-15)[47–51] and thus expand the infused cell product, which is enriched for tumor antigen–reactive T cells. The most potent antigens may be patient-specific or private mutations in proteins that are processed and presented effectively through the class I (and probably also class II) antigen processing machinery to the expanded population of therapeutic T cells.[52] Broader application of this modality still faces many challenges, including safely accessible tumor for the preparation of TIL cells, the risks and toxicities of the lymphodepleting regimen (and whether it can be replaced by exogenous delivery of homeostatic cytokine), identification of the optimal postinfusion regimen for expansion and survival of effective cytotoxic T cells and achievement of memory responses, and manipulation of the immunosuppressive tumor microenvironment that continues to deliver hostile signals even to the infused highly cytotoxic TIL product.[53–56] Other forms of adoptive T-cell therapies are also under investigation, including antigen-specific peripheral blood–derived cells expanded ex vivo and reinfused to lymphodepleted patients followed by cytokines and checkpoint-blocking antibodies. The role for more elaborate strategies such as genetically modified T cells expressing selected T-cell receptors or immunoglobulin chains with specificity for tumor antigen has not been extensively explored but may face challenges because of the single-antigen reactivity of these effectors, the potential requirement for costimulatory molecules with excessive toxicities because of off-target effects, the potential for autoimmunity caused by cross-reactivity with nonmelanoma normal tissues, and the efficiency of melanoma escape from such focused therapies.[52,56,57]

Vaccines and Cytokines

Although vaccines developed for established cancer or for the prevention of relapse in the postsurgical adjuvant setting are intended to trigger either a de novo immune response or enhance an existing but ineffective one (break tolerance), their failure is likely caused by multiple factors, including not only the thymic (central) deletion of self-antigen–specific T-cell receptor–bearing lymphocytes but also peripheral tolerance via the wide spectrum of suppressive mechanisms detailed earlier. Many patients have circulating lymphocytes or TIL with reactivity against tumor-associated antigens that could be therapeutic under optimal conditions,[58] and it is also likely that the adaptive antitumor immune response can be enhanced by interventions that stimulate innate immunity (NK cells and DCs) as well as adaptive responses. NK cells exert an antigen-nonspecific response that includes cytotoxicity and cytokine production but has little to no immunologic memory, and molecules that stimulate T-cell responses may induce negative signaling in NK cells through their vast array of inhibitory receptors and limited stimulatory receptors. However, along with several subpopulations of DCs, NK cells also contribute to the elaboration of potent adaptive responses that include the most critical element: antigen-specific immunologic memory. Cytokines such as the interferons, particularly class I IFN-α, and selected interleukins such as IL-2 and IL-15, stimulate not only T cells but also NK cells, inducing cytokine production, cytotoxicity, and cell proliferation.[48,59] The cytokines differ in their relative ability to bind and activate their receptors on target cells, many of them sharing receptor subunits and partially overlapping signaling functions, and some may activate and expand suppressive cells (eg, IL-2[60]) or memory responses (eg, IL-7 and IL-15).[61] Thus, the design of any immunotherapeutic strategy for melanoma must attempt to optimize those functions that promote early antitumor responses as well as antigen-specific persistence and memory responses. Recent data suggest that the extension of T-cell responses to antigens not targeted by the primary therapeutic intervention (antigen or epitope spread) may also be critical for effective and long-lived responses and should be a goal of immunotherapy strategies for melanoma (Chapuis and colleagues, manuscript submitted, 2014). Because cytokines are easy to produce and prepare for human administration, and their target cells, immunologic functions, and clinical management are well understood, the exploitation of cytokine-based immunotherapies remains of great interest in immunotherapy for melanoma but is more likely to be of value for its contribution to carefully designed combinations than as single-agent therapies. Among the most important questions to build into study design include the impact of T_{reg}-blocking or T_{reg}-depleting strategies,[62] the potential and pitfalls of immune checkpoint blockade targeting not only CTLA4 and the PD-1/PD-L1 axis but also the immunomodulatory receptors TIM-3 and LAG-3,[63,64] and the optimal use of homeostatic cytokines and/or lymphodepletion strategies.

Escape from effective antigen-specific T-cell responses can also result from the mutational or epigenetically controlled loss of MHC molecules, antigen/immunogenic peptides, and costimulatory molecules required for the recognition and response by cytotoxic effectors of optimally processed and presented antigen on both antigen-presenting cells and tumor cells.[65] Mediators of inflammation such as TNF-α may mediate changes in effective antigen presentation through dedifferentiation programs in melanoma cells that may be reversible with agents that alter gene expression as well as with blocking antibodies, another strategy that may be of value in the design of clinical trials.[66]

Special Immunotherapy Designs Based on Modulation of the Tumor Microenvironment

Lesional immunotherapy

Intralesional immunotherapy has been of interest for many years, in part because of the long-standing interest in immunotherapy for this disease, the availability of agents like bacille Calmette-Guérin (BCG), interferons, IL-2, and granulocyte-monocyte colony-stimulating factor (GM-CSF), and the frequent accessibility of lesions for injection (and sometimes the need for symptom palliation of bulky or unresectable metastases). The goals of lesional therapy are 2-fold and include the regression of the injected mass and the establishment of a strong and persistent systemic immune response that can control established distant metastases and prevent the occurrence of new lesions. Despite decades of efforts dedicated to these objectives, researchers have to date had to deal with the same dilemma as many other efforts to derive systemic benefit from locoregional therapies: frequent benefit at the injection site(s) with little to no systemic impact.[67] Nevertheless, rapidly expanding understanding of the cellular and molecular components of the tumor microenvironment are providing insights into new targets and surrogate end points that may lead to greater success, particularly with combinatorial strategies such as injection of immunomodulatory molecules, including antibodies that block immune checkpoints or deplete T_{reg}.[68,69] One of the newest approaches has been the use of modified human herpesviruses engineered to reduce their pathogenicity, enhance their expression in tumor cells, and express GM-CSF, which can confer potent antigenic properties on the tumor cells and turn them into a potent tumor vaccine to induce an effective local and systemic antitumor immune response.[70] Ongoing randomized trials will determine whether this method of delivering potent immunomodulatory signals directly into the tumor microenvironment can achieve the goals of overcoming many of the suppressive and inhibitory signals detailed earlier and result in vaccination of the patient with melanoma with potent and durable local and systemic antitumor effects.

Radiation therapy

The use of radiotherapy to palliate melanoma has been challenged by the poor radioresponsiveness of this tumor, probably in large part because of the myriad of mechanisms for DNA repair and protection against apoptosis. Radiotherapy is known to cause lymphopenia and potential immunosuppression because of its effects on lymphocytes as they circulate through the radiation portal. However, in some models, immune responses are important for the optimal antitumor effects of radiotherapy[71] and selected dose schedules of focal radiation have been shown to induce potent immunomodulatory effects that may be additive or even synergistic with systemic immunotherapies and can also produce tumor regression at a distance from the irradiated site (the so-called abscopal effect). The mechanisms of this abscopal effect of tumor radiotherapy have been the focus of intense recent investigation, which has led to the observation that although apoptosis of tumor cells induced by radiotherapy does not typically provide an inflammatory or immunogenic stimulus, certain doses and schedules can induce local acute inflammation, which is the danger signal necessary to achieve strong innate responses that contribute to antigen-specific adaptive T-cell responses with increased expression of antigen, epitope spread, and costimulatory molecules. The precise mechanisms for these reactions seem to involve a highly orchestrated cascade of damage-associated reactions in DCs, initiated by the translocation of calreticulin to the cell membrane, which induces a phagocytic signal to local DCs, an autophagy program that further signals to DCs and provides additional inflammatory mediators and ultimately the release of high-mobility group box 1 protein that synergizes with DC-activating receptors (**Fig. 9**).[72,73]

Based on a series of recent clinical observations of such abscopal effects in melanoma treated systemically with either ipilimumab or IL-2, and an elegant investigation of the cellular and humoral immune responses to the important cancer-testis antigen NY-ESO-I underlying a clinical rescue response to radiotherapy and reinstitution of ipilimumab in a patient with ipilimumab-refractory metastatic melanoma,[74] several groups of investigators have initiated clinical trials to better define the essential variable. Most of the reports have featured either stereotactic ablative radiotherapy or other types of hypofractionated, large-dose-per-fraction radiotherapy, and current trials are directed at radiotherapy dose and fractions, choice of systemic immunotherapy, and immunologic correlates of benefit[75] (see also http://clinicaltrials.gov/ct2/show/NCT01449279?term=knox+and+melanoma&rank=4; http://clinicaltrials.gov/ct2/show/NCT01497808?term=rengan+and+melanoma&rank=1).

SUMMARY

The immune system plays an essential role across the natural history of melanoma, from the benign or premalignant nevus, through the radial and vertical growth phases of melanoma, to lymphatic and hematogenous routes of dissemination and in the pre-metastatic and metastatic tumor microenvironment. In parallel with rapid advances in elucidating the molecular biology of all melanoma variants have been important developments in the understanding of tumor and host immunology, with potential for highly effective therapeutic strategies along the natural history continuum. The tools are currently available to make a meaningful impact on the severe toll taken by this challenging disease and are likely to expand further with ongoing investigations.

REFERENCES

1. Kanavy HE, Gerstenblith MR. Ultraviolet radiation and melanoma. Semin Cutan Med Surg 2011;30:222–8.
2. Sahu RP, Turner MJ, DaSilva SC, et al. The environmental stressor ultraviolet B radiation inhibits murine antitumor immunity through its ability to generate platelet-activating factor agonists. Carcinogenesis 2012;33:1360–7.
3. Ullrich SE, Byrne SN. The immunologic revolution: photoimmunology. J Invest Dermatol 2012;132:896–905.
4. Berwick M, Armstrong BK, Ben-Porat L, et al. Sun exposure and mortality from melanoma. J Natl Cancer Inst 2005;97:195–9.
5. Taube JM, Anders RA, Young GD, et al. Colocalization of inflammatory response with B7-h1 expression in human melanocytic lesions supports an adaptive resistance mechanism of immune escape. Sci Transl Med 2012;4:127ra37.
6. Schreiber RD, Old LJ, Smyth MJ. Cancer immunoediting: integrating immunity's roles in cancer suppression and promotion. Science 2011;331:1565–70.
7. Boni A, Cogdill AP, Dang P, et al. Selective BRAFV600E inhibition enhances T-cell recognition of melanoma without affecting lymphocyte function. Cancer Res 2010;70:5213–9.
8. Sumimoto H, Imabayashi F, Iwata T, et al. The BRAF-MAPK signaling pathway is essential for cancer-immune evasion in human melanoma cells. J Exp Med 2006;203:1651–6.
9. Frederick DT, Piris A, Cogdill AP, et al. BRAF inhibition is associated with enhanced melanoma antigen expression and a more favorable tumor microenvironment in patients with metastatic melanoma. Clin Cancer Res 2013;19:1225–31.
10. Liu C, Peng W, Xu C, et al. BRAF inhibition increases tumor infiltration by T cells and enhances the antitumor activity of adoptive immunotherapy in mice. Clin Cancer Res 2013;19:393–403.
11. Koya RC, Mok S, Otte N, et al. BRAF inhibitor vemurafenib improves the anti-tumor activity of adoptive cell immunotherapy. Cancer Res 2012;72:3928–37.
12. Cooper ZA, Frederick DT, Juneja VR, et al. BRAF inhibition is associated with increased clonality in tumor-infiltrating lymphocytes. Oncoimmunology 2013;2:e26615.
13. Wilmott JS, Scolyer RA, Long GV, et al. Combined targeted therapy and immunotherapy in the treatment of advanced melanoma. Oncoimmunology 2012;1:997–9.

14. Zitvogel L, Galluzzi L, Smyth MJ, et al. Mechanism of action of conventional and targeted anticancer therapies: reinstating immunosurveillance. Immunity 2013; 39:74–88.
15. Gao C, Kozlowska A, Nechaev S, et al. TLR9 signaling in the tumor microenvironment initiates cancer recurrence after radiotherapy. Cancer Res 2013;73: 7211–21.
16. Liu F, Cao J, Wu J, et al. Stat3-targeted therapies overcome the acquired resistance to vemurafenib in melanomas. J Invest Dermatol 2013;133:2041–9.
17. Angell H, Galon J. From the immune contexture to the Immunoscore: the role of prognostic and predictive immune markers in cancer. Curr Opin Immunol 2013; 25:261–7.
18. Gajewski TF. Failure at the effector phase: immune barriers at the level of the melanoma tumor microenvironment. Clin Cancer Res 2007;13:5256–61.
19. Gajewski TF, Woo SR, Zha Y, et al. Cancer immunotherapy strategies based on overcoming barriers within the tumor microenvironment. Curr Opin Immunol 2013;25:268–76.
20. Spranger S, Spaapen RM, Zha Y, et al. Up-regulation of PD-L1, IDO, and T(regs) in the melanoma tumor microenvironment is driven by CD8(+) T cells. Sci Transl Med 2013;5:200ra116.
21. Spranger S, Gajewski T. Rational combinations of immunotherapeutics that target discrete pathways. J Immunother Cancer 2013;1:16.
22. Pradere JP, Dapito DH, Schwabe RF. The Yin and Yang of Toll-like receptors in cancer. Oncogene 2013. [Epub ahead of print].
23. Lattanzi L, Rozera C, Marescotti D, et al. IFN-alpha boosts epitope cross-presentation by DCs via modulation of proteasome activity. Immunobiology 2011;216:537–47.
24. Respa A, Bukur J, Ferrone S, et al. Association of IFN-gamma signal transduction defects with impaired HLA class I antigen processing in melanoma cell lines. Clin Cancer Res 2011;17:2668–78.
25. Hervas-Stubbs S, Mancheno U, Riezu-Boj JI, et al. CD8 T cell priming in the presence of IFN-alpha renders CTLs with improved responsiveness to homeostatic cytokines and recall antigens: important traits for adoptive T cell therapy. J Immunol 2012;189:3299–310.
26. Fratta E, Sigalotti L, Colizzi F, et al. Epigenetically regulated clonal heritability of CTA expression profiles in human melanoma. J Cell Physiol 2010;223:352–8.
27. Paraiso KH, Haarberg HE, Wood E, et al. The HSP90 inhibitor XL888 overcomes BRAF inhibitor resistance mediated through diverse mechanisms. Clin Cancer Res 2012;18:2502–14.
28. Brandner JM, Haass NK. Melanoma's connections to the tumour microenvironment. Pathology 2013;45:443–52.
29. Braeuer RR, Watson IR, Wu CJ, et al. Why is melanoma so metastatic? Pigment Cell Melanoma Res 2014;27:19–36.
30. Das S, Sarrou E, Podgrabinska S, et al. Tumor cell entry into the lymph node is controlled by CCL1 chemokine expressed by lymph node lymphatic sinuses. J Exp Med 2013;210:1509–28.
31. Negin B, Panka D, Wang W, et al. Effect of melanoma on immune function in the regional lymph node basin. Clin Cancer Res 2008;14:654–9.
32. Mohos A, Sebestyen T, Liszkay G, et al. Immune cell profile of sentinel lymph nodes in patients with malignant melanoma – FOXP3+ cell density in cases with positive sentinel node status is associated with unfavorable clinical outcome. J Transl Med 2013;11:43.

33. Umansky V, Sevko A. Tumor microenvironment and myeloid-derived suppressor cells. Cancer Microenviron 2013;6:169–77.
34. Vallacchi V, Vergani E, Camisaschi C, et al. Transcriptional profiling of melanoma sentinel nodes identify patients with poor outcome and reveal an association of CD30+ T lymphocytes with progression. Cancer Res 2014;74(1):130–40.
35. Messaoudene M, Fregni G, Fourmentraux-Neves E, et al. Mature cytotoxic CD56bright/CD16+ natural killer cells can infiltrate lymph nodes adjacent to metastatic melanoma. Cancer Res 2014;74(1):81–92.
36. Ross AL, Sanchez MI, Grichnik JM. Molecular nevogenesis. Dermatol Res Pract 2011;2011:463184.
37. Kubica AW, Brewer JD. Melanoma in immunosuppressed patients. Mayo Clin Proc 2012;87:991–1003.
38. Casey SC, Bellovin DI, Felsher DW. Noncanonical roles of the immune system in eliciting oncogene addiction. Curr Opin Immunol 2013;25:246–58.
39. Atsumi T, Singh R, Sabharwal L, et al. Inflammation amplifier, a new paradigm in cancer biology. Cancer Res 2014;74(1):8–14.
40. Chen DS, Mellman I. Oncology meets immunology: the cancer-immunity cycle. Immunity 2013;39:1–10.
41. Kawakami Y, Robbins PF, Wang RF, et al. The use of melanosomal proteins in the immunotherapy of melanoma. J Immunother 1998;21:237–46.
42. Becker JC, Andersen MH, Hofmeister-Muller V, et al. Survivin-specific T-cell reactivity correlates with tumor response and patient survival: a phase-II peptide vaccination trial in metastatic melanoma. Cancer Immunol Immunother 2012;61:2091–103.
43. Kyte JA, Gaudernack G, Dueland S, et al. Telomerase peptide vaccination combined with temozolomide: a clinical trial in stage IV melanoma patients. Clin Cancer Res 2011;17:4568–80.
44. Filipazzi P, Pilla L, Mariani L, et al. Limited induction of tumor cross-reactive T cells without a measurable clinical benefit in early melanoma patients vaccinated with human leukocyte antigen class I-modified peptides. Clin Cancer Res 2012;18:6485–96.
45. Kruit WH, Suciu S, Dreno B, et al. Selection of immunostimulant AS15 for active immunization with MAGE-A3 protein: results of a randomized phase II study of the European Organisation for Research and Treatment of Cancer Melanoma Group in Metastatic Melanoma. J Clin Oncol 2013;31:2413–20.
46. Ulloa-Montoya F, Louahed J, Dizier B, et al. Predictive gene signature in MAGE-A3 antigen-specific cancer immunotherapy. J Clin Oncol 2013;31:2388–95.
47. Wang LX, Li R, Yang G, et al. Interleukin-7-dependent expansion and persistence of melanoma-specific T cells in lymphodepleted mice lead to tumor regression and editing. Cancer Res 2005;65:10569–77.
48. Waldmann TA. The biology of interleukin-2 and interleukin-15: implications for cancer therapy and vaccine design. Nat Rev Immunol 2006;6:595–601.
49. Overwijk WW, Schluns KS. Functions of gammaC cytokines in immune homeostasis: current and potential clinical applications. Clin Immunol 2009;132:153–65.
50. Lugli E, Goldman CK, Perera LP, et al. Transient and persistent effects of IL-15 on lymphocyte homeostasis in nonhuman primates. Blood 2010;116:3238–48.
51. Dudley ME, Yang JC, Sherry R, et al. Adoptive cell therapy for patients with metastatic melanoma: evaluation of intensive myeloablative chemoradiation preparative regimens. J Clin Oncol 2008;26:5233–9.

52. Robbins PF, Lu YC, El-Gamil M, et al. Mining exomic sequencing data to identify mutated antigens recognized by adoptively transferred tumor-reactive T cells. Nat Med 2013;19:747–52.

53. Rosenberg SA, Yang JC, Sherry RM, et al. Durable complete responses in heavily pretreated patients with metastatic melanoma using T-cell transfer immunotherapy. Clin Cancer Res 2011;17:4550–7.

54. Radvanyi LG, Bernatchez C, Zhang M, et al. Specific lymphocyte subsets predict response to adoptive cell therapy using expanded autologous tumor-infiltrating lymphocytes in metastatic melanoma patients. Clin Cancer Res 2012;18:6758–70.

55. Besser MJ, Shapira-Frommer R, Itzhaki O, et al. Adoptive transfer of tumor-infiltrating lymphocytes in patients with metastatic melanoma: intent-to-treat analysis and efficacy after failure to prior immunotherapies. Clin Cancer Res 2013;19:4792–800.

56. Robbins PF, Morgan RA, Feldman SA, et al. Tumor regression in patients with metastatic synovial cell sarcoma and melanoma using genetically engineered lymphocytes reactive with NY-ESO-1. J Clin Oncol 2011;29:917–24.

57. Yeh S, Karne NK, Kerkar SP, et al. Ocular and systemic autoimmunity after successful tumor-infiltrating lymphocyte immunotherapy for recurrent, metastatic melanoma. Ophthalmology 2009;116(5):981–9.e1.

58. Lee PP, Yee C, Savage PA, et al. Characterization of circulating T cells specific for tumor-associated antigens in melanoma patients. Nat Med 1999;5:677–85.

59. Sosinowski T, White JT, Cross EW, et al. CD8alpha+ DC trans presentation of IL-15 to naive CD8+ T cells produces antigen-inexperienced T cells in the periphery with memory phenotype and function. J Immunol 2013;190:1936–47.

60. Amado IF, Berges J, Luther RJ, et al. IL-2 coordinates IL-2-producing and regulatory T cell interplay. J Exp Med 2013;210:2707–20.

61. Cieri N, Camisa B, Cocchiarella F, et al. IL-7 and IL-15 instruct the generation of human memory stem T cells from naive precursors. Blood 2013;121(4): 573–84.

62. Jacobs JF, Nierkens S, Figdor CG, et al. Regulatory T cells in melanoma: the final hurdle towards effective immunotherapy? Lancet Oncol 2012;13(1):e32–42.

63. Legat A, Speiser DE, Pircher H, et al. Inhibitory receptor expression depends more dominantly on differentiation and activation than "exhaustion" of human CD8 T cells. Front Immunol 2013;4:455.

64. Woo SR, Turnis ME, Goldberg MV, et al. Immune inhibitory molecules LAG-3 and PD-1 synergistically regulate T-cell function to promote tumoral immune escape. Cancer Res 2012;72:917–27.

65. Khong HT, Wang QJ, Rosenberg SA. Identification of multiple antigens recognized by tumor-infiltrating lymphocytes from a single patient: tumor escape by antigen loss and loss of MHC expression. J Immunother 2004;27:184–90.

66. Landsberg J, Kohlmeyer J, Renn M, et al. Melanomas resist T-cell therapy through inflammation-induced reversible dedifferentiation. Nature 2012;490: 412–6.

67. Hersey P, Gallagher S. Intralesional immunotherapy for melanoma. J Surg Oncol 2013;109:320–6.

68. Marabelle A, Kohrt H, Sagiv-Barfi I, et al. Depleting tumor-specific Tregs at a single site eradicates disseminated tumors. J Clin Invest 2013;123:2447–63.

69. Marabelle A, Kohrt H, Levy R. Intratumoral anti-CTLA-4 therapy: enhancing efficacy while avoiding toxicity. Clin Cancer Res 2013;19:5261–3.

70. Senzer NN, Kaufman HL, Amatruda T, et al. Phase II clinical trial of a granulocyte-macrophage colony-stimulating factor-encoding, second-generation oncolytic herpesvirus in patients with unresectable metastatic melanoma. J Clin Oncol 2009;27:5763–71.

71. Burnette BC, Liang H, Lee Y, et al. The efficacy of radiotherapy relies upon induction of type I interferon-dependent innate and adaptive immunity. Cancer Res 2011;71(7):2488–96.

72. Kalbasi A, June CH, Haas N, et al. Radiation and immunotherapy: a synergistic combination. J Clin Invest 2013;123:2756–63.

73. Lauber K, Ernst A, Orth M, et al. Dying cell clearance and its impact on the outcome of tumor radiotherapy. Front Oncol 2012;2:116.

74. Postow MA, Callahan MK, Barker CA, et al. Immunologic correlates of the abscopal effect in a patient with melanoma. N Engl J Med 2012;366(10):925–31.

75. Seung SK, Curti BD, Crittenden M, et al. Phase 1 study of stereotactic body radiotherapy and interleukin-2–tumor and immunological responses. Sci Transl Med 2012;4(137):137ra174.

Vaccines and Melanoma

Patrick A. Ott, MD, PhD[a,b,c,d,*], Edward F. Fritsch, PhD[a,e],
Catherine J. Wu, MD[a,d,f], Glenn Dranoff, MD[a,d,f]

KEYWORDS

- Melanoma • Vaccine • Immunotherapy • Neoantigen

KEY POINTS

- The potential for therapeutic efficacy of a melanoma vaccine has been evident preclinically for many years.
- In patients with melanoma, vaccines have resulted in the induction of immune responses, although clinical benefit has not been clearly documented.
- The recent achievements with immune-checkpoint blockade, such as anti–CTLA-4 and anti–PD-1/PD-L1 in melanoma and other cancers, have illustrated that immunotherapy can be a powerful tool in cancer therapy.
- With increased understanding of tumor immunity, the limitations of many previous cancer vaccination approaches have become evident.
- Rapid progress in technologies that enable better vaccine design raise the expectation that these limitations can be overcome, thus leading to a clinically effective melanoma vaccine in the near future.

INTRODUCTION

Vaccination against melanoma represents an effort to stimulate an antitumor immune response that is directed either against an established tumor in patients with unresectable metastatic disease, or against micrometastatic disease in patients who are at high risk for recurrence after surgical resection. In both situations, the host has already failed the task of cancer immunosurveillance. The reasons for this failure are either the complete lack of an antimelanoma immune response or tumor-mediated immune evasion, caused by numerous mechanisms that cancers can elaborate. A successful antitumor vaccine therefore will induce a de novo immune response or boost an ineffective existing response, reprogramming the (failed) immune response by providing it

[a] Department of Medical Oncology, Dana-Farber Cancer Institute, 450 Brookline Avenue, Boston, MA 02215, USA; [b] Melanoma Disease Center, Dana-Farber Cancer Institute, 450 Brookline Avenue, Boston, MA 02215, USA; [c] Center for Immuno-Oncology, Dana-Farber Cancer Institute, 450 Brookline Avenue, Boston, MA 02215, USA; [d] Department of Medicine, Brigham and Women's Hospital, Harvard Medical School, 75 Francis Street, Boston, MA 02215, USA; [e] Broad Institute of Harvard and MIT, 7 Cambridge Center, Cambridge, MA 02142, USA; [f] Cancer Vaccine Center, Dana-Farber Cancer Institute, 450 Brookline Avenue, Boston, MA 02215, USA
* Corresponding author. Melanoma Disease Center, Center for Immuno-Oncology, Dana-Farber Cancer Institute, Harvard Medical School, 450 Brookline Avenue, Boston, MA 02215-5450.
E-mail address: Patrick_Ott@DFCI.harvard.edu

Hematol Oncol Clin N Am 28 (2014) 559–569
http://dx.doi.org/10.1016/j.hoc.2014.02.008
0889-8588/14/$ – see front matter © 2014 Elsevier Inc. All rights reserved.

with new targets and stronger stimulation (**Fig. 1**). Differences among strategies relate to the vehicle used to deliver the antigenic target, the antigenic target itself, the number of targets provided, and the appropriate immune-stimulating context (adjuvant). Checkpoint blockade, an antigen-independent immunotherapy, is designed to overcome 1 or more mechanisms of immune evasion, and provides exciting synergistic opportunities to strengthen vaccine therapy. Vaccination strategies offer the capacity for potentiated adaptive immune activation, antigen(s)/target specificity, multiarm immune engagement, and the realization of durable, effective immunologic memory, a hallmark of effective immunity.

No other tumor has been more thoroughly investigated with different vaccine approaches than melanoma. This article first summarizes prior efforts undertaken over the last 20 years, which demonstrated promise but were lacking in broad clinical activity. Further described are exciting new approaches that leverage recent technological advances with important biological insights to yield potential advances in this field.

PREVIOUS VACCINE APPROACHES IN MELANOMA: SOME PROMISE, BUT LIMITED CLINICAL ACTIVITY

Immunogens

Most vaccine approaches to date have used whole proteins or peptide fragments as the immunogen, which must be delivered to professional antigen-presenting cells

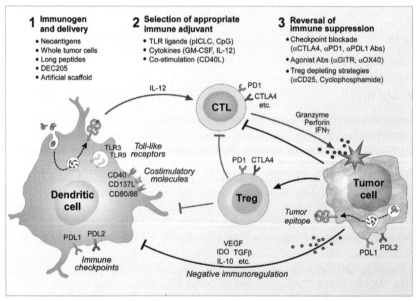

Fig. 1. Important features of an effective vaccine. (1) An immunogen that is capable of inducing tumor-specific T cells, rather than tolerance to "self." (2) The appropriate immune adjuvant that will provide the necessary inflammatory context, leading to activation of professional antigen presenting cells such as dendritic cells. (3) Reversal of immunosuppressive mechanisms such as checkpoint blockade (anti–CTLA-4, anti–PD-1/PD-L1), deletion/suppression of regulatory T cells (Treg), inhibition of immunosuppressive factors (anti-VEGF, anti-IDO, and so forth). CTL, cytotoxic T lymphocyte; CTLA-4, cytotoxic T-lymphocyte antigen-4; GM-CSF, granulocyte-macrophage colony-stimulating factor; IDO, indoleamine 2,3-dioxygenase; IL, interleukin; PD1, programmed death 1; PDL1, programmed death 1 ligand; TGF, transforming growth factor; VEGF, vascular endothelial growth factor.

(APCs) such as dendritic cells (DCs), usually in conjunction with an immune-stimulating adjuvant to serve as an effective vaccine. The objective is antigen uptake, processing, and cross-presentation by APCs to effect priming of naïve T cells or stimulation of memory T cells. The appropriate immune adjuvant will provide the danger signal, promoting immune pathways analogous to those activated in response to bacterial or viral infection. Key considerations when designing an effective vaccine include format (ie, whole protein vs peptide), route of delivery, and choice of adjuvant. Regarding the former, factors include cost (advantage: peptide), in vivo stability (advantage: peptide), and breadth of antigenic selection (advantage: protein). A significant limitation to peptide vaccines is their restriction to specific human leukocyte antigen (HLA) haplotypes. Most vaccine developers to date have focused on peptides that bind to the predominant HLA allele (HLA-A2) to capture the largest target population possible with a single vaccine. Unfortunately, this strategy excludes a vast pool of potentially immunogenic peptides and a considerable proportion of melanoma patients. This drawback could partially be addressed by using longer peptides (containing more than 1 epitope) or the use of multiple peptides, but as yet no such research has been conducted.

Tumor-associated antigens (TAA) are developmental, differentiation, or growth-promoting proteins that are frequently overexpressed or somewhat specifically expressed by tumors. Much of cancer vaccinology for the past 20 years has focused on inducing or identifying T cells that recognize such proteins.

The first TAA for melanoma, MAGE-1, was uncovered in 1991, and the capacity to generate cytotoxic T lymphocytes that recognize the protein was simultaneously demonstrated.[1] Following its discovery, vaccines specifically targeting MAGE-1, in addition to other subsequently identified antigenic targets, rapidly emerged.[2,3] The first clinical trial targeting a TAA focused on the differentiation antigen glycoprotein 100 (gp100).[4] Popular melanoma targets have since included additional gp100 epitopes,[5] MART-1,[6] MAGE-1,[1] MAGE-3,[7] tyrosinase,[8] and NY-ESO-1.[9]

Tumor-specific antigens (TSAs), derived from viral proteins or tumor-specific genetic mutations found in tumors, provide a recent opportunity to overcome many of the aforementioned immunogen issues, and will be discussed in more detail.

Clinical trials with TAA vaccines

No peptide or protein vaccine has demonstrated a clear improvement in overall survival in melanoma patients to date. For the most part, melanoma vaccines have targeted TAAs such as described above.

Small, single-arm studies At the National Cancer Institute surgery branch 323 subjects, almost all with metastatic melanoma, received peptide vaccines on a variety of different protocols. The peptides were derived from various TAAs including MART-1, gp100, tyrosinase, TRP-2, NY-ESO-1, MAGE-1/3, Her2/neu, or telomerase proteins.[10] Except for 15 patients who received peptides pulsed on DCs, peptides were emulsified in incomplete Freund adjuvant (IFA). Only 9 of these 323 subjects had a partial response and 2 had a complete response, resulting in an overall objective response rate of 2.9%. Of note, most of the responders had metastatic disease confined to skin and lymph nodes. Peptide vaccine studies in melanoma patients using multiple different epitopes, single peptide and multipeptide strategies, and different adjuvants such as granulocyte-macrophage colony-stimulating factor (GM-CSF), and low-dose interleukin (IL)-2 have produced similar results: low objective tumor response rates, generally from lower than 5% up to 10%, with variable effects on the immune response.[11,12]

Larger, comparative studies In a phase 2 cooperative group trial, 121 previously treated metastatic melanoma patients received 3 HLA-A2 restricted peptides (MART-1, gp100M, and tyrosinase) either alone or in combination with GM-CSF or interferon (IFN)-α, respectively. Six objective responses were observed, and a T-cell response measured by IFN-γ ELISPOT against at least 1 of the 3 peptides was seen in 26 of 75 (35%) patients with serial samples available.[13] Patients with immune responses had improved overall survival (21.3 vs 13.4 months; P = .046).

In a phase 3 trial, stage IV melanoma patients were treated with a modified gp100 peptide with increased binding affinity to HLA-A2 (gp100M) in combination with high-dose IL-2 versus IL-2 alone.[14] The objective tumor response rate was higher in the IL-2/gp100M combination arm in comparison with IL-2 alone (16 vs 6%, P = .03), and the progression-free survival was longer (2.2 vs 1.6 months, P = .008). There was also a trend toward improved overall survival (17.8 vs 11.1 months; P = .06). Noteworthy is that the objective response rate of 6% in the IL-2 arm is markedly lower than the 16% reported historically with this drug.[15] Only a few patients in the gp100M + IL-2 arm developed gp100-specific T cells in the peripheral blood, and there was no correlation between gp100-specific peripheral T cells and clinical responses. The lack of correlation of clinical responses and documented immune responses targeting the vaccine suggest lack of vaccine efficacy.

In a series of 3 phase 2 studies conducted by the Cytokine Working Group, 132 HLA-A2–positive advanced melanoma patients received the gp100M peptide combined with high-dose IL-2 given on variable schedules.[16] Given the strikingly similar response rates with gp100 plus IL-2 in the phase 2 and 3 trials and historical data with IL-2 alone (~15%), it appears that the clinical benefit seen with gp100 plus IL-2 is mostly driven by the high-dose IL-2 and not an effect of the peptide vaccine.[15] This finding is also in line with the phase 3 experience using the anti–cytotoxic T-lymphocyte antigen 4 (CTLA-4) antibody ipilimumab and gp100 in previously treated metastatic melanoma patients.[17] In this trial, no difference in response rate or overall survival was seen between ipilimumab + gp100 when compared with ipilimumab alone. Together, these results suggest that gp100 is an ineffective vaccine as currently administered.

Full-length proteins may provide a more comprehensive spectrum of tumor epitopes for presentation to DCs. MAGE-A3 is a cancer testis antigen overexpressed in approximately 65% of melanomas. A recombinant MAGE-A3 vaccine consists of full-length MAGE-A3 protein fused to protein D (a lipoprotein on the surface of *Haemophilus influenzae* B) and a polyhistidine tail. This vaccine, given with the immune adjuvant ASO2B, consisting of a saponin/lipid-A emulsion combined with TLR4 and TLR9 agonists, is currently being tested in a prospective, randomized phase 3 study in patients with high-risk resected, MAGE-A3 positive melanoma. The coprimary end point of disease-free survival (DFS) was not met according to a recent announcement by the study's sponsor, Glaxo Smith Kline.

Recombinant Viral Vector–Based Vaccines

Viral vectors encoding tumor antigens take advantage of immune responses against viral components, resulting in an adjuvant effect that can augment the antitumor-directed T-cell response. In melanoma, a viral-based vaccine approach that has been tested in phase 2 and 3 clinical trials consists of a second-generation herpes virus engineered to selectively replicate in and lyse tumor cells and to express GM-CSF, thereby attracting DCs into the tumor microenvironment (OncoVex^GM−CSF; BioVex, Cambridge, MA). Based on promising clinical activity in a multi-institutional phase 2 study in patients with unresectable stage IIIC or IV melanoma (8 complete and 5 partial responses in 50 patients), 436 patients with unresectable stage IIIB, IIIC, and IV melanoma were randomized 2:1 to receive either intratumoral OncoVex^{GM-CSF} or GM-CSF given subcutaneously.[18,19] In an interim analysis reported at the annual meeting of the American Society of Clinical Oncology 2013, the primary end point of increased durable response rate of OncoVex^{GM-CSF} over GM-CSF was met, and a trend toward improved overall survival in patients treated with vaccine was observed.[19]

Whole Cell–Based Vaccines

A theoretical advantage of using whole tumor cells for vaccination is the broad spectrum of TAAs and mutated antigens potentially available for recognition and attack by immune cells. Vaccination with autologous tumors appears to be most suitable for this approach; a limitation is the difficulty of harvesting and preparing tumor tissue from individual patients. Irradiated melanoma cells harvested from metastatic lesions and engineered to secrete GM-CSF induced tumor necrosis and infiltration with T lymphocytes and plasma cells in metastatic sites of melanoma patients. Vaccination sites showed infiltration with T cells, DCs, and macrophages.[20] In a follow-up study, patients with advanced melanoma previously vaccinated with irradiated autologous GM-CSF–secreting melanoma cells received ipilimumab after an interval of several years. Of note, metastatic melanoma lesions in 3 of 3 melanoma patients with previous vaccine exhibited extensive tumor necrosis with lymphocyte and granulocyte infiltrates, whereas no tumor necrosis was seen in 4 of 4 melanoma patients previously immunized with defined melanosomal antigens.[21] A separate study, in which patients with metastatic melanoma were treated with ipilimumab 1 to 4 months after treatment with irradiated autologous GM-CSF–secreting melanoma cells, showed a linear relationship between the extent of tumor necrosis in posttreatment biopsies and the ratio of intratumoral CD8$^+$ T cells and FoxP3$^+$ Tregs.[22]

M-Vax (AVAX Technologies, Philadelphia, PA) is an autologous whole-cell melanoma vaccine consisting of irradiated tumor cells treated with the hapten dinitrofluorobenzene (DNP). Six of 97 patients with advanced melanoma who received M-Vax after a low dose of cyclophosphamide in a phase 2 trial had a complete or partial response; 5 patients had a mixed tumor response. The median overall survival was 21.4 months in responders and 8.7 months in nonresponders ($P = .010$).[23] Based on these data, a phase 3 trial was initiated randomizing M-Vax versus placebo (2:1) given with cyclophosphamide, low-dose IL-2, and bacillus Calmette-Guérin (BCG).

Allogeneic whole-cell vaccines derived from tumor cell lines or individual tumors from other patients have the advantage that they can be produced for off-the-shelf use. A prominent example is the allogeneic GM-CSF–secreting prostate carcinoma cell vaccine termed GVAX (Cell Genesys, South San Francisco, CA), which showed encouraging tumor activity in phase 1/2 trials,[24,25] but ultimately failed because of lack of clinical efficacy in 2 phase 3 trials.[26] Similarly, an allogeneic whole tumor cell vaccine comprising 3 melanoma cell lines known as Canvaxin appeared to show an overall survival benefit in a nonrandomized phase 2 trial, in which 150 completely resected stage IV melanoma patients vaccinated with Canvaxin lived longer than 113 matched, nonvaccinated controls. Nevertheless, a prospective phase 3 trial randomizing Canvaxin plus BCG versus BCG alone, enrolling more than 1500 patients with fully resected stage III or stage IV melanoma, was stopped early because of a low likelihood of demonstrating an overall survival benefit in the vaccine arm.

NEW STRATEGIES

Several features, lacking in most melanoma vaccines to date, are critical for the induction of effective clinical antitumor responses: (1) an antigen and delivery system that is highly specific to the tumor with no cross-reactivity to self-antigens, resulting in maximal immunogenicity and avoiding autoimmunity; (2) an effective immune adjuvant that provides a stimulatory immune context, thereby activating APCs such as DCs; and (3) a strategy to counteract immunosuppressive mechanisms (see **Fig. 1**). Technological advances such as massively parallel sequencing and novel biomaterials, in addition to the emergence of new agents such as immune-checkpoint blocking antibodies, have enabled the design of tumor vaccines that incorporate these features and are more physiologically relevant. The combination of these new reagents promises to generate effective responses that will build on the already encouraging signal that has been seen with checkpoint inhibition alone. The following sections describe 2 such novel approaches that are currently under clinical trial at the authors' institution: (1) NeoVax in patients with high-risk melanoma, and (2) WDVAX in patients with unresectable metastatic melanoma.

NeoVax: A New Concept for Antigen Selection Coupled with an Effective Immune Adjuvant

Most antigens used for vaccination against tumors are either overexpressed or selectively expressed tumor-associated antigens. The immunogenicity of these types of antigens is limited by the downmodulating effects of central tolerance through thymic deletion, in addition to peripheral tolerance mechanisms. Recent advances in cancer genomics and immunology have provided new tools to overcome these limitations. NeoVax is a novel approach to personalized vaccine that may overcome some of the shortcomings of previous melanoma vaccines.

Choice of antigen: neoantigens

Massively parallel sequencing technology allows sequencing of the entire genome or exome of a tumor and identification of all mutations by comparing the information with matched normal tissue cells. Intense and ever more comprehensive tumor-sequencing efforts have demonstrated that individual tumors contain a host of patient-specific mutations that alter the protein-coding content of many genes,[27] enabling the identification and use of a new class of immunogens termed neoantigens.[28,29] These mutations range from single amino acid changes (caused by missense mutations) to addition of long regions of novel amino acid sequence owing to frame shifts, read-through of termination codons, or translation of intron regions (novel open reading frame mutations; neoORFs). Such altered proteins are, to the immune system, distinct from self and analogous to foreign proteins, rendering them less sensitive to the immune-dampening effects of self-tolerance (**Fig. 2**). Furthermore, these targets are exquisitely tumor specific, being found exclusively in tumor cells. Several studies in both animals and humans have demonstrated that mutated gene products can encode for epitopes effective in inducing an immune response.[30,31] Importantly, spontaneous tumor regression or long-term survival were found to correlate in small numbers of patients with CD8[+] T-cell responses to mutated epitopes.[32,33] Furthermore, escape from host immunosurveillance (immunoediting) can be tracked in some cases to alterations in expression of dominant mutated antigens.[34,35]

Choice of delivery: long peptides

Most peptide vaccines have nearly exclusively consisted of short peptides, based on the minimum length of peptides (usually 8–10 amino acids) needed to bind the major histocompatibility complex I molecule. Recent work has shown that such peptides can be tolerogenic rather than stimulatory,[36] because they are capable of direct binding to the HLA molecule on the surface of nonprofessional APCs, including B and T cells, resulting in tolerance. Long peptides, which are approximately 20 to 30 amino acids

Native antigens   Neoantigens

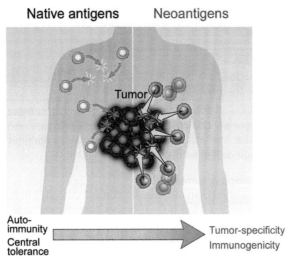

Fig. 2. Neoantigens are a novel class of antigens encoded by the unique mutations specific to each patient's tumor. Tumor neoantigens (*right, blue*) are specific to tumor cells and are not subject to central tolerance (ie, deletion of their cognate antigen-specific T cells in the thymus). The result of this should be optimal immunogenicity and tumor specificity of the induced T-cell response, potentially comparable with the T-cell response to a foreign antigen such as from a virus or bacteria. By contrast, native antigens such as overexpressed or selectively expressed antigens commonly used in cancer vaccines are at the other end of the spectrum of tumor specificity, resulting in a higher likelihood of self-tolerance and autoimmunity (*left, red*).

in length, have been shown to produce more robust and more durable immune responses.[37,38] Long peptides require internalization, processing, and cross-presentation to bind to HLA molecules, all of which only occur in professional APCs such as DCs. Long peptides therefore necessitate presentation of the peptide by professional APCs, a critical step for the induction of a strong antitumor immune response.

Choice of adjuvant: the TLR-3 agonist poly-ICLC

Toll-like receptors (TLRs) belong to the family of pattern recognition receptors (PRRs), which recognize conserved motifs shared by many microorganisms, termed pathogen-associated molecular patterns (PAMPS). Recognition of PAMPS leads to the activation of the innate and adaptive immune systems. Key functions of DCs, including upregulation of costimulation markers, lymph node trafficking, phagocytosis, and cytokine production, are enhanced on activation by TLR stimulation. The TLR-3 agonist poly-ICLC is a synthetically prepared double-stranded RNA consisting of polyI and polyC stabilized by the addition of polylysine and carboxymethyl-cellulose. Poly-ICLC activates TLR3 and MDA5, complementary pathways leading to DC and natural killer (NK) cell activation, and production of a "natural mix" of type I interferons, cytokines, and chemokines. Preclinical studies in rodents and nonhuman primates demonstrated that poly-ICLC enhances virus, tumor, and autoantigen-specific T-cell responses, emphasizing its effectiveness as a vaccine adjuvant. A placebo-controlled study in healthy human volunteers recently showed similar transcriptional expression profiles of signal transduction canonical pathways, including those of the innate immune system, after either treatment with GMP-grade poly-ICLC (Hiltonol; Oncovir, Washington, DC) or vaccination with the highly effective yellow fever vaccine YF17D.[39]

WDVAX: A Scaffold Vaccine Incorporating Autologous Whole Tumor Cells, GM-CSF, and CpG into a Unique Delivery System

Novel biomaterials provide an opportunity to deliver the critical components of a tumor vaccine in a spatiotemporally controlled fashion, establishing an environment that is maximally supportive for the induction of an effective tumor immune response. WDVAX takes advantage of this technology.

Choice of antigen: autologous tumor cells

The authors have previously shown that vaccination with lethally irradiated autologous tumor cells can induce strong immune responses. Specifically, this vaccine elicited dense DC, macrophage, granulocyte, and lymphocyte infiltrates at the injection sites in 19 of 26 evaluable patients with melanoma, and 18 of 25 evaluable patients with lung cancer. Metastatic lesions resected after vaccination showed brisk, T-lymphocyte and plasma-cell infiltrates with tumor necrosis in 10 of 16 patients with melanoma and in 3 of 6 patients with lung cancer.

Choice of adjuvant: tumor cell–secreted GM-CSF in combination with the TLR-9 agonist oligodeoxynucleotide containing unmethylated cytosine and guanine

Vaccination with autologous tumor cells established safety, feasibility, and biologic activity, but antitumor activity in melanoma patients was low. One explanation for the insufficient clinical efficacy is the dual role of GM-CSF during the generation of an immune response identified in the authors' previous studies (autologous tumor cells are engineered by adenovirus-mediated gene transfer to secrete GM-CSF), which found that the homeostatic function of GM-CSF is to maintain immune tolerance through supporting the activities of regulatory T cells (Tregs).[40] The concurrent provision of a second signal, such as the TLR-9 agonist oligodeoxynucleotide containing unmethylated cytosine and guanine (CpG), downregulates the GM-CSF tolerance pathway and switches GM-CSF activity toward immune stimulation, with the induction of T-helper (Th)1, Th17, and CD8$^+$ T cells. Hence, codelivery of GM-CSF with CpG might lead to the sustained induction of cytotoxic T cells while dampening the generation of Tregs, thereby enhancing tumor destruction.

Choice of delivery: a novel material engineered scaffold

To capitalize on the improved understanding of GM-CSF biology, in collaboration with colleagues at the Wyss Institute for Biologically Inspired Engineering at Harvard University, the authors have developed a novel material engineered scaffold, consisting of a macroporous polylactide-coglycolide (PLG) matrix polymer. This scaffold allows delivery of immunostimulatory agents in vivo with precise spatial and temporal control. In addition to serving as a drug-delivery device, PLG represents a physical, antigen-presenting structure to which DCs (in addition to other immune cells and soluble factors) may be recruited and activated. In murine tumor models, the subcutaneous implantation of PLG scaffolds incorporating GM-CSF protein, CpG, and tumor-cell lysates creates a microenvironment in which the appropriate signals for dendritic cell antigen presentation and the induction of antitumor T cells can be maintained for at least 2 weeks. Under these conditions, robust levels of antitumor immunity were achieved, resulting in the regression of established B16 melanomas.[41,42]

SUMMARY AND OUTLOOK

Despite decades of intense investigation, a melanoma vaccine that induces effective cytotoxic T-cell responses and is capable of controlling or eradicating melanoma has been elusive. However, increased understanding of tumor immunity has led to the recognition that most of the approaches taken in the past were limited through weak immune adjuvants, poor choice of tumor antigen, or delivery of the vaccine. The recent successes with immune checkpoint blockade in melanoma and other cancers, leading to durable tumor responses in a considerable proportion of patients, have highlighted the potential of immunotherapy in melanoma. These insights and advances, coupled with the rapid progress in many areas relevant to effective vaccine design such as sequencing technology, biomaterials, and immune adjuvants, provide new opportunities for the successful development of a clinically effective melanoma vaccine. NeoVax, featuring a novel class of immunogens based on individual tumor mutations, and WDVAX, providing a unique delivery system by taking advantage of a novel material engineered scaffold, are examples of innovative vaccine design in melanoma. Both technologies are currently under clinical investigation in patients with high-risk (NeoVax) and advanced melanoma (WDVAX) at the authors' institution. These new strategies, either alone or in combination with immune checkpoint blockade or other synergistic immune stimulants will, it is hoped, lead the way toward future successful melanoma vaccines.

REFERENCES

1. van der Bruggen P, Traversari C, Chomez P, et al. A gene encoding an antigen recognized by cytolytic T lymphocytes on a human melanoma. Science 1991; 254:1643–7.
2. Cormier JN, Salgaller ML, Prevette T, et al. Enhancement of cellular immunity in melanoma patients immunized with a peptide from MART-1/Melan A. Cancer J Sci Am 1997;3:37–44.
3. Marchand M, van Baren N, Weynants P, et al. Tumor regressions observed in patients with metastatic melanoma treated with an antigenic peptide encoded by gene MAGE-3 and presented by HLA-A1. Int J Cancer 1999;80:219–30.
4. Rosenberg SA, Yang JC, Schwartzentruber DJ, et al. Immunologic and therapeutic evaluation of a synthetic peptide vaccine for the treatment of patients with metastatic melanoma. Nat Med 1998;4:321–7.
5. Kawakami Y, Eliyahu S, Delgado CH, et al. Identification of a human melanoma antigen recognized by tumor-infiltrating lymphocytes associated with in vivo tumor rejection. Proc Natl Acad Sci U S A 1994;91:6458–62.
6. Kawakami Y, Eliyahu S, Delgado CH, et al. Cloning of the gene coding for a shared human melanoma antigen recognized by autologous T cells infiltrating into tumor. Proc Natl Acad Sci U S A 1994;91:3515–9.
7. Chaux P, Vantomme V, Stroobant V, et al. Identification of MAGE-3 epitopes presented by HLA-DR molecules to CD4(+) T lymphocytes. J Exp Med 1999;189: 767–78.
8. Brichard V, Van Pel A, Wolfel T, et al. The tyrosinase gene codes for an antigen recognized by autologous cytolytic T lymphocytes on HLA-A2 melanomas. J Exp Med 1993;178:489–95.
9. Zeng G, Touloukian CE, Wang X, et al. Identification of CD4+ T cell epitopes from NY-ESO-1 presented by HLA-DR molecules. J Immunol 2000;165:1153–9.
10. Rosenberg SA, Yang JC, Restifo NP. Cancer immunotherapy: moving beyond current vaccines. Nat Med 2004;10:909–15.

11. Slingluff CL Jr, Petroni GR, Yamshchikov GV, et al. Clinical and immunologic results of a randomized phase II trial of vaccination using four melanoma peptides either administered in granulocyte-macrophage colony-stimulating factor in adjuvant or pulsed on dendritic cells. J Clin Oncol 2003;21: 4016–26.

12. Slingluff CL Jr, Petroni GR, Olson WC, et al. Effect of granulocyte/macrophage colony-stimulating factor on circulating CD8+ and CD4+ T-cell responses to a multipeptide melanoma vaccine: outcome of a multicenter randomized trial. Clin Cancer Res 2009;15:7036–44.

13. Kirkwood JM, Lee S, Moschos SJ, et al. Immunogenicity and antitumor effects of vaccination with peptide vaccine+/-granulocyte-monocyte colony-stimulating factor and/or IFN-alpha2b in advanced metastatic melanoma: Eastern Cooperative Oncology Group Phase II Trial E1696. Clin Cancer Res 2009;15:1443–51.

14. Schwartzentruber DJ, Lawson DH, Richards JM, et al. gp100 peptide vaccine and interleukin-2 in patients with advanced melanoma. N Engl J Med 2011; 364:2119–27.

15. Atkins MB, Lotze MT, Dutcher JP, et al. High-dose recombinant interleukin 2 therapy for patients with metastatic melanoma: analysis of 270 patients treated between 1985 and 1993. J Clin Oncol 1999;17:2105–16.

16. Sosman JA, Carrillo C, Urba WJ, et al. Three phase II cytokine working group trials of gp100 (210M) peptide plus high-dose interleukin-2 in patients with HLA-A2-positive advanced melanoma. J Clin Oncol 2008;26:2292–8.

17. Hodi FS, O'Day SJ, McDermott DF, et al. Improved survival with ipilimumab in patients with metastatic melanoma. N Engl J Med 2010;363:711–23.

18. Senzer NN, Kaufman HL, Amatruda T, et al. Phase II clinical trial of a granulocyte-macrophage colony-stimulating factor-encoding, second-generation oncolytic herpesvirus in patients with unresectable metastatic melanoma. J Clin Oncol 2009;27:5763–71.

19. Andtbacka RH, CF, Amatruda T, et al. OPTiM: a randomized phase III trial of talimogene laherparepvec (T-VEC) versus subcutaneous (SC) granulocyte-macrophage colony-stimulating factor (GM-CSF) for the treatment (tx) of unresected stage IIIB/C and IV melanoma. J Clin Oncol 2013;31(Suppl): [Abstract LBA9008].

20. Soiffer R, Lynch T, Mihm M, et al. Vaccination with irradiated autologous melanoma cells engineered to secrete human granulocyte-macrophage colony-stimulating factor generates potent antitumor immunity in patients with metastatic melanoma. Proc Natl Acad Sci U S A 1998;95:13141–6.

21. Hodi FS, Schmollinger JC, Soiffer RJ, et al. ATP6S1 elicits potent humoral responses associated with immune-mediated tumor destruction. Proc Natl Acad Sci U S A 2002;99:6919–24.

22. Hodi FS, Butler M, Oble DA, et al. Immunologic and clinical effects of antibody blockade of cytotoxic T lymphocyte-associated antigen 4 in previously vaccinated cancer patients. Proc Natl Acad Sci U S A 2008;105:3005–10.

23. Berd D, Sato T, Cohn H, et al. Treatment of metastatic melanoma with autologous, hapten-modified melanoma vaccine: regression of pulmonary metastases. Int J Cancer 2001;94:531–9.

24. Small EJ, Sacks N, Nemunaitis J, et al. Granulocyte macrophage colony-stimulating factor–secreting allogeneic cellular immunotherapy for hormone-refractory prostate cancer. Clin Cancer Res 2007;13:3883–91.

25. Higano CS, Corman JM, Smith DC, et al. Phase 1/2 dose-escalation study of a GM-CSF-secreting, allogeneic, cellular immunotherapy for metastatic hormone-refractory prostate cancer. Cancer 2008;113:975–84.

26. Copier J, Dalgleish A. Whole-cell vaccines: a failure or a success waiting to happen? Curr Opin Mol Ther 2010;12:14–20.
27. Wood LD, Parsons DW, Jones S, et al. The genomic landscapes of human breast and colorectal cancers. Science 2007;318:1108–13.
28. Heemskerk B, Kvistborg P, Schumacher TN. The cancer antigenome. EMBO J 2013;32:194–203.
29. Hacohen N, Fritsch EF, Carter TA, et al. Getting Personal with Neoantigen-Based Therapeutic Cancer Vaccines. Cancer Immunol Res 2013;1:OF10–4.
30. Buckwalter MR, Srivastava PK. "It is the antigen(s), stupid" and other lessons from over a decade of vaccitherapy of human cancer. Semin Immunol 2008;20: 296–300.
31. Sensi M, Anichini A. Unique tumor antigens: evidence for immune control of genome integrity and immunogenic targets for T cell-mediated patient-specific immunotherapy. Clin Cancer Res 2006;12:5023–32.
32. Karanikas V, Colau D, Baurain JF, et al. High frequency of cytolytic T lymphocytes directed against a tumor-specific mutated antigen detectable with HLA tetramers in the blood of a lung carcinoma patient with long survival. Cancer Res 2001;61: 3718–24.
33. van Rooij N, van Buuren MM, Philips D, et al. Tumor exome analysis reveals neoantigen-specific T-cell reactivity in an ipilimumab-responsive melanoma. J Clin Oncol 2013;31:e439–42.
34. Matsushita H, Vesely MD, Koboldt DC, et al. Cancer exome analysis reveals a T-cell-dependent mechanism of cancer immunoediting. Nature 2012;482:400–4.
35. DuPage M, Mazumdar C, Schmidt LM, et al. Expression of tumour-specific antigens underlies cancer immunoediting. Nature 2012;482:405–9.
36. Bijker MS, van den Eeden SJ, Franken KL, et al. CD8+ CTL priming by exact peptide epitopes in incomplete Freund's adjuvant induces a vanishing CTL response, whereas long peptides induce sustained CTL reactivity. J Immunol 2007;179:5033–40.
37. Welters MJ, Kenter GG, Piersma SJ, et al. Induction of tumor-specific CD4+ and CD8+ T-cell immunity in cervical cancer patients by a human papillomavirus type 16 E6 and E7 long peptides vaccine. Clin Cancer Res 2008;14:178–87.
38. Kenter GG, Welters MJ, Valentijn AR, et al. Phase I immunotherapeutic trial with long peptides spanning the E6 and E7 sequences of high-risk human papillomavirus 16 in end-stage cervical cancer patients shows low toxicity and robust immunogenicity. Clin Cancer Res 2008;14:169–77.
39. Gaucher D, Therrien R, Kettaf N, et al. Yellow fever vaccine induces integrated multilineage and polyfunctional immune responses. J Exp Med 2008;205: 3119–31.
40. Jinushi M, Nakazaki Y, Dougan M, et al. MFG-E8-mediated uptake of apoptotic cells by APCs links the pro- and antiinflammatory activities of GM-CSF. J Clin Invest 2007;117:1902–13.
41. Ali OA, Huebsch N, Cao L, et al. Infection-mimicking materials to program dendritic cells in situ. Nat Mater 2009;8:151–8.
42. Ali OA, Emerich D, Dranoff G, et al. In situ regulation of DC subsets and T cells mediates tumor regression in mice. Sci Transl Med 2009;1:8ra19.

Interferon, Interleukin-2, and Other Cytokines

Elizabeth I. Buchbinder, MD*, David F. McDermott, MD

KEYWORDS

- Melanoma • Cytokines • Interferon • Interleukin-2 • Interleukin-21
- Granulocyte-macrophage colony–stimulating factor

KEY POINTS

- Interferon-α has immune-modulating effects and when used at high dosages in the adjuvant setting has an impact in preventing recurrence in high-risk melanoma patients.
- Interleukin-2 plays a complex role in the immune system and when given at high dosages to patients with metastatic melanoma a subset achieve a long-term durable complete response.
- The use of cytokines in the treatment of melanoma continues to evolve as does their role in combination with other immune-modulating agents and targeted therapies in the future of melanoma treatment.

CYTOKINES

Cytokines are a complex group of naturally occurring glycoproteins produced when the immune system is activated by an infection, foreign antigen, or self-antigen. The antitumor effects of cytokines are likely mediated through immunomodulation, antiproliferative activity, and inhibition of angiogenesis. Melanoma has proved to be one of the most immunogenic malignancies based on documented cases of spontaneous regression and its higher prevalence in immunocompromised patients. This evidence of immunogenicity has led to the testing of numerous cytokines including interferon (IFN)-α, IFN-γ, granulocyte-macrophage colony–stimulating factor (GM-CSF), interleukin (IL)-2, IL-4, IL-6, IL-12, IL-18, and IL-21 in patients with advanced melanoma.

INTERFERON

In 1957 Isaacs and Lindenmann[1] were studying the influenza virus and discovered that incubation of heated virus with chick chorioallantoic membrane led to release

Division of Hematology/Oncology, Beth Israel Deaconess Medical Center, 330 Brookline Avenue, Boston, MA 02215, USA
* Corresponding author.
E-mail address: ebuchbin@bidmc.harvard.edu

Hematol Oncol Clin N Am 28 (2014) 571–583
http://dx.doi.org/10.1016/j.hoc.2014.02.001
0889-8588/14/$ – see front matter © 2014 Elsevier Inc. All rights reserved.

of a previously unknown factor. This factor interfered with growth of live virus in fresh pieces of membrane and was named "interferon." In parallel, Yasuichi Nagano was discovering IFN while exploring antiviral activity that occurred after injecting inactivated vaccinia virus into rabbit skin.[2]

Subsequently, IFNs were found to be produced in many animal cells and tissues. Ten mammalian IFN species have been discovered. Of these eight are found in humans, six are type I (IFN-α, IFN-β, IFN-ε, IFN-κ, IFN-ω, and IFN-ν), one is type II (IFN-γ), and one is type III (IFN-λ).[3,4] IFN was purified from human fibroblasts and the mRNAs responsible for its production were isolated.[5,6] A full length copy of the IFN sequence was found leading to the ability to produce and purify a recombinant IFN-α2 that expanded opportunities for its use in research and clinical trials.

The actions of IFNs are mediated by interaction with the receptors IFNAR1 and IFNAR2.[7] These receptors are multichain complexes that use several signaling pathways within the cells. One of the pathways activated through the action of IFN is the JAK-STAT pathway.[8]

Treatment with IFNα2b has numerous effects on the immune system. It leads to the downregulation of intercellular adhesion molecule and the upregulation of HLA-DR expression, which may modulate tumor cell-host immune response. In addition natural killer cell function, T-cell function, and subset distribution are modulated in patients treated with IFN.[9] In addition it can lead to the induction and/or activation of proapoptotic genes and proteins, such as TRAIL, caspases, Bak, and Bax, and repression of antiapoptotic genes, such as Bcl-2 and IAP.[10]

IFN-α has multiple effects in a variety of malignancies and has been the most broadly evaluated clinically. There are three commercially available isoforms that differ by one to two amino acids: IFN-α2a (Roche), IFN-α2b (Merck), and IFN-α2c (Boehringer Ingelheim). IFN has been approved for the treatment of hairy cell leukemia, relapsing-remitting multiple sclerosis, malignant melanoma, follicular lymphoma, condylomata acuminate (genital warts), AIDS-related Kaposi sarcoma, and chronic hepatitis B and C.

Initial Use in Melanoma

As with all antineoplastics the first testing of IFNs in melanoma was in the metastatic disease setting. In 1978, the American Cancer Society initiated a multicenter trial testing IFN-α in patients with metastatic melanoma. Forty-five patients were enrolled among whom there was one partial responder and minimal responses in two others.[11,12] A similar study was performed by Retsas and colleagues[13] in which 17 patients with melanoma were treated with IFN-α and one partial response was seen.

Studies continued as more dosing information became available. Several phase I/II studies were performed with very similar results. In these trials there were 2 responses out of 15 patients, 4 responses out of 23 patients, and 3 responses out of 20 patients.[12] Tumor response rates around 16% were observed with some late responders. It is unknown if there is a survival benefit for IFN in the metastatic setting because no randomized trials comparing it with cytotoxic therapy or supportive care have been performed. Most of the responders had a low tumor volume.[14] This led to the hypothesis that the greatest benefit of IFN-α would be in patients with microscopic residual disease.

Adjuvant Testing

Randomized phase III trials have been performed testing both high-dose IFN-α2b and pegylated (PEG) IFN-α2b in the adjuvant setting in high-risk melanoma patients (**Table 1**). The first trial was Eastern Cooperative Group E1684, a randomized

Table 1
Summary of adjuvant trials of high-dose interferon treatment of melanoma

Trial	Patient Number	Population	Dose	Relapse-free Survival	Overall Survival
ECOG 1684[15]	287	T4 (>4.0 mm) and/or Nx (regional LN metastasis)	20 MIU/m² 5x/wk for 1 mo, then 10 MIU/m² 3x/wk for 48 wk vs observation	$P = .004$	$P = .046$
ECOG 1690[16]	642	T4 and/or Nx	20 MIU/m² 5x/wk for 1 mo, then 10 MIU/m² 3x/wk for 48 wk vs 3 MIU/m² 3x/wk for 3 y vs observation	$P = .05$ $P = .17$	NS NS
ECOG 1694[18]	880	T4 and/or Nx	20 MIU/m² 5x/wk for 1 mo then 10 MIU/m² 3x/wk for 48 wk vs GM2-KLH/QS-21 vaccine	$P = .0027$	$P = .0147$
EORTC 18991[22]	1256	TxNx	6 µg/kg weekly for 8 wk then 3 µg/kg weekly for 5 y vs observation	$P = .01$	NS

controlled study of 287 patients with T4 or N1 melanoma. Patients were given IFN-α2b, 20 MU/m²/d intravenously for 1 month followed by 10 MU/m²/d three times per week subcutaneously for 48 weeks versus observation. In this study a significant prolongation of relapse-free survival (RFS) ($P = .0023$) was observed with an increase from 1.0 to 1.7 years disease-free survival. In addition a significant prolongation in overall survival (OS) ($P = .0237$) was also observed with an increase from 2.8 to 3.8 years. The benefit of therapy was greatest among patients with lymph node involvement.[15]

Based on the positive results from E1684 the decision was made to move forward with a comparison of high- and low-dose IFN in an Intergroup trial. E1690 was a three-arm prospective, randomized trial of patients with IIB and III melanoma. A total of 642 patients were enrolled and randomized to high-dose IFN at the same doses as E1984, low-dose IFN (3 MU/m²/d three times per week subcutaneously for 2 years), or observation. This trial showed a RFS benefit for the high-dose IFN arm by Cox multivariable analysis ($P = .03$). However, there was no significant RFS benefit seen for the low-dose arm. In addition there was no OS benefit comparing either the high-dose or low-dose arm with observation. The investigators concluded that these results may have been confounded by the high proportion of patients who received IFN-α2b at progression in the observation arm.[16]

Vaccination is another adjuvant therapy being explored for use in melanoma treatment. The ganglioside GM2 is a serologically well-defined melanoma antigen that has shown efficacy when combined with various adjuvants.[17] Intergroup E1694 compared high-dose IFN alfa-2b versus vaccination with GM2 conjugate. A total of 880 patients with stage IIB/III melanoma were randomized to each treatment arm. The trial was closed early after an interim analysis indicated inferiority of GM2 compared with IFN. IFN had a significant RFS ($P = .0015$) and OS benefit ($P = .009$) compared with the GM2 conjugate vaccine (**Table 2**).[18]

Three large meta-analyses of the published results of IFN-based trials in the adjuvant setting were performed with similarly mixed results. The first analysis by Wheatley and colleagues[19] included 12 randomized controlled trials and showed a significant

Table 2 Summary of meta-analysis of adjuvant trials of high-dose interferon treatment of melanoma				
Meta-Analysis	Number of Trials	RFS	OS	Comments
Wheatley et al,[19] 2003	12	$P = .000003$	$P = .1$	Did not include E1684, increased benefit at higher dose
Wheatley et al,[20] 2007	13	$P = .00006$	$P = .008$	13% risk reduction in RFS; 10% risk reduction in OS
Mocellin et al,[21] 2010	14	$P<.001$	$P = .002$	18% risk reduction in RFS; 11% risk reduction in OS

Abbreviations: OS, overall survival; RFS, relapse-free survival.

RFS benefit ($P = .000003$) and unclear OS benefit ($P = .1$). This meta-analysis did not include E1694 because of the control arm being vaccine and suggested an increased benefit for IFN at increased doses.

The second two meta-analyses showed a risk reduction in RFS and OS for IFN therapy. The first by Wheatley and colleagues[20] included 13 randomized controlled trials and showed a 13% risk reduction in RFS and a 10% risk reduction in OS. The final meta-analysis by Mocellin and colleagues[21] from 2010 showed an 18% risk reduction in RFS and an 11% risk reduction in OS. Overall these meta-analyses showed a consistent benefit to the use of IFN in the adjuvant setting for high-risk melanoma.

PEG-IFN

To further reduce the toxicity associated with high-dose IFN there was an effort to see if PEG-IFN alfa-2b would facilitate prolonged exposure with reduced toxicity. In EORTC 18991, a total of 1256 patients with resected stage III melanoma were randomly assigned to observation versus PEG-IFN-α2b at 6 µg/kg per week for 8 weeks followed by 3 µg/kg per week for an intended duration of 5 years. There was a statistical difference in RFS between the two groups ($P = .01$). However, there was no difference in OS between the two groups.[22] Based on these results PEG-IFN alfa-2b was approved by the Food and Drug Administration in 2011.

A post hoc meta-analysis of EORTC trials showed that tumor stage and ulceration were predictive factors for the efficacy of adjuvant IFN/PEG-IFN therapy. The efficacy was lower in stage III-N2 patients with ulceration and uniformly absent in patients without ulceration.[23] EORTC 18081 is currently enrolling patients with ulcerated primaries and no nodal disease to 2 years of PEG-IFN versus placebo to confirm this effect.

Toxicity

IFN is a difficult treatment to tolerate and up to 50% of the initial patients in E1684 required a dose reduction or treatment discontinuation. Efforts have been made to improve compliance with therapy and some centers have been able to get 90% of their patients, who do not have early relapse, through 1 year of therapy.[18] However, the toxicity is clearly a limiting factor to adoption and continuation of IFN.

The predominant side effects seen in trials include myelotoxicity, elevation of liver enzymes, nausea and vomiting, flulike symptoms, and neuropsychiatric symptoms. Within the spectrum of flulike symptoms patients often report fevers, chills, anorexia, weight loss, diarrhea, rash, and fatigue. These symptoms can often be managed with supportive care or a dose reduction. However, they are often unacceptable to melanoma patients who tend to be younger and need to continue working.

Patient selection for treatment with IFN is important. It should only be considered in patients with a risk of relapse greater than 30%. In addition it should be avoided in patients with a history of significant heart disease, liver toxicity, or depression.

Adjuvant Dosing and Schedule

Based on the low number of patients in the original trials that were able to complete a full year of therapy the possibility of a shorter course has been explored. The Hellenic Cooperative Oncology group conducted a noninferiority phase III trial to evaluate the efficacy and safety of 4 weeks versus 42 weeks of high-dose IFN in patients with stage IIB, IIC, and III melanoma. This trial showed no significant difference in OS and RFS between the two different regimens.[24]

E1697 assessed the benefit of 4 weeks high-dose IFN compared with observation in patients with intermediate- and high-risk melanomas. The trial was terminated early after 1150 patients were enrolled because an interim analysis showed no improvement in RFS or OS for 4 weeks high-dose IFN versus observation.[25] Based on these results 1 year of high-dose adjuvant IFN remains the standard adjuvant therapy for appropriate patients.

Predicting Response

Unfortunately, adjuvant therapy for melanoma continues to have a limited benefit with substantial toxicity. Attempts to identify patients who would have the highest benefit from adjuvant IFN have been ongoing. It has been observed that patients who exhibit symptoms of autoimmunity are more likely to respond to IFN. Such immune toxicities include hypothyroidism, hyperthyroidism, the antiphospholipid-antibody syndrome, and vitiligo.

Studies to look at the role of autoimmunity in these patients have been ongoing. In particular Gogas and colleagues[26] evaluated 200 patients who were part of a larger randomized trial to look for markers of response. Serum was tested for antithyroid, antinuclear, anti-DNA, and anticardiolipin antibodies, and patients were examined for vitiligo. The development of autoimmunity was an independent prognostic marker for improved RFS and OS ($P<.001$).

Further study to uncover why certain patients are more likely to develop autoimmunity than others is ongoing. To date no genetic marker or molecular profile that consistently correlates with IFN response has been found.

Future Directions

As newer immunomodulatory agents and targeted therapy emerge in the metastatic melanoma setting these agents are being transitioned into the adjuvant setting. Novel treatments are being compared with high-dose IFN or placebo. ECOG 1609 is a large trial currently accruing patients to a comparison of high-dose IFN versus two doses of ipilimumab in patients at high risk for recurrence. Enrollment to this trial is ongoing.

Despite controversy and limited adoption, IFN is the standard of care for adjuvant treatment of patients with high-risk melanoma. It remains to be seen if IFN will have a continued role in the future of melanoma treatment.

IL-2

IL-2 was initially discovered in 1976 when medium obtained from stimulated lymphocytes was found to lead to the growth of T lymphocytes.[27] It was initially called T-cell growth factor but subsequently named "interleukin-2" because it was produced by and acted on leukocytes. In 1983 the cDNA for IL-2 was isolated allowing for the production of recombinant IL-2 and its use in the laboratory and clinic.[28]

The effects of IL-2 are mediated through the IL-2 receptor, a class I cytokine receptor.[29] IL-2 boosts the natural killer compartment, augments the cytotoxicity of human monocytes, induces T-helper function, and increases reactivity of cytotoxic T lymphocytes.[30] In addition, incubation of human lymphocytes with IL-2 leads to the generation of cells capable of lysing tumor cells. These cells were named lymphokine-activated killer cells (LAK) and target tumor cells specifically without lysing normal cells. The systemic administration of IL-2 to tumor-bearing mice was found to lead to the generation of LAK cells and mediate regression of pulmonary metastasis and subcutaneous tumor implants.[31]

Initial Studies

Although initial studies involving IL-2 alone were disappointing, when combined with systemic administration of autologous LAK cells regression was observed in 11 of 25 patients with metastatic cancer.[32] A complete regression was observed in one patient with melanoma and this was sustained.

In animal models it was observed that dosing IL-2 until toxic effects precluded further administration was most effective. Based on this a high-dose IL-2 regimen was developed in which IL-2 was administered by short intravenous infusion every 8 hours, with or without LAK cells until toxic effects prevented further administration. In a study of 157 patients with solid malignancies treated with IL-2 with or without LAK cells there were nine total complete responses, two of which were in patients with melanoma.[33]

A subsequent randomized clinical trial was performed to evaluate whether the administration of LAK cells in conjunction with high-dose IL-2 alters response and survival rates compared with high-dose IL-2 alone. Although a trend for improved survival was observed in patients with melanoma treated with the combination the benefit was insufficient to justify the continued addition of LAK cells to the IL-2 treatment regimen.[34]

Studies in Melanoma

Phase II clinical trials of high-dose IL-2 therapy in melanoma were conducted between 1985 and 1993 and produced responses in up to 20% of patients. An analysis of eight of these trials, involving 270 patients, yielded an objective response rate of 16% with 6% complete responses and 10% partial responses. It was noted during this study that those patients with a complete response remained progression-free indicating very durable responses (**Fig. 1**).[35]

Follow-up analysis of the 270 patients treated with IL-2 confirmed the durability of responses with no patient relapsing who had achieved a response in excess of 30 months.[36] High-dose IL-2 administered at 600,000 to 720,000 units per kilogram by bolus intravenous infusion every 8 hours on Days 1 to 5 and 15 to 19 received Food and Drug administration approval for the treatment of patients with advanced melanoma in January of 1998. Treatment courses were repeated at 8- to 12-week intervals in responding patients. Unfortunately, the toxicity of this regimen limits its use to selected patients with excellent organ function. In addition, the treatment can only be given in well-established treatment centers with experience giving IL-2 therapy.

IL-2 Combined with Chemotherapy

Biochemotherapy, or the combination of IL-2 with cytotoxic chemotherapy, has been extensively evaluated. Initial phase II trials produced responses in approximately 50%

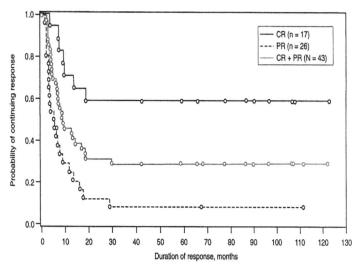

Fig. 1. Response duration curves for the 37 responding patients in the 270-patient cohort of high-dose IL-2–treated patients with advanced melanoma. CR, complete response; PR, partial response. (*Data from* Atkins MB, Lotze MT, Dutcher JP, et al. High-dose recombinant interleukin 2 therapy for patients with metastatic melanoma: analysis of 270 patients treated between 1985 and 1993. J Clin Oncol 1999;17:2110.)

of patients with 10% achieving durable complete responses. Early phase III trials failed to confirm the benefit initially seen in a more selected group of patients and were limited by toxicity.

An EORTC trial compared IFN alfa-2a and IL-2 with or without cisplatin in 138 patients. The response rate was higher in the biochemotherapy arm (33% vs 18%); however, there was no statistically significant difference in OS between the two arms.[37] The intergroup trial E3695 compared concurrent CVD (cisplatin, vinblastine, and dacarbazine) plus IL-2 and IFN to CVD alone in 395 patients. Although median progression-free survival was significantly longer for the biochemotherapy there was no OS advantage.[38]

Based on the results to date it has been concluded that biochemotherapy offers no significant advantage over cytotoxic chemotherapy or IL-2 alone. However, it may still play a role as a bridge to immunotherapy in patients with rapidly progressive disease who do not have time for the delayed responses seen with immunotherapy.

IL-2 Combined with Other Cytokines

During the administration of IL-2 an increase in Treg activity and frequency has been observed suggesting that IL-2 may lead to immune tolerance rather than antitumor immunity in some patients.[39] This suggests that it activates immune responses and participates in a negative feedback loop to limit immune responses. Based on this, combinations with more selective immunostimulatory cytokines have been performed. Combination trials with IL-4 and IL-6 have been disappointing but investigations with IL-12 and IL-18 showed some initial promise.

IL-2 Combined with Vaccines

One attractive approach for improving response rates to IL-2 is the use of vaccines to target the immune stimulation. Vaccination with the gp100 peptide vaccine showed very high rates of circulating T cells capable of recognizing and targeting melanoma cells. As a result gp100 was combined with IL-2 in several promising phase II trials and a large phase III trial.[40] The phase III trial showed an improved overall clinical response of 16% versus 6% and a longer OS (17.8 vs 11.1 months). The vaccine caused minimal additional toxicity beyond that seen with IL-2 alone. Some skin reactions and arrhythmias were observed.

The gp100 vaccine did not add additional efficacy when combined with CTLA4 inhibition with ipilimumab. These mixed results may be representative of different effects on the immune system. However, at this time it remains unclear if use of the gp100 vaccine outside of clinical trials will become a new standard of care.

Other IL-2 Combinations

The combination of IL-2 with tumor-infiltrating lymphocytes showed promise in tumor models and is being tested within the National Cancer Institute Surgery Branch. Studies involving the administration of clonally expanded, tumor antigen-specific CD8[+] lymphocytes and IL-2 following chemotherapy and radiation-induced lymphodepletion have showed encouraging activity in patients with refractory melanoma.[41]

IL-2 therapy is also being combined with molecularly targeted therapy. There are trials ongoing combining IL-2 with BRAF-targeted agents. The future will likely bring further combinations as more targeted agents are found to have activity against metastatic melanoma.

Toxicity

High-dose IL-2 therapy is toxic and must be administered in the inpatient setting. Fortunately the side effects are dose dependent and largely predictable and reversible. Common side effects include fever, chills, myalgias, diarrhea, nausea, anemia, thrombocytopenia, hepatic dysfunction, myocarditis, and confusion. Capillary leak induced by IL-2 leads to fluid retention, hypotension, prerenal azotemia, and occasionally myocardial infarction.[42] IL-2 patients are also predisposed to infection. Early studies with the drug were associated with 2% to 4% mortality.[35] The mortality has dropped to less than 1% at experienced treatment centers with the routine use of antibiotic prophylaxis, more extensive cardiac screening, and better patient selection.[43]

Patient Selection

The safe administration of high-dose IL-2 should only be considered in patients without significant cardiac disease and exercise-induced ischemia on a stress test. In addition they should have adequate renal, hepatic, and pulmonary function. Patients should be screened for central nervous system metastasis and not treated in the setting of neurologic disease.[43]

Given the high toxicity of IL-2 and the low number of patients achieving a durable benefit there has been extensive effort to better identify those patients most likely to respond. A retrospective analysis of 374 patients with melanoma treated with high-dose IL-2 at the National Cancer Institute showed no difference in response based on prior therapy or laboratory parameters. However, 53.6% of patients with only subcutaneous and/or cutaneous metastasis responded, compared with 12.4% of patients with disease at other sites.[44] This analysis also showed an increased response in patients who developed lymphocytosis, vitiligo, and abnormal thyroid function tests immediately after therapy.

The association of autoimmune phenomena with clinical benefit from cytokine therapy has also been reported in the use of IFN and CTLA4 antibody administration.

This suggests that benefit from these therapies may be limited to patients capable of mounting an immune response to self-antigens and may help focus these therapies in the future. Analysis of pretreatment gene expression profiles showed that tumor responsiveness was correlated with genes related to T-cell regulation. This suggests that immune responsiveness might be predetermined by a tumor microenvironment more prone to immune recognition.[45]

In recent years, correlation of IL-2 response with melanoma driver mutations has been performed. In a study of 208 patients it was observed that there was a significant difference in response rates based on mutation status: NRAS, 47%; BRAF, 23%; and WT/WT, 12%.[46] This analysis also showed a negative link between elevated lactate dehydrogenase and progression-free survival and OS, with a trend toward a decreased response rate.

Efforts are ongoing to identify factors that can easily be tested within the tumor tissue or blood to predict for response. An analysis of biopsied melanoma from patients before and after IL-2 treatment is currently underway through the Cytokine Working Group with results expected within the next few years.

OTHER CYTOKINES
IL-21

Interleukin-21 is a member of the IL-2 cytokine family, which leads to enhancement of adaptive T-cell immunity, antibody production, activation of natural killer cell subtypes, and opposition to suppressive effects mediated by regulatory T cells.[47] IL-21 showed activity in preclinical models and phase I trials in melanoma.

A phase II study of IL-21 by Petrella and coworkers[48] showed a 22.5% overall response rate with 9 partial responses out of 40 patients enrolled. The OS was found to be 12.4 months. It remains to be seen if IL-21 plays a role in the future treatment of melanoma.

GM-CSF

GM-CSF was initially approved for clinical use in chemotherapy-induced neutropenia; however, it also has immunotherapeutic potential. Administration of irradiated melanoma cells expressing GM-CSF in mice with established tumors improved their survival by 40% to 60%.[49] The activity of GM-CSF is related to its ability to activate macrophages and dendritic cells. Natural killer cells also play a role in GM-CSF immune responses.[50]

GM-CSF–secreting tumor vaccines showed synergy with ipilimumab treatment in preclinical models. In E1608 ipilimumab and GM-CSF were compared with ipilimumab alone in the treatment of 245 patients with melanoma. The combination showed a benefit in OS with less high-grade adverse events in patients receiving combination therapy.[51]

Another promising role for GM-CSF in melanoma is intralesional injection.[52] Multiple trials using autologous tumor vaccines engineered to secrete GM-CSF have shown biologic activity. Talimogene laherparepvec (T-VEC) is an immunotherapy derived from herpes simplex virus type-1 designed to selectively replicate within tumors and produce GM-CSF. In a phase III trial comparing T-VEC with GM-CSF it was observed that T-VEC had a statistically significant improvement in durable response rate with an objective response rate of 26% compared with 6% with GM-CSF.[53]

The role of T-VEC and GM-CSF in the treatment of melanoma is sure to evolve in the near future. At this time T-VEC is an interesting option for patients with extensive in-transit disease or those who cannot tolerate systemic therapy.

SUMMARY

Cytokine therapies have wide potential in the treatment of melanoma. At this time only IFN and IL-2 are routinely used in the clinic. IFN is approved for use in the adjuvant setting and has been shown to help decrease recurrence rate and improve survival. However, its use is controversial given the high toxicity and limited benefit. IL-2 has proven efficacy in a small subset of patients where it produces a prolonged durable response. The toxicity of IL-2 limits its use to experienced centers and appropriate patients. Studies are ongoing to further define the role of cytokines within the therapeutic landscape and they will likely remain a critical component of curative strategies in melanoma.

REFERENCES

1. Isaacs A, Lindenmann J. Virus interference. I. The interferon. Proc R Soc Lond B Biol Sci 1957;147:258–67.
2. Ozato K, Uno K, Iwakura Y. Another road to interferon: Yasuichi Nagano's journey. J Interferon Cytokine Res 2007;27:349–52.
3. Pestka S, Krause CD, Walter MR. Interferons, interferon-like cytokines, and their receptors. Immunol Rev 2004;202:8–32.
4. Pestka S. The interferons: 50 years after their discovery, there is much more to learn. J Biol Chem 2007;282:20047–51.
5. Knight E Jr, Hunkapiller MW, Korant BD, et al. Human fibroblast interferon: amino acid analysis and amino terminal amino acid sequence. Science 1980;207: 525–6.
6. Weissenbach J, Chernajovsky Y, Zeevi M, et al. Two interferon mRNAs in human fibroblasts: in vitro translation and Escherichia coli cloning studies. Proc Natl Acad Sci U S A 1980;77:7152–6.
7. Krause CD, Pestka S. Historical developments in the research of interferon receptors. Cytokine Growth Factor Rev 2007;18:473–82.
8. Darnell JE Jr, Kerr IM, Stark GR. Jak-STAT pathways and transcriptional activation in response to IFNs and other extracellular signaling proteins. Science 1994;264:1415–21.
9. Kirkwood JM, Richards T, Zarour HM, et al. Immunomodulatory effects of high-dose and low-dose interferon a2b in patients with high-risk resected melanoma: the E2690 laboratory corollary of intergroup adjuvant trial E1690. Cancer 2002; 95:1101–12.
10. Clemens MJ. Interferons and apoptosis. J Interferon Cytokine Res 2003;23: 277–92.
11. Krown SE, Burk MW, Kirkwood JM, et al. Human leukocyte (alpha) interferon in metastatic malignant melanoma: the American Cancer Society phase II trial. Cancer Treat Rep 1984;68:723–6.
12. Kirkwood JM, Ernstoff MS. Interferons in the treatment of human cancer. J Clin Oncol 1984;2:336–51.
13. Retsas S, Priestman TJ, Newton KA, et al. Evaluation of human lyphoblastoid interferon in advanced malignant melanoma. Cancer 1982;51:273–6.
14. Creagan ET, Ahmann DL, Frytak S, et al. Recombinant leukocyte A interferon (rIFN-aA) in the treatment of disseminated malignant melanoma. Analysis of complete and long-term responding patients. Cancer 1986;58:2576–8.
15. Kirkwood JM, Strawderman MH, Ernstoff MS, et al. Interferon alfa-2b adjuvant therapy of high-risk resected cutaneous melanoma: the Eastern Cooperative Oncology Group Trial EST 1684. J Clin Oncol 1996;14:7–17.

16. Kirkwood JM, Ibrahim JG, Sondak VK, et al. High- and low-dose interferon alfa-2b in high risk melanoma: first analysis of intergroup trial E1690/S9111/C9190. J Clin Oncol 2000;18:2444–58.
17. Livingston PO, Wong GYC, Adluri S, et al. Improved survival in stage III melanoma patients with GM2 antibodies: a randomized trial of adjuvant vaccination with GM2 ganglioside. J Clin Oncol 1994;12:1036–44.
18. Kirkwood JM, Ibrahim JG, Sosman JA, et al. High-dose interferon alfa-2b significantly prolongs relapse-free and overall survival compared with the GM2-KLH/QS-21 vaccine in patients with resected stage IIB-III melanoma: results of intergroup trial E1694/S9512/C509801. J Clin Oncol 2001;19:2370–80.
19. Wheatley K, Ives N, Hancock B, et al. Does adjuvant interferon-α for high-risk melanoma provide a worthwhile benefit? A meta-analysis of randomized trials. Cancer Treat Rev 2003;29:241–52.
20. Wheatley K, Ives N, Eggermont A, et al, International Malignant Melanoma Collaborative Group. Interferon-α as adjuvant therapy for melanoma: an individual patient data meta-analysis of randomized trials [abstract]. J Clin Oncol 2007; 25:8526.
21. Mocellin S, Pasquali S, Rossi CF, et al. Interferon alpha adjuvant therapy in patients with high-risk melanoma: a systematic review and meta-analysis. J Natl Cancer Inst 2010;102:493–501.
22. Eggermont AM, Suciu S, Santinami M, et al. Adjuvant therapy with pegylated interferon alfa-2b versus observation alone in resected stage III melanoma: final results of EORTC 18991, a randomized phase III trial. Lancet 2008;372: 117–26.
23. Eggermont AM, Suciu S, Tesori A, et al. Ulceration and stage are predictive of interferon efficacy in melanoma: results of the phase III adjuvant trials EORTC 18952 and EORTC 18991. Eur J Cancer 2012;48:218–25.
24. Pectasides D, Dafni U, Bafaloukos D, et al. Randomized phase III study of 1 month versus 1 year of adjuvant high-dose interferon alfa-2b in patients with resected high-risk melanoma. J Clin Oncol 2009;27:939–44.
25. Agarwala SS, Lee SJ, Flaherty LE, et al. Randomized phase III trial of high-dose interferon alfa-2b (HDI) for 4 weeks induction only in patients with intermediate- and high-risk melanoma (Intergroup trial E1697). J Clin Oncol 2011; 29(Suppl) [abstract 8505].
26. Gogas H, Ioannovich J, Dafni U, et al. Prognostic significance of autoimmunity during treatment of melanoma with interferon. N Engl J Med 2006;16:709–18.
27. Morgan DA, Ruscetti FW, Gallo R. Selective in vitro growth of T lymphocytes for normal human bone marrows. Science 1976;193:1007–8.
28. Taniguchi T, Matsui H, Fujita T, et al. Structure and expression of cloned cDNA for human interleukin-2. Nature 1983;302:305–10.
29. Waldmann TA, Tsudo M. Interleukin-2 receptors: biology and therapeutic potentials. Hosp Pract (Off Ed) 1987;22:77–84, 93–4.
30. Foa R, Guarini A, Gansbacher B. IL2 treatment for cancer: from biology to gene therapy. Br J Cancer 1992;66:992–8.
31. Rosenberg SA, Mule JJ, Speiss PJ, et al. Regression of established pulmonary metastases and subcutaneous tumor mediated by the systemic administration of high-dose recombinant interleukin 2. J Exp Med 1985;161:1169–88.
32. Rosenberg SA, Lotze MT, Muul LM, et al. Observations on the systemic administration of autologous lymphokine-activated killer cells and recombinant interleukin-2 to patients with metastatic cancer. N Engl J Med 1985;313: 1485–92.

33. Rosenberg SA, Lotze MT, Muul LM, et al. A progress report on the treatment of 157 patients with advanced cancer using lymphokine activated killer cells and interleukin-2 or high-dose interleukin-2 alone. N Engl J Med 1987;316: 889–97.

34. Rosenberg SA, Lotze MT, Yang JC, et al. Prospective randomized trial of high-dose interleukin-2 alone or in conjunction with lymphokine-activated killer cells of the treatment of patients with advanced cancer. J Natl Cancer Inst 1993; 85:622–32.

35. Atkins MB, Lotze MT, Dutcher JP, et al. High-dose recombinant interleukin 2 therapy for patients with metastatic melanoma: analysis of 270 patients treated between 1985 and 1993. J Clin Oncol 1999;17:2105–16.

36. Atkins MB, Kunkel L, Sznol M, et al. High-dose recombinant interleukin-2 therapy in patients with metastatic melanoma: long-term survival update. Cancer J Sci Am 2006;6(Suppl 1):11–4.

37. Atkins MB, Hsu J, Lee S, et al. Phase III trial comparing concurrent biochemotherapy with cisplatin, vinblastine, dacarbazine, interleukin-2, and interferon alfa-2b with cisplatin, vinblastine, and dacarbazine alone in patients with metastatic malignant melanoma (E3695): a trial coordinated by the Eastern Cooperative Oncology Group. J Clin Oncol 2008;10:5748–54.

38. O'Day SJ, Atkins MB, Baosberg P, et al. Phase II multicenter trial of maintenance biotherapy after induction concurrent biochemotherapy for patients with metastatic melanoma. J Clin Oncol 2009;27:6207–12.

39. Atkins MB. Cytokine-based therapy and biochemotherapy for advanced melanoma. Clin Cancer Res 2006;12:2353s–8s.

40. Schwarzentruber DJ, Lawson DH, Richards JM, et al. gp100 peptide vaccine and interleukin-2 in patients with advanced melanoma. N Engl J Med 2011; 364:2119–27.

41. Dudley ME, Jang JC, Sherry R, et al. Adoptive cell therapy for patients with metastic melanoma: evaluation of intensive myeloablative chemoradiation preparative regimens. J Clin Oncol 2008;26:5233–9.

42. Margolin K. The clinical toxicities of high-dose interleukin-2. In: Atkins M, editor. Therapeutic applications of interleukin-2. New York: Marcel Dekker Inc; 1993. p. 331–62.

43. Kammula US, White DE, Rosenberg SA, et al. Trends in the safety of high dose bolus interleukin-2 administration in patients with metastatic cancer. Cancer 1998;83:797–805.

44. Phan GQ, Attia P, Steinberg SM, et al. Factors associated with response to high-dose interleukin-2 in patients with metastatic melanoma. J Clin Oncol 2001;19: 3477–82.

45. Wang E, Miller LD, Ohnmacht GA, et al. Prospective molecular profiling of melanoma metastasis suggests classifiers of immune responsiveness. Cancer Res 2002;62:3581–6.

46. Joseph RW, Sullivan RJ, Harrell R, et al. Correlation of NRAS mutations with clinical response to high-dose IL-2 in patients with advanced melanoma. J Immunother 2012;35:66–72.

47. Davis ID, Skak K, Smyth MJ, et al. Interleukin-21 signaling: functions in cancer and autoimmunity. Clin Cancer Res 2007;13:6926–32.

48. Petrella TM, Tozer R, Belanger K, et al. Interleukin-21 has activity in patients with metastatic melanoma: a phase II study. J Clin Oncol 2012;30:3396–401.

49. Dranoff G, Jaffee E, Lazenby A, et al. Vaccination with irradiated tumor cells engineered to secrete murine granulocyte-macrophage colony stimulating factor

stimulates potent, specific, and long-lasting anti-tumor immunity. Proc Natl Acad Sci U S A 1993;90:3539–43.

50. Armstrong CA, Botella R, Galloway TH, et al. Antitumor effects of granulocyte-macrophage colony stimulating factor production by melanoma cells. Cancer Res 1996;56:2191–8.

51. Hodi SF, Lee SJ, McDermott DF, et al. Multicenter, randomized phase II trial of GM-CSF (GM) plus ipilimumab (Ipi) versus Ipi alone in metastatic melanoma: E1608. J Clin Oncol 2013;31(Suppl) [abstract CRA9007].

52. Ridolfi L, Ridolfi R. Preliminary experiences of intralesional immunotherapy in cutaneous metastatic melanoma. Hepatogastroenterology 2002;49:335–9.

53. Andtbacka RH, Collichio FA, Amatruda T, et al. OPTiM: a randomized phase III trial of talimogene laherparepvec (T-VEC) versus subcutaneous (SC) granulocyte-macrophage colony-stimulating factor (GM-CSF) for the treatment of unresected stage IIIB/C and IV melanoma. J Clin Oncol 2013;31(Suppl) [abstract LBA9008].

Immune Checkpoint Blockade

Jarushka Naidoo, MB, BCh, BAO[a],*, David B. Page, MD[a], Jedd D. Wolchok, MD, PhD[b,c]

KEYWORDS

- Ipilimumab • Tremelimumab • Nivolumab • Immunotherapy • Checkpoint inhibitor
- Anti–PD-1 • Anti–PD-L1 • Anti-CTLA4

KEY POINTS

- Cytotoxic T-lymphocyte antigen 4 (CTLA-4) and programmed death 1 (PD-1) are immune checkpoint molecules. These co-inhibitory molecules on the surface of T-cells and self-cells regulate T-cell function by shutting down an immune stimulus.
- Ipilimumab is an anti-CTLA4 antibody that reinvigorates an antitumor T-cell response. It is a therapy approved by the Food and Drug Administration for first-line treatment of metastatic melanoma.
- Nivolumab and MK-3475 are anti–PD-1 antibodies, and MPDL3280A is an antibody that blocks the ligand of PD-1, PD-L1. These agents have demonstrated promising results in the treatment of advanced melanoma in early-phase studies.
- Immune-related response criteria are a novel set of radiologic criteria used to define response to immunotherapeutic agents.
- Immune-related adverse events are side effects of immunotherapeutic agents associated with cytokine release and immune infiltration of organs.

INTRODUCTION

The immune system performs the vital function of defense against foreign antigens. In doing so, it requires a variety of checks and balances to protect against self-antigens while assuring appropriate activation against foreign antigens.[1] These checks and balances consist of immune-activating and inhibiting receptors and ligands expressed by T-cells and other immune cell subsets. Antigen recognition by T-cells occurs through

---

Disclosures: None.

Conflicts of Interest: None (J. Naidoo, D.B. Page); Consultant to MedImmune, Merck, GlaxoSmithKline and Bristol Myers-Squibb (J.D. Wolchok).

[a] Department of Medicine, Memorial Sloan-Kettering Cancer Center, 1275 York Avenue, New York, NY 10065, USA; [b] Melanoma and Immunotherapy Service, Department of Medicine, Memorial Sloan-Kettering Cancer Center, 1275 York Avenue, New York, NY 10065, USA; [c] Ludwig Center for Cancer Immunotherapy, Memorial Sloan-Kettering Cancer Center, 1275 York Avenue, New York, NY 10065, USA

* Corresponding author.

E-mail address: naidooj@mskcc.org

http://dx.doi.org/10.1016/j.hoc.2014.02.002
0889-8588/14/$ – see front matter © 2014 Elsevier Inc. All rights reserved.
hemonc.theclinics.com

the engagement of the T-cell receptor (TCR) and peptide major histocompatibility complexes (MHC), as well as co-stimulation through CD28 binding to either B7-1 (CD80) or B7-2 (CD86) on antigen-presenting cells (APCs).[2] Several of these molecules also play a role in T-cell activity in chronic infections and in cancer.[3] CD28 is thus the first checkpoint in T-cell activation, as it responds to the expression of CD80/CD86 on an APC. Cytotoxic T-lymphocyte antigen 4 (CTLA-4) is a co-inhibitory molecule that acts at this checkpoint. CTLA-4 binds with high affinity to CD80/CD86, and can block T-cell activation by direct competition with CD80/CD86 and by downstream CTLA-4–mediated inhibitory signaling.[4]

Immune checkpoints thus refer to a group of molecules on the surface of both self-cells and cells of the immune system that send a co-inhibitory stimulus, and in so doing attenuate an immune response (**Fig. 1**).[5] Therefore, monoclonal antibodies that bind and block the inhibitory actions of CTLA-4 might promote antigen-mediated T-cell activation.[6] Melanoma is a cancer type with known immunogenic properties. The T-cell stimulatory cytokine interleukin-2 is already a Food and Drug Administration (FDA)-approved drug licensed for the treatment of this disease, and has been known to produce rare but durable long-term responses in both melanoma and renal cell carcinoma (RCC).[7] These diseases thus provide the first ports of call for the development of further immunotherapies.[8] Examples of immune checkpoints with potential therapeutic benefit include: CTLA-4, programmed death 1 (PD-1), lymphocyte activation gene 3 (LAG-3), and T-cell immunoglobulin and mucin protein 3 (TIM-3), as detailed in **Fig. 1**.[5]

CTLA-4 INHIBITORS

The most well-known and widely studied immune checkpoint is CTLA-4.

Preclinical Studies with CTLA-4

CTLA-4 is a molecule expressed on the surface of CD-4 and CD-8 T-cells, and is a member of the CD28/immunoglobulin superfamily (IGSF).[5] CTLA-4 competes with

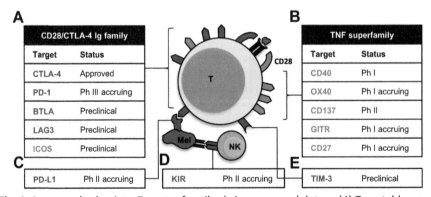

Fig. 1. Immune checkpoints. Targets of antibody immune modulators. (*A*) Targetable members of the CD28/CTLA-4 immunoglobulin superfamily include cytotoxic T-lymphocyte antigen 4 (CTLA-4), programmed cell death protein 1 (PD-1), B- and T-cell attenuator (BTLA), lymphocyte activation gene 3 (LAG3), and inducible T-cell costimulator (ICOS). (*B*) Targetable members of the tumor necrosis factor (TNF) superfamily include CD40, OX40, CD137/4-1BB, glucocorticoid-induced TNFR-related protein (GITR), and CD27. (*C*) Programmed cell death ligand 1 (PD-L1). (*D*) Killer inhibitory receptor (KIR). (*E*) T-cell immunoglobulin- and mucin-containing domain 3 (TIM3). (*From* Page DB, Postow MA, Callahan MK, et al. Immune modulation in cancer with antibodies. Annu Rev Med 2014;65:191; with permission.)

CD28 to bind to ligands B7-1 (CD80) and B7-2 (CD86) on APCs.[1] CTLA-4 mediates an inhibitory signal, thereby dampening T-cell responses in the tumor microenvironment (TME). CTLA-4 is also expressed on $CD25^+FOXP3^+$ T-regulatory cells (Tregs), and plays a pivotal role in the function of Tregs and in the CD4:CD8 ratio in the TME.[3] CTLA-4 blockade has also been shown to deplete intratumoral Tregs.[9] CTLA4 knockout mice demonstrate an increase in activated T-cells after 3 to 4 weeks, which manifests clinically as pancreatitis, myocarditis, and T-cell infiltration of the liver, heart, and lungs of the mice.[10,11] When CTLA-4 signaling is blocked, protein tyrosine kinases FYN, LCK, and ZAP-70 are activated.[12] To control T-cell activation CTLA-4 recruits 2 phosphatases, SHP2 and PP2A, which control these protein tyrosine kinases.[12] CTLA-4 activation of SHP2 results in dephosphorylation of the CD3z chain, dampening the signal from the TCR. CTLA-4 recruitment of PP2A inhibits Akt phosphorylation, further dampening the TCR signal.[12]

Blocking the action of CTLA-4 with an anti–CTLA-4 antibody was first studied in transplantable tumor models of colon carcinoma (51BLim10), fibrosarcoma (Sa1 N and CSA1 M), ovarian cancer (OV-HM), and prostate cancer (TRAMPC1).[6,13,14] In these models, the blocking of CTLA-4 caused primary shrinkage of tumors and protected the mice against tumor rechallenge. Thus it was initially postulated that blocking CTLA-4 could induce durable control of tumors in humans.

Ipilimumab

Ipilimumab is a fully humanized immunoglobulin (Ig)G1 monoclonal antibody that binds to and inhibits the action of CTLA-4. In an initial trial of 17 patients with unresectable melanoma treated with ipilimumab, there were 2 partial responses (PRs) at the starting dose of 3 mg/kg administered as a single dose.[15] These responses were durable, with the only notable adverse event (AE) being a mild rash.[15] Ipilimumab was then combined with a glycoprotein (gp)100 peptide vaccine in a phase I clinical trial, where 14 patients with advanced melanoma were treated with 3 mg/kg of ipilimumab followed by a gp100 peptide vaccine. Three patients responded to treatment, including 2 complete responses (CRs). However, more than 3 subjects experienced grade 3 and 4 AEs that appeared to be immune-related, including dermatitis, enterocolitis, hypophysitis, and hepatitis.[16] A dose-response relationship was demonstrated in a double-blind phase II trial of ipilimumab monotherapy administered at 3 dose levels in 217 patients with advanced melanoma. These patients received 0.3, 3, or 10 mg/kg of antibody every 3 weeks for 4 doses. If patients experienced stable disease (SD) or a response to therapy, and tolerated treatment, they subsequently received maintenance 12-weekly ipilimumab. A response rate (RR) of 11% and a median overall survival (OS) of 14 months were reported in the 10 mg/kg group. This dose is thus considered to be the optimum one, although it is also associated with the greatest rate of immune-related (ir) AEs.[17]

Ipilimumab is now an FDA-approved therapy for metastatic melanoma (Yervoy; Bristol Myers-Squibb, New York, NY). FDA approval of ipilimumab was based on the results of 2 phase III randomized controlled trials (RCTs) that demonstrated an OS benefit with ipilimumab.[18,19] A phase III trial of pretreated patients with advanced melanoma was a 3-arm study that compared ipilimumab at a dose of 3 mg/kg with or without gp100 peptide vaccine, with the gp100 peptide vaccine alone. The median OS in the ipilimumab and ipilimumab/gp100 groups was 10.1 versus 10.0 months, respectively, compared with 6.4 months with gp100 alone (hazard ratio [HR] 0.68, $P<.001$).[18] The first-line phase III RCT compared ipilimumab/dacarbazine with dacarbazine/placebo, at an ipilimumab dose of 10 mg/kg, followed by maintenance ipilimumab or placebo every 12 weeks.[19] This trial demonstrated an improvement in median OS in the combination arm (11.2 vs 9.1 months). Of note, higher survival rates were seen in the ipilimumab/dacarbazine group at 1 year (47.3% vs 36.3%), 2 years (28.5% vs 17.9%), and 3 years (20.8% vs 12.2%) (HR for death 0.72; P<.001). The median duration of response was 19.3 months with the combination and 8.1 months with dacarbazine alone.[19] AEs of all grades were more common in the combination arm, most notably in elevations of levels of alanine aminotransferase (ALT) (33.2% vs 5.6%) and aspartate aminotransferase (AST) (29.1% vs 5.6%), diarrhea (36.4% vs 24.7%), pruritus (29.6% vs 8.8%), and rash (24.7% vs 6.8%). Grade 3 or 4 AEs were noted in 56.3% of patients in the combination arm, compared with 27.5% of those receiving dacarbazine/placebo (P<.001).

The potential benefit of reinduction ipilimumab has also not been fully elucidated. In the ipilimumab/gp100 trial reported by Hodi and colleagues,[18] 31 patients were reinduced. Nineteen percent (n = 6/31) of patients demonstrated a treatment response, and 48% (n = 15/31) had SD. The benefit of reinduction ipilimumab will be investigated in a trial comparing this agent with investigator's choice of chemotherapy (NCT00495066).

Tremelimumab

Tremelimumab is an inhibitory human IgG2 monoclonal antibody against CTLA-4.[20] Tremelimumab has been investigated in 9 clinical studies as a single agent, with a total of more than 1000 patients having received this agent. Early-phase studies with tremelimumab demonstrated a 6% to 10% RR, with durable responses lasting for more than 170 days.[21,22] Tremelimumab was compared with investigator's choice chemotherapy in a phase III study in advanced melanoma, at a dose of 15 mg/kg every 3 months.[23] This study demonstrated a median duration of response of 35.8 months, compared with 13.7 months with combination chemotherapy (P = .0011), but did not demonstrate an OS benefit. This finding can potentially be explained by the exclusion of patients with an elevated level of lactate dehydrogenase onto this study, crossover of patients to ipilimumab, and the possibility of suboptimal dose and schedule.

Adverse Events

A spectrum of AEs associated with CTLA-4 inhibitors are well described, and are termed irAEs. irAEs relate to the mode of action of these agents, which can lead to the development of a CD-4 and CD-8 T-cell inflammatory infiltration of solid organs, and increased serum inflammatory cytokines.[24] irAEs can occur at any time point during ipilimumab therapy and can range in severity from mild to fatal, and in onset from slow to sudden.[24] Management is aimed at correctly identifying the irAE, grading the toxicity based on National Cancer Institute common toxicity criteria of AEs, and initiating early treatment with supportive care or steroid medications. The incidence of grade 3 or higher irAEs in published studies ranges from 5% to 25%, and is dose related.[18,25] The most common irAEs are dermatitis (pruritus, rash), enterocolitis, endocrinopathies (hypophysitis, thyroiditis), liver abnormalities (elevated serum liver tests, hepatitis), and uveitis. In the trial reported by Hodi and colleagues,[18] the most frequent AEs were rash (30%), pruritus (33%), diarrhea (33%), colitis (8%), endocrine abnormalities (9%), AST/ALT elevations (2%), and hepatitis (1%). irAEs with tremelimumab in the study reported by Ribas and colleagues[23] were similar to those of ipilimumab, such as colitis, rash, vitiligo, hepatitis, and autoimmune endocrinopathies.

Management of irAEs

Management algorithms have emerged for irAEs such as diarrhea/colitis. Grade I diarrhea is managed with oral hydration, an American Dietary Association colitis diet, and loperamide. Diarrhea of grade 2 or greater can be managed with oral budesonide, oral steroids, intravenous methylprednisolone, and, occasionally, infliximab. In a post hoc analysis of patients with colitis of grade 3 or higher, 90% of patients received corticosteroids, and 14% of these patients received further immunosuppression with infliximab.[26] Median time until resolution of diarrhea was 2 weeks.[27] Colitis-associated mortality was associated with management delays, failure to withhold ipilimumab, and an inadequate antidiarrheal regimen.[26] In a series of 15 reported cases of ipilimumab-related colitis requiring infliximab, treatment was effective within 3 days in most subjects.[28] Administration of corticosteroids has not been associated with changes in survival or duration of response to anti–CTLA-4 therapy.[29] The use of effective management algorithms have reduced life-threatening complications, with bowel perforations occurring in fewer than 1% of patients (**Table 1**).[5]

Evaluating Response with CTLA-4 Inhibitors

When analyzing the Kaplan-Meier survival curves of the 2 phase III studies reported by the groups of Hodi and Robert,[18,19] a characteristic shape of the survival curves is noted. First, the survival curves overlap until approximately 4 months, after which the ipilimumab arm diverges, and subsequently plateaus. This pattern indicates that a subset of patients achieves a benefit, and that this benefit is durable. Long-term follow-up of patients treated on earlier-phase studies with ipilimumab confirms durable responses, with 4-year OS ranging from 13.8% to 49.5% at various doses of ipilimumab.[31] It is with this in mind that Wolchok and colleagues[32] first described the immune-related response criteria (irRC) tailored toward evaluating response to

Table 1
Trials of CTLA-4 inhibitors in malignant melanoma

Agent	Study Design	No. of Patients	Response	Survival (mo)	Grade 3/4 Adverse Events
Ipilimumab	Phase III Ipilumumab + gp100 vs gp100[18]	676	6% ORR 14% SD (ipi + gp100)	6.0 vs 10.0	Overall (ipi + gp100) 17% Colitis 1% Diarrhea 5% Endocrinopathy 1% Abnormal LFTs 1%
	Phase III Ipilimumab + dacarbazine vs dacarbazine[19]	502	—	11.2 vs 9.1	Overall (ipi + dacarb) 42% High ALT 21% High AST 17% Diarrhea/colitis 6% Pruritus 2%
Tremelimumab	Phase III Treme vs physician's choice chemotherapy[23]	655	10.7% (treme) 9.8% (chemo)	12.6 vs 10.7	Overall 52% Diarrhea 15% Fatigue 6% Nausea 4% Vomiting 4%
	Phase II Treme + pegIFN α2b[30]	37	24% ORR 38% SD	21.0 overall survival	Neutropenia 16% Diarrhea 11% Abnormal LFTs 11%

Abbreviations: ALT, alanine aminotransferase; AST, aspartate aminotransferase; dacarb, dacarbazine; gp, glycoprotein; ipi, ipilimumab; LFTs, liver function tests; ORR, objective response rate; pegIFN, pegylated interferon; SD, stable disease; treme, tremelimumab.

From Page DB, Postow MA, Callahan MK, et al. Immune modulation in cancer with antibodies. Annu Rev Med 2014;65:188; with permission.

immunotherapeutic agents. These criteria are based on the rationale that immunotherapies generate an antitumor effect with response kinetics distinct from those of cytotoxic chemotherapy. Antitumor responses with immunotherapeutic agents may be delayed; in some patients, lesions may enlarge before ultimately shrinking, perhaps related to the underlying immune mechanism of T-cell activation and tumoral infiltration. Patients may also achieve SD with slow tumor regression over time. The irRC thus recommend interval imaging at least 4 weeks apart to aid in the confirmation of progression. In determining SD or PR, new lesions are allowed in the context of overall decreases in tumor burden.[32] In contrast to traditional World Health Organization criteria, new non-measurable lesions do not define progression in irRC criteria. Because of these response patterns, patients who experience a clinically insignificant progression of disease often continue to receive therapy until progression is confirmed on subsequent imaging.

ANTI–PD-1 ANTIBODIES
Preclinical Studies

PD-1 (CD279) is a transmembrane molecule on T lymphocytes, B lymphocytes, and monocytes that acts as an immune checkpoint. When PD-1 is stimulated, the immune response mediated by these cells is inhibited.[33] The PD-1 signaling pathway is mediated by the binding of PD-1 to ligands PD-L1 and PD-L2 on APCs, as well as PD-L1 binding to the co-stimulatory molecule B7-1.[34] The term "programmed death" was given to this molecule on its identification in 1992 as a gene upregulated in T-cell hybridoma undergoing cell death.[35] The structure of PD-1 consists of an IGSF domain, a transmembrane domain, an intracellular domain containing an immunoreceptor tyrosine-based inhibitory motif, and an immunoreceptor tyrosine-based switch motif (ITSM). The inhibitory function of PD-1 is lost when the ITSM is mutated, suggesting that this tyrosine plays a primary functional role.[36] During PD-1 pathway activation, PD-1 can recruit phosphatases SHP-1 and SHP-2, and causes dephosphorylation of the CD3z chain.[37,38] PD-1 and CTLA-4 therefore mediate their effects through slightly different mechanisms, as PD-1 inhibits Akt activation via the phosphoinositide 3-kinase (PI3K) pathway, whereas CTLA-4 inhibits Akt independent of PI3K.[39] PD-1 knockout mice demonstrate elevated serum IgG2b and IgA levels, and develop a lupus-like syndrome and dilated cardiomyopathy.[40,41] These side effects appear less frequently and later in life in PD-1 knockout mice than in CTLA-4 knockout mice.

Nivolumab

Nivolumab (BMS-936558; anti–PD-1 monoclonal antibody [mAb]) is a fully human monoclonal IgG4 antibody that binds to the PD-1 cell-surface membrane receptor. Sosman and colleagues[42] initially investigated nivolumab in a phase I study of 107 patients with metastatic melanoma. Patients received doses from 0.1 to 10 mg/kg, and demonstrated an overall response rate (ORR) of 31%, with an RR of 41% in the 3 mg/kg group. Excellent durability of responses was seen, with 61% 1-year and 44% 2-year survival rates.[43] Treated-related AEs included fatigue, rash, diarrhea, and pruritus. Grade 3 and 4 toxicities were reported in 21% of patients, with an incidence of 1% to 3% in fatigue, diarrhea, nausea, and anemia. The antitumor effect of PD-1 receptor blockade by nivolumab has been investigated in several tumor types. Results from a phase I/II study reported by Topalian and colleagues[44] indicate that nivolumab is active in multiple tumor types. Treatment-related pneumonitis was reported in 3% (n = 9) of these patients, and accounted for 3 patient deaths in this study, none of which had melanoma. Nivolumab monotherapy at a dose of 3 mg/kg is currently being studied in phase III clinical trials in advanced melanoma, RCC, and non–small lung carcinoma (NSCLC). In melanoma, a first-line study of the 3 mg/kg dose of nivolumab is currently being studied in a comparison with dacarbazine (NCT01721772). Successful reinduction therapy with nivolumab has been described in a patient with melanoma who achieved a PR, followed by a period of SD for 16 months off treatment.[45] Reinduction resulted in a successful response after relapse in this patient.

MK-3475

MK-3475 is a humanized monoclonal IgG4 PD-1 antibody. A phase I dose-escalation study involving patients with multiple solid tumor types demonstrated the safety of this agent at the dose levels 1 mg/kg, 3 mg/kg, and 10 mg/kg administered every 2 weeks, and no maximum tolerated dose was identified.[46] In addition, clinical responses were observed at all the dose levels. MK-3475 was studied as a single agent in patients with advanced melanoma, in both patients who had previously received ipilimumab and those who had not. A phase I study reported by Hamid and colleagues[47] tested 2 doses, 2 and 10 mg/kg, given every 2 or 3 weeks. The immune-related responses in patients who had and had not received prior ipilimumab were identical, at 56%, in patients who received the 10 mg/kg dose every 2 weeks. Responses were 22% and 33% in patients who received the 3-weekly 10 mg/kg dose with and without prior ipilimumab, respectively. Seventy-nine percent (n = 107) of patients reported treatment-related AEs of all grades, and 13% reported grade 3 or 4 AEs. Pneumonitis occurred in 4% of patients, with no cases of grade 3 or 4 events. A phase II trial of this agent at 2 dose levels in comparison with chemotherapy is currently in accrual (NCT01704287.) The large experience with MK-3475 reports RRs close to 50%, and, again, excellent response durability.[47]

ANTI–PD-L1 ANTIBODIES
Preclinical Studies

PD-L1 is a transmembrane molecule that acts as a ligand for PD-1, and is expressed on hematopoietic and nonhematopoietic cells, T-cells, B-cells, macrophages, natural killer (NK) cells, dendritic cells (DCs), and mast cells.[48,49] PD-L1 expression has also been noted on the cardiac endothelium, lung, small intestine, keratinocytes, islet cells of the pancreas, and syncytiotrophoblasts in the placenta. PD-L1 expression is dynamic, and can be influenced in pattern and degree of expression by other immune mediators such as type I and type II interferons. PD-L2 expression is found nearly exclusively on hematopoietic cells. PD-L1 is also heterogeneously expressed on solid tumors such as melanoma, NSCLC, and urothelial, ovarian, breast, cervical, pancreatic, and gastric cancers as well as glioblastoma.[50–55] PD-L1 expression has been demonstrated to correlate with poor clinical outcome in some cancers, and may be a predictive marker for response to PD-1/PD-L1–directed therapy.[33,55]

MPDL3280A

MPDL3280A is a human mAb containing an engineered Fc portion that targets PD-L1. In a phase I trial of single-agent MPDL3280A administered to 45 patients with advanced melanoma, an RR of 26% (n = 9/35) was observed, and progression-free survival (PFS) at 24 weeks was 35%.[56] The incidence of grade 3 and 4 AEs was 33%, and included hyperglycemia (7%), elevated ALT (7%), and elevated AST (4%). No cases of grades 3 to 5 pneumonitis were reported, and no treatment-related deaths occurred.

MEDI4736

MEDI4736 is a human mAb of the IgG1κ subclass that inhibits binding of PD-L1 to PD-1 and B7-1.[57] In a xenograft model, MEDI4736 inhibited human tumor growth via a T-cell–dependent mechanism. Moreover, an anti-mouse PD-L1 antibody demonstrated improved survival in a syngeneic tumor model when given as monotherapy, and resulted in complete tumor regression in more than 50% of treated mice when given with chemotherapy.[57] NCT01693562 is the first-time-in-human study of single-agent MEDI4736 aimed at evaluating the safety, tolerability, and pharmacokinetics of this agent in subjects with advanced solid tumors. This phase I study has a classic 3 + 3 dose-escalation phase, followed by an expansion phase in various malignancies, including melanoma, NSCLC, and pancreatic cancer (**Table 2**).

MUCOSAL MELANOMA

Mucosal melanoma is a type of cutaneous melanoma usually found at the head and neck, vulvovagina, or anorectal mucosa.[59] Relapse rates after surgery are high, with a significant number of patients needing systemic therapy. The potential role of immune checkpoint inhibition in mucosal melanoma has yet to be elucidated. Postow and colleagues[60] reported a multicenter retrospective case series of 33 patients with mucosal melanoma treated with ipilimumab. Thirty patients were assessable by irRC at 12 weeks, 1 patient sustained an irCR, 1 patient had an irPR, 6 had irSD, and 22 had immune-related progressive disease. irAEs consisted of 18% (n = 6) with rash, 9% (n = 3) with diarrhea, 3% (n = 1) with thyroiditis, 3% (n = 1) with grade 3 hepatitis, and 3% (n = 1) with grade 2 hypophysitis. Median OS was 6.4 months (range 1.8–26.7 months). Response rates from single-institution studies of biochemotherapy with cisplatin, vinblastine, dacarbazine, interleukin-2, and interferon-α in mucosal melanoma demonstrate responses of approximately 36% to 47%.[61–63] These rates are lower than those seen with ipilimumab in this study.[60]

UVEAL MELANOMA

Uveal melanoma is a rare subtype of melanoma, accounting for 3% to 5% of all cutaneous melanomas. Fifty percent of cases metastasize, and contribute to a median survival of 12 months.[64] The uveal region of the eye is an immunologically privileged area,

Table 2
Trials of anti–PD-1/PD-L1 drugs in malignant melanoma

Agent	Study Design	No. of Patients	Response	Survival	Grade 3/4 Adverse Events
Nivolumab (Anti–PD-1)	Phase I[44]	107	31% ORR	16.8 mo median OS	Overall 21% Lymphopenia 3% Fatigue 3% Diarrhea 2%
MK3475 (Anti–PD-1)	Phase I	135	37% ORR	>7 mo median PFS	Overall 13% Rash 2% Abnormal LFTs 1% Pruritus 1% Diarrhea 1%
MPDL3280A (Anti–PD-L1)	Phase I[58]	45	26% ORR	—	Overall 33% High AST 7% High ALT 7% Hyperglycemia 7%

Abbreviations: ORR, objective response rate; OS, overall survival; PFS, progression-free survival.
From Page DB, Postow MA, Callahan MK, et al. Immune modulation in cancer with antibodies. Annu Rev Med 2014;65:188; with permission.

and therefore provides a physiologic rationale for the therapeutic use of immune checkpoint inhibitors.[65] Uveal melanomas are also known to exhibit increased expression of immunogenic cancer antigens such as gp100, melanoma-associated antigen (MAGE), melanoma antigen recognized by T-cells (MART-1), and tyrosinase-related protein 1 (TRP-1).[66,67] Luke and colleagues[65] reported a retrospective series of 39 patients with metastatic uveal melanoma who received ipilimumab in 4 academic centers. Thirty-four patients received a dose of 3 mg/kg and 5 patients received 10 mg/kg of ipilimumab. At week 12, ipilimumab demonstrated a 2.6% RR and 46% disease control rate. irAEs were observed in 28 patients (71.8%), with 7 (17.9%) grade 3 and 4 events, mostly in those who received the 10-mg/kg dose. Median OS was 9.6 months (95% confidence interval: 6.3–13.4 months).[65]

IDENTIFYING A BIOMARKER
Prognostic Markers

Absolute lymphocyte count (ALC) at 7 weeks ($\geq$1000 cells/μL) and the magnitude increase in ALC with ipilimumab have been demonstrated to correlate with improved OS in patients treated with ipilumumab.[68,69] Baseline absolute eosinophil count and relative eosinophil count have also been associated with improved survival.[70] Moreover, it is hypothesized that quantifying the number, type, and location of tumor-infiltrating lymphocytes (TILs) in a primary tumor can represent an "immunoscore," whereby a higher immunoscore is a good prognostic factor.[71] This hypothesis has been tested in breast cancer, whereby the percentage of lymphocytic infiltrate from 481 triple-negative breast cancer samples from patients enrolled in adjuvant studies E1199 and E2197 demonstrated prognostic value.[72] This concept has been tested in other studies of breast cancer and colorectal cancer, but has yet to be validated for solid tumors such as melanoma.

Predictive Biomarkers

No predictive biomarkers for response to therapy have been confirmed for immune checkpoint inhibitors. In the original phase I trial of nivolumab reported by Topalian and colleagues,[44] 101 patients with pre-treatment biopsies were evaluated for PD-L1 expression by immunohistochemistry (IHC). Patients with tumors expressing PD-L1 had an ORR of 44%, versus 17% in patients with PD-L1–negative tumors.[44] In a phase I study of more than 300 patients with multiple solid tumors who received single-agent MPDL3280A, more than 90 immune-related markers were evaluated in paired tumor samples obtained at baseline and during treatment.[73] Of 140 patients who were evaluated, 11 of 38 patients had metastatic melanoma. Elevated PD-L1 expression by IHC in baseline samples was associated with response to treatment, with PD-L1–positive tumors exhibiting a 36% ORR (n = 3/36), compared with 13% (n = 9/67) in PD-L1 negative tumors. A T-cell gene signature of CD8, EOMES, interferon-γ, and granzyme A was also associated with response to MPDL3280A.[73] On-treatment samples in responders demonstrated increased PD-L1 expression, and a T-helper pathway 1 dominant immune infiltrate of CD8$^+$ T-cells. PD-L1 expression is being prospectively evaluated as a biomarker in a phase III trial comparing nivolumab with chemotherapy in melanoma (NCT01721746).

Immunoprofiling

Ascierto and colleagues[74] propose that characteristics of the TMEs could potentially predict response to immune checkpoint inhibitors. A retrospective study in patients treated with ipilimumab suggests that clinical activity is related to increased expression of immune-related genes such as FoxP3 and indoleamine 2,3-dioxygenase (IDO) at baseline, as well as an increase in TILs between a baseline biopsy and a biopsy obtained at week 4.[75] Myeloid-derived suppressor cells (MDSC) are a different type of immune cell that can be detected in both primary and metastatic lesions. These cells could play a potential role in melanoma progression and the prediction of response to ipilimumab.[76] Immunoprofiling will take into account the expression of surface receptors on immune cells in addition to other immune factors such as cytokines. A 12-chemokine gene expression signature incorporating CCL2, CCL3, CCL4, CCL5, CCL8, CCL18, CCL19, CCL21, CXCL9, CXCL10, CXCL11, and CXCL13 has recently demonstrated an association with improved patient outcomes in both colorectal cancer and melanoma.[77]

NOVEL IMMUNE CHECKPOINTS

Several other immune checkpoint targets are in preclinical and early clinical development. New agents attempt to target other immunomodulatory receptors on T-cells, as well as proteins on the surface of other immune cells. NK cells possess killer Ig-like receptors (KIRs) on their surface, which, when activated by binding to human leukocyte antigen class I molecules on APCs such as tumor cells, deliver an inhibitory signal that prevents NK-cell–mediated cytotoxicity.[78] Blocking this signal with the use of anti-KIR antibodies could thus reinvigorate an antitumor response.

OX40 is a co-stimulatory receptor found on the surface of B-cells and T-cells that potentiates TCR signaling, and can encourage proliferation and survival of these immune cells.[79] Curti and colleagues[80] performed a phase I study in which an mAb that acts as an OX40 agonist was administered to patients with advanced solid tumors, including melanoma. After 1 cycle of therapy with anti-OX40 mAb, patients demonstrated tumor shrinkage of at least 1 metastatic lesion in 12 of 30 subjects.[80]

Glucocorticoid-induced tumor necrosis factor family receptor (GITR) is a co-stimulatory molecule present on T-cells, particularly Tregs and TILs. Blocking of GITR with agonist monoclonal rat antimouse GITR antibody (DTA-1) induced autoimmunity, and demonstrated reinvigoration of an exhausted T-cell response in mouse models.[81] A humanized agonist antihuman GITR mAb (TRX518) that acts in a similar fashion to DTA-1 has been found to enhance co-stimulation in human lymphocytes in vitro. A dose-escalation phase I clinical trial of this agent has been recently initiated (NCT1239134).

CD-137 (4-1BB) is a surface protein present on activated T-cells, with corresponding ligands found on macrophages, activated B-cells, and DCs.[82] Antibodies that are agonists of CD137 and CD137 ligand enhance the co-stimulatory signal on T-cells.[83] Both humanized and chimeric mAbs against CD137 have been produced (urelumab, PF-05082566). Urelumab has demonstrated activity in phase I and II studies; however, severe hepatotoxicity has been reported with this agent.[84,85] Other immune targets in early clinical development include anti–LAG-3, anti–TIM-3, CD69, transforming growth factor β, and interleukin-10.[86]

SUMMARY

Immunotherapy has long been questioned as a viable strategy in the fight against cancer. The therapeutic success and FDA approval of the immune checkpoint inhibitor ipilimumab for the treatment of metastatic malignant melanoma has created a renaissance in immunotherapy for cancer. Not only did this drug demonstrate efficacy and durability in this disease, but it also created a wealth of knowledge in the understanding of the role the immune system plays in cancer, and called into question the methods by which clinicians assess a cancer's response and manage the toxicities observed with novel treatments. Ipilimumab has set a precedent for a new generation of immune checkpoint inhibitors such as nivolumab and MK-3475, and the targeting of immune checkpoint ligands with anti–PD-L1 antibody therapy. Furthermore, the discovery and therapeutic targeting of more novel checkpoint molecules such as KIR and GITR strengthen the argument that these agents are here to stay. Clinical trials have moved on to combining immune checkpoint inhibitors with standard therapies such as radiation, chemotherapy, and targeted therapy, thus supporting a new wave of research in melanoma, and potential continued successes for science, medicine, and patients.

REFERENCES

1. Avogadri F, Yuan J, Yang A, et al. Modulation of CTLA-4 and GITR for cancer immunotherapy. Curr Top Microbiol Immunol 2011;344:211–44.
2. Linsley PS, Ledbetter JA. The role of the CD28 receptor during T cell responses to antigen. Annu Rev Immunol 1993;11:191–212.
3. Nirschl RJ, Drake CG. Coexpression of immune checkpoint molecules: signalling pathways and implications for cancer immunotherapy. Clin Cancer Res 2013;19:4917–24.
4. Van der Merwe PA, Bodian DL, Daenke S, et al. CD80 (B7-1) binds both CD28 and CTLA-4 with a low affinity and very fast kinetics. J Exp Med 1997;185: 393–403.
5. Page DB, Postow MA, Callahan MK, et al. Immune modulation in cancer with antibodies. Annu Rev Med 2014;65:185–202.
6. Leach DR, Krummel MF, Allison JP. Enhancement of antitumor immunity by CTLA-4 blockade. Science 1996;271:1734–6.
7. Haddad H, Rini B. Current treatment considerations in metastatic renal cell carcinoma. Curr Treat Options Oncol 2012;13:212–29.
8. Drake CG, Lipson EJ, Brahmer JR. Breathing new life into immunotherapy: review of melanoma, lung and kidney cancer. Nat Rev Clin Oncol 2014;11: 24–37.
9. Peggs KS, Quezada SA, Chambers CA, et al. Blockade of CTLA-4 on both effector and regulatory T cell compartments contributes to the antitumor activity of anti-CTLA-4 antibodies. J Exp Med 2009;206:1717–25.
10. Tivol EA, Borriello F, Schweitzer AN, et al. Loss of CTLA-4 leads to massive lymphoproliferation and fatal multiorgan tissue destruction, revealing a critical negative regulatory role of CTLA-4. Immunity 1995;3:541–7.
11. Waterhouse P, Penninger JM, Timms E, et al. Lymphoproliferative disorders with early lethality in mice deficient in Ctla-4. Science 1995;270:985–8.
12. Marengere LE, Waterhouse P, Duncan GS, et al. Regulation of T cell receptor signaling by tyrosine phosphatase SYP association with CTLA-4. Science 1996;272:1170–3.
13. Kwon ED, Hurwitz AA, Foster BA, et al. Manipulation of T cell costimulatory and inhibitory signals for immunotherapy of prostate cancer. Proc Natl Acad Sci U S A 1996;94:8099–103.
14. Yang YF, Zou JP, Mu J, et al. Enhanced induction of antitumor T-cell responses by cytotoxic T lymphocyte-associated molecule-4 blockade: the effect is manifested only at the restricted tumor-bearing stages. Cancer Res 1997;57: 4036–41.

15. Tchekmedyian S, Glaspy J, Korman A, et al. MDX-010 (human anti-CTLA4): a phase I trial in malignant melanoma. In: Programs and abstracts of The American Society of Clinical Oncology Annual Meeting. Orlando, Florida, May 18–21, 2002 [abstract: 56].

16. Phan GQ, Yang JC, Sherry RM, et al. Cancer regression and autoimmunity induced by cytotoxic T lymphocyte-associated antigen 4 blockade in patients with metastatic melanoma. Proc Natl Acad Sci U S A 2003;100:8372–7.

17. Wolchok JD, Neyns B, Linette G, et al. Ipilimumab monotherapy in patients with pretreated advanced melanoma: a randomised, double-blind, multicentre, phase 2, dose-ranging study. Lancet Oncol 2010;11:155–64.

18. Hodi FS, O'Day SJ, McDermott DF, et al. Improved survival with ipilimumab in patients with metastatic melanoma. N Engl J Med 2010;363:711–23.

19. Robert C, Thomas L, Bondarenko I, et al. Ipilimumab plus dacarbazine for previously untreated metastatic melanoma. N Engl J Med 2011;364:2517–26.

20. Ribas A, Hanson DC, Noe DA, et al. Review tremelimumab (CP-675,206), a cytotoxic T lymphocyte associated antigen 4 blocking monoclonal antibody in clinical development for patients with cancer. Oncologist 2007;12: 873–83.

21. Ribas A, Camacho LH, Lopez-Berestein G, et al. Antitumor activity in melanoma and anti-self responses in a phase I trial with the anti-cytotoxic T lymphocyte-associated antigen 4 monoclonal antibody CP-675,206. J Clin Oncol 2005;25: 8968–77.

22. Kirkwood JM, Lorigan P, Hersey P, et al. Phase II trial of tremelimumab (CP-675,206) in patients with advanced refractory or relapsed melanoma. Clin Cancer Res 2010;16:1042–8.

23. Ribas A, Kefford R, Marshall MA, et al. Phase III randomized clinical trial comparing tremelimumab with standard-of-care chemotherapy in patients with advanced melanoma. J Clin Oncol 2013;31:616–22.

24. Fecher LA, Agarwala SS, Hodi FS, et al. Ipilimumab and its toxicities: a multidisciplinary approach. Oncologist 2013;18:733–43.

25. O'Day SJ, Maio M, Chiarion-Sileni V, et al. Efficacy and safety of ipilimumab monotherapy in patients with pretreated advanced melanoma: a multicenter single-arm phase II study. Ann Oncol 2010;21:1712–7.

26. Weber JS, Dummer R, de Pril V, et al. Patterns of onset and resolution of immune-related adverse events of special interest with ipilimumab: detailed safety analysis from a phase 3 trial in patients with advanced melanoma. Cancer 2013;119:1675–82.

27. O'Day S, Weber JS, Wolchok JD, et al. Effectiveness of treatment guidance on diarrhea and colitis across ipilimumab studies. Presented at the American Society of Clinical Oncology Annual Meeting, Chicago, June 3–7, 2012.

28. Pages C, Gornet JM, Monsel G, et al. Ipilimumab-induced acute severe colitis treated by infliximab. Melanoma Res 2013;23:227–30.

29. Downey SG, Klapper JA, Smith FO, et al. Prognostic factors related to clinical response in patients with metastatic melanoma treated by CTL-associated antigen-4 blockade. Clin Cancer Res 2007;13:6681–8.

30. Tarhini AA, Cherian J, Moschos SJ, et al. Safety and efficacy of combination immunotherapy with interferon alfa-2b and tremelimumab in patients with stage IV melanoma. J Clin Oncol 2012;30:322–8.

31. Wolchok JD, Weber JS, Maio M, et al. Four-year survival rates for patients with metastatic melanoma who received ipilimumab in phase II clinical trials. Ann Oncol 2013;24:2174–80.

32. Wolchok JD, Hoos A, O'Day S, et al. Guidelines for the evaluation of immune therapy activity in solid tumors: immune-related response criteria. Clin Cancer Res 2009;15:7412–20.

33. Keir ME, Butte MJ, Freeman GJ, et al. PD-1 and its ligands in tolerance and immunity. Annu Rev Immunol 2008;26:677–704.

34. Butte MJ, Keir ME, Phamduy TB, et al. Programmed death-1 ligand 1 interacts specifically with the B7-1 costimulatory molecule to inhibit T cell responses. Immunity 2007;27:111–22.

35. Ishida Y, Agata Y, Shibahara K, et al. Induced expression of PD-1, a novel member of the immunoglobulin gene superfamily, upon programmed cell death. EMBO J 1992;11:3887–95.

36. Okazaki T, Maeda A, Nishimura H, et al. PD-1 immunoreceptor inhibits B cell receptor-mediated signaling by recruiting src homology 2-domain containing tyrosine phosphatase 2 to phosphotyrosine. Proc Natl Acad Sci U S A 2001; 98:13866–71.

37. Chemnitz JM, Parry RV, Nichols KE, et al. SHP-1 and SHP-2 associate with immunoreceptor tyrosine-based switch motif of programmed death 1 upon primary human T cell stimulation, but only receptor ligation prevents T cell activation. J Immunol 2004;173:945–54.

38. Sheppard KA, Fitz LJ, Lee JM, et al. PD-1 inhibits T-cell receptor induced phosphorylation of the ZAP70/CD3zeta signalosome and downstream signaling to PKC theta. FEBS Lett 2004;574:37–41.

39. Parry RV, Chemnitz JM, Frauwirth KA, et al. CTLA-4 and PD-1 receptors inhibit T-cell activation by distinct mechanisms. Mol Cell Biol 2005;25:9543–53.

40. Nishimura H, Minato N, Nakano T, et al. Immunological studies on PD-1 deficient mice: implication of PD-1 as a negative regulator for B cell responses. Int Immunol 1998;10:1563–72.

41. Nishimura H, Okazaki T, Tanaka Y, et al. Autoimmune dilated cardiomyopathy in PD-1 receptor-deficient mice. Science 2001;291:319–22.

42. Sosman J, Sznol M, McDermott D, et al. Clinical activity and safety of anti-programmed death-1 (PD-1) (BMS-936558/MDX-1106/ONO-4538) in patients with advanced melanoma. Ann Oncol 2012;23(Suppl) [abstract: 11090].

43. Sznol M, Kluger HM, Hodi FS, et al. Survival and long-term follow-up of safety and response in patients with advanced melanoma in a phase I trial of nivolumab (anti-PD-1; BMS-936558; ONO-4538). In: Programs and abstracts of the Annual Meeting of The American Society of Clinical Oncology. Chicago, Illinois, May 31-June 4, 2013 [abstract: CRA9006].

44. Topalian SL, Hodi FS, Brahmer JR, et al. Safety, activity, and immune correlates of anti-PD-1 antibody in cancer. N Engl J Med 2012;366:2443–54.

45. Lipson EJ, Sharfman WH, Drake CG, et al. Durable cancer regression off-treatment and effective reinduction therapy with an anti-PD-1 antibody. Clin Cancer Res 2013;19:462–8.

46. Patnaik A, Kang SP, Tolcher AW, et al. Phase I study of MK-3475 (anti-PD-1 monoclonal antibody) in patients with advanced solid tumors. J Clin Oncol 2012;30(Suppl):2512.

47. Hamid O, Robert C, Daud A, et al. Safety and tumor responses with lambrolizumab (Anti-PD-1) in melanoma. N Engl J Med 2013;369:134–44.

48. Freeman GJ, Long AJ, Iwai Y, et al. Engagement of the PD-1 immunoinhibitory receptor by a novel B7 family member leads to negative regulation of lymphocyte activation. J Exp Med 2000;192:1027–34.

49. Ishida M, Iwai Y, Tanaka Y, et al. Differential expression of PD-L1 and PD-L2, ligands for an inhibitory receptor PD-1, in the cells of lymphohematopoietic tissues. Immunol Lett 2002;84:57–62.

50. Strome SE, Dong H, Tamura H, et al. B7-H1 blockade augments adoptive T-cell immunotherapy for squamous cell carcinoma. Cancer Res 2003;63:6501–5.

51. Inman BA, Sebo TJ, Frigola X, et al. PD-L1 (B7-H1) expression by urothelial carcinoma of the bladder and BCG-induced granulomata: associations with localized stage progression. Cancer 2007;109:1499–505.

52. Nomi T, Sho M, Akahori T, et al. Clinical significance and therapeutic potential of the programmed death-1 ligand/programmed death-1 pathway in human pancreatic cancer. Clin Cancer Res 2007;13:2151–7.

53. Wu C, Zhu Y, Jiang J, et al. Immunohistochemical localization of programmed death-1 ligand-1 (PD-L1) in gastric carcinoma and its clinical significance. Acta Histochem 2006;108:19–24.

54. Parsa AT, Waldron JS, Panner A, et al. Loss of tumor suppressor PTEN function increases B7-H1 expression and immunoresistance in glioma. Nat Med 2007; 13:84–8.

55. Hamanishi J, Mandai M, Iwasaki M, et al. Programmed cell death 1 ligand 1 and tumor-infiltrating CD8_ T lymphocytes are prognostic factors of human ovarian cancer. Proc Natl Acad Sci U S A 2007;104:3360–5.

56. Hamid O, Sosman JA, Lawrence DP, et al. Clinical activity, safety, and biomarkers with MPDL32801A, an engineered anti-PDL1 antibody in patients with locally advanced or metastatic malignant melanoma. J Clin Oncol 2013; 31(Suppl) [abstract: 9010].

57. Stewart RA, Morrow M, Chordoge M. MEDI4736: delivering effective blockade of immunosuppression to enhance tumour rejection: monoclonal antibody discovery and preclinical development. Cancer Res 2011;71(Suppl 1) [abstract: LB-158].

58. Herbst RS, Gordon MS, Fine GD, et al. A study of MPDL3280A, an engineered PD-L1 antibody in patients with locally advanced or metastatic tumors. In: Programs and abstracts of the Annual Meeting of The American Society of Clinical Oncology. Chicago, Illinois, May 31-June 4, 2013 [abstract: 3000].

59. Patel SG, Prasad ML, Escrig M, et al. Primary mucosal malignant melanoma of the head and neck. Head Neck 2002;24:247–57.

60. Postow MA, Luke JJ, Bluth MJ, et al. Ipilimumab for patients with advanced mucosal melanoma. Oncologist 2013;18:726–32.

61. Bartell HL, Bedikian AY, Papadopoulos NE, et al. Biochemotherapy in patients with advanced head and neck mucosal melanoma. Head Neck 2008;30:1592–8.

62. Harting MS, Kim KB. Biochemotherapy in patients with advanced vulvovaginal mucosal melanoma. Melanoma Res 2004;14:517–20.

63. Kim KB, Sanguino AM, Hodges C, et al. Biochemotherapy in patients with metastatic anorectal mucosal melanoma. Cancer 2004;100:1478–83.

64. Singh AD, Topham A. Incidence of uveal melanoma in the United States: 1973-1997. Ophthalmology 2003;110:956–61.

65. Luke JJ, Callahan MK, Postow MA, et al. Clinical activity of ipilimumab for metastatic uveal melanoma: a retrospective review of the Dana-Farber Cancer Institute, Massachusetts General Hospital, Memorial Sloan-Kettering Cancer Center, and University Hospital of Lausanne experience. Cancer 2013;119:3687–95.

66. de Vries TJ, Trancikova D, Ruiter DJ, et al. High expression of immunotherapy candidate proteins gp100, MART-1, tyrosinase and TRP-1 in uveal melanoma. Br J Cancer 1998;78:1156–61.

67. Luyten GP, van der Spek CW, Brand I, et al. Expression of MAGE, gp100 and tyrosinase genes in uveal melanoma cell lines. Melanoma Res 1998;8:11–6.
68. Ku GY, Yuan J, Page DB, et al. Single-institution experience with ipilimumab in advanced melanoma patients in the compassionate use setting: lymphocyte count after 2 doses correlates with survival. Cancer 2010;116: 1767–75.
69. Postow MA, Chasalow SD, Yuan J, et al. Evaluation of the absolute lymphocyte count as a biomarker for melanoma patients treated with the commercially available dose of ipilimumab (3 mg/kg). In: Programs and abstracts of the Annual Meeting of the American Society of Clinical Oncology. Chicago, Illinois, June 1–5, 2012 [abstract: 8575].
70. Schindler K, Harmankaya K, Postow MA, et al. Pretreatment levels of absolute and relative eosinophil count to improve overall survival (OS) in patients with metastatic melanoma under treatment with ipilimumab, an anti-CTLA-4 antibody. In: Programs and abstracts of the Annual Meeting of the American Society of Clinical Oncology. Chicago, Illinois, May 31-June 4, 2013 [abstract: 9024].
71. Galon J, Pagès F, Marincola FM, et al. The immune score as a new possible approach for the classification of cancer. J Transl Med 2012;10:1.
72. Adams S, Gray R, Demaria S, et al. Towards and immunoscore for triple negative breast cancer (TNBC): lymphocytic infiltrate predicts outcome. In: Programs and abstracts of the 28th Society for Immunotherapy in Cancer Annual Meeting. National Harbor, Maryland, November 8–10, 2013. p. 55 [oral abstract].
73. Kohrt H, Kowanetz M, Gettinger S, et al. Intratumoral characteristics of tumor and immune cells at baseline and on-treatment correlated with clinical responses to MPDL3280A, an engineered antibody against PD-L1. In: Programs and abstracts of the 28th Society for Immunotherapy in Cancer Annual Meeting. National Harbor, Maryland, November 8–10, 2013. p. 53. [oral abstract].
74. Ascierto PA, Capone M, Urba WJ, et al. The additional facet of immunoscore: immunoprofiling as a possible predictive tool for cancer treatment. J Transl Med 2013;11:54.
75. Hamid O, Schmidt H, Nissan A, et al. A prospective phase II trial exploring the association between tumor microenvironment biomarkers and clinical activity of ipilimumab in advanced melanoma. J Transl Med 2011;9:204.
76. Ascierto PA, Kalos M, Schaer DA, et al. Biomarkers for immunostimulatory monoclonal antibodies in combination strategies for melanoma and other tumor types. Clin Cancer Res 2013;19:1009–20.
77. Messina JL, Fenstermacher DA, Eschrich S, et al. 12-Chemokine gene signature identifies lymph node-like structures in melanoma: potential for patient selection for immunotherapy? Sci Rep 2012;2:765.
78. Parham P. MHC class I molecules and KIRs in human history, health and survival. Nat Rev Immunol 2005;5:201–14.
79. Mallett S, Fossum S, Barclay AN. Characterization of the MRC OX40 antigen of activated CD4 positive T lymphocytes—a molecule related to nerve growth factor receptor. Embo J 1990;9:1063–8.
80. Curti BD, Kovacsovics-Bankowski M, Morris N, et al. OX40 is a potent immune-stimulating target in late-stage cancer patients. Cancer Res 2013;73: 7189–98.
81. Cohen AD, Schaer DA, Liu C, et al. Agonist anti-GITR monoclonal antibody induces melanoma tumor immunity in mice by altering regulatory T cell stability and intra-tumor accumulation. PLoS One 2010;5:10436.

82. Lin W, Voskens CJ, Zhang X, et al. Fc dependent expression of CD137 on human NK cells: insights into "agonistic" effects of anti-CD137 monoclonal antibodies. Blood 2008;112:699–707.

83. Kroon HM, Li Q, Teitz-Tennenbaum S, et al. 4-1BB costimulation of effector T cells for adoptive immunotherapy of cancer: involvement of Bcl gene family members. J Immunother 2007;30:406–16.

84. Sznol M, Hodi FS, Margolin K, et al. Phase I study of BMS-663513, a fully human anti-CD137 agonist monoclonal antibody, in patients with advanced cancer. J Clin Oncol 2008;26(Suppl) [abstract: 3007].

85. Ascierto PA, Simeone E, Sznol M, et al. Clinical experiences with anti-CD137 and anti-PD1 therapeutic antibodies. Semin Oncol 2010;37:508–16.

86. Melero I, Grimaldi AM, Perez-Gracia JL, et al. Clinical development of immunostimulatory monoclonal antibodies and opportunities for combination. Clin Cancer Res 2013;19:997–1008.

Combinatorial Approach to Treatment of Melanoma

Michelle T. Ashworth, MD[a], Adil I. Daud, MD[b],*

KEYWORDS

- Melanoma • BRAF • Mitogen-activated extracellular kinase • Immunotherapy
- Combination therapy • Targeted therapy

KEY POINTS

- In the unprecedented circumstance of multiple effective and well-tolerated treatments approved by the US Food and Drug Administration for patients with advanced melanoma, the next logical step is exploration of combination therapy.
- Cytotoxic therapies, including targeted therapies, increase antigen presentation and in many cases create a favorable environment for the action of immune therapy.
- Response to the combination of targeted therapy and immunotherapy may vary by tumor genotype (eg, concurrent PTEN loss).
- Exploration of combination therapy should be explored in a clinical trial setting because of possible unanticipated adverse effects, and to maximize scientific understanding through correlative studies.

INTRODUCTION

The past several years have seen a rapid increase in effective and tolerable treatment options for patients with advanced melanoma across the major modalities in systemic therapy: options have progressed from cytotoxic chemotherapy to targeted therapy to dramatic improvements in immunotherapy. Despite multiple clinical trials of various combination regimens, cytotoxic chemotherapy has not proved effective in increasing overall survival but can lead to an objective response in a fraction of patients. In the past, trials of biochemotherapy (cytokine therapy plus chemotherapy) regimens in advanced melanoma have not shown improved overall survival compared with chemotherapy.[1,2] Targeted therapy has an excellent response rate in BRAF V600[E/K]-mutant

Funding Sources: University of California, San Francisco (M.T. Ashworth); nil (A.I. Daud).
Conflict of Interest: Nil.
[a] Hematology/Oncology, University of California, San Francisco, 505 Parnassus Avenue, M1286 MS1270, San Francisco, CA 94143, USA; [b] Melanoma Clinical Research, UCSF Helen Diller Family Comprehensive Cancer Center, 1600 Divisadero Street, San Francisco, CA 94115, USA
* Corresponding author. Department of Cutaneous Oncology, University of California, San Francisco, 1600 Divisadero Street, Box 1770, San Francisco, CA 94115.
E-mail address: adaud@medicine.ucsf.edu

Hematol Oncol Clin N Am 28 (2014) 601–612
http://dx.doi.org/10.1016/j.hoc.2014.03.002
0889-8588/14/$ – see front matter © 2014 Elsevier Inc. All rights reserved.

advanced melanoma: up to 76% when given as combination BRAF plus mitogen-activated extracellular kinase inhibition, but the duration of response is limited, with the longest median time to progression so far reported being 9.4 months.[3] Immunotherapy with new anti-PD1 antibodies has shown a response rate greater than or equal to 30%, with even higher response rates when given in combination[4] with anti-CTLA4 antibody ipilimumab (Yervoy), and responses have been durable in most patients. A next step in achieving both a higher overall response rate and a prolonged duration of response for patients with advanced melanoma is exploration of combination systemic therapy regimens across treatment types: chemotherapy, targeted therapy, and immunotherapy.

COMBINATION IMMUNOTHERAPY PLUS CHEMOTHERAPY
Rationale

Cytotoxic chemotherapy can act in 2 complementary ways: direct damage and death of cancer cells, and the attraction and activation of cytotoxic immune cells. Cell death triggered by treatment with chemotherapy has been shown to be immunogenic and to lead to dendritic cell activation and subsequent activation of tumor antigen–specific T cells.[5–7] After administration of dacarbazine (DTIC), activation of genes involved in cytokine production, leukocyte activation, immune response, and cell motility have been observed, changes thought to create a favorable environment for tumor antigen–specific CD8+ T-cell responses.[8] In another study, a low dose of melphalan (Alkeran) was shown to induce tumor expression of chemokines that lead to enhanced recruitment of tumor-reactive T cells[9] and improved response to anti-CTLA4 therapy.[10] In addition, in examination of pretreatment biopsy specimens, a tumor microenvironment with infiltrate featuring CD8+ T cells has been associated with an improved response rate to chemotherapy.[11]

Clinical Trials

Phase II to III trials have shown early evidence of tolerability and efficacy with the combination of ipilimumab with cytotoxic drugs such as alkylating agents dacarbazine and temozolomide, which is also active in the central nervous system, or fotemustine, a drug that is available in Europe (**Table 1**).

Table 1
Ipilimumab plus cytotoxic chemotherapy

Regimen	Phase	N	ORR (%)	PFS	OS (%)
Ipilimumab plus dacarbazine vs ipilimumab[12]	II	35 vs 37	14.3 vs 5.4	No difference	14.3 mo vs 11.4 mo; 1-y OS, 62 vs 45; 2-y OS, 24 vs 21; 3-y OS, 20 vs 9
Ipilimumab plus dacarbazine vs dacarbazine[13]	III	196 vs 218	38 vs 26; 4 CR, 34 PR, and 45 SD vs 2 CR, 24 PR, 50 SD	No difference	1-y OS, 47.3 vs 36.3; 2-y OS, 28.5 vs 17.9; 3-y OS, 20.8 vs 12.2
Ipilimumab plus temozolomide[14,15]	II	64	28.1; 10 CR, 8 PR	5.1 mo	NR
Ipilimumab plus fotemustine[16,17]	II	86	irORR 29.1; 5 CR, 20 PR	irPFS, 5.3 mo	1-y OS, 51.8

Abbreviations: CR, complete response; irPFS, immune-related progression-free survival; N, number of treated patients; NR, not reported; ORR, overall response rate; OS, median overall survival; PFS, median progression-free survival; PR, partial response; irORR, immune-related overall response rate.

COMBINATION IMMUNOTHERAPY PLUS TARGETED THERAPY
Rationale

The combination of targeted therapy and immunotherapy seems to be symmetric: high response rate and rapid onset of action in targeted therapy, with hope of long-term response to slower-acting immunotherapy. There is no evidence that patients with BRAF[V600E] mutations are less likely to respond to immunotherapy.[18] Vemurafenib (Zelboraf) and the biochemically similar compound PLX4720 have been shown to have a cytotoxic effect in melanoma,[19] and as previously discussed with chemotherapy, drugs with cytotoxic effect can enhance immune activity. BRAF inhibition has been shown to enhance T-cell recognition of melanoma cells and not interfere with lymphocyte functioning.[20] Review of tumor biopsies from patients treated with BRAF inhibitors vemurafenib or dabrafenib (Tafinlar) showed enhanced melanoma antigen expression and a more favorable tumor microenvironment in patients with metastatic melanoma.[21,22] Response to ipilimumab is linked to an immune-active tumor microenvironment.[23]

Preclinical testing of combination immunotherapy plus targeted therapy has been done in the context of an anti-CTLA4 monoclonal antibody plus PLX4720 (vemurafenib precursor) in an immune-competent mouse model of BRAF[V600E]/PTEN$^{-/-}$ mutant melanoma. In contrast with the observed cytotoxicity of BRAF inhibitors reported in human patients with melanoma,[19] treatment in this mouse model does not cause cell death but leads to decreased tumor proliferation.[24] Decreased tumor-resident lymphocyte frequencies were observed after treatment with PLX4720 (decreased CD45+ leukocytes, CD8+ T cells, CD4+ T cells, T_{regs}; no change in B-lymphocytes; slightly increased natural killer cells, myeloid-derived suppressor cells, macrophages), along with decrease in visible inflammation at tumor sites. These changes in T-lymphocyte frequencies were not found elsewhere in the mouse tissues (lymph nodes or spleen) or in similarly treated mice with BRAF-WT tumors, arguing against a direct effect of PLX4720 on the T cells. No synergy was observed in the combination of PLX4720 and anti-CTLA4 monoclonal antibody (mAb) in this study. Concurrent treatment with PLX4720 and the anti-CTLA4 mAb did not restore the intratumoral immune milieu. In a group of human patients with BRAF[V600E] mutations treated with dabrafenib, those with concurrent PTEN loss had decreased median progression-free survival.[25,26] One interpretation of this may be that, in patients with PTEN loss, a tendency for BRAF inhibitors to have a more cytostatic than cytotoxic effect may lead to decreased efficacy, and there may also be a deleterious effect on the immune tumor microenvironment that decreases the likelihood of response to anti-CTLA therapy. It should also be noted that PLX4720 has a less dramatic effect in mouse models than vemurafenib does in human melanoma. This observation needs further examination in clinical trials of the combination of BRAF inhibitors and the anti-PD1 antibodies, with studies of the correlation between observed clinical responses, tumor genetics, and lymphocyte profiling.

Ipilimumab Plus Vemurafenib

A recent phase I study of concurrent vemurafenib plus ipilimumab showed dose-limiting toxicity of grade III to IV hepatotoxicity in 50% of patients and asymptomatic liver function tests increases that were reversible with dose interruption or administration of corticosteroids,[27] and the study was closed to further accrual. Efficacy outcomes were not reported. The investigators recommend well-designed clinical trials to examine future combinations even of approved therapies with nonoverlapping toxicities and separate mechanisms of action.

SEQUENTIAL THERAPY
Rationale

In clinical oncology, combination regimens are often developed to maximize response, but these can be limited by overlapping toxicities, and patients often proceed from one regimen sequentially to another at the time of progression of disease or end of tolerability. As targeted therapies, anti-CTLA4 antibodies, and anti-PD1/PDL1 antibody drugs, have all been under development during recent years, and patients have been treated sequentially, going from one clinical trial to another.

As monotherapy (eg, choosing between available open clinical trials) has often been the only option at a given point in a patient's care, targeted therapy may be the first option chosen for its high response rate and rapid onset of action; for example, in a patient presenting with widely metastatic disease or bulky symptomatic disease causing pain or threatening organ function, whereas immune therapy may be chosen in advance for patients with a low burden of disease who are able to tolerate a delayed onset of action and trade a lower response rate for the opportunity for a long-term response.

Experience and Next Directions

An dichotomy of response has been revealed in patients at the time of discontinuation of BRAF inhibitor therapy. A retrospective review of 28 patients first treated with a BRAF inhibitor (vemurafenib or dabrafenib) followed by ipilimumab reported that 43% of the patients experienced rapid progression of disease when the BRAF inhibitor was discontinued, and this prevented successful completion of planned treatment with ipilimumab.[28,29] However, in another series of patients, a proportion were observed to have tumor shrinkage at the time of discontinuation of BRAF inhibitor.[30] The response to BRAF inhibitors can be rescued in some patients with reinitiation of treatment after an interruption.[31] This finding has led to exploration of intermittent dosing of BRAF inhibitors in an effort to delay or overcome resistance.[32] A strategy of continuous targeted therapy followed by abrupt discontinuation of treatment at time of progression and then initiation of immunotherapy is unlikely to be successful in many patients, and combination strategies (with or without intermittent dosing of BRAF inhibitor) are more likely to yield long-lasting benefits.

Sequential Therapy Versus Combination Therapy

As multiple agents are approved by the US Food and Drug Administration, and combination therapies are explored in ongoing clinical trials, there will be keen interest in the outcomes of efficacy and tolerability/toxicity. There will also be practical questions of cost, because each individual agent will be patent protected for the near future. Overall, a combination that provides a rapid, deep, and prolonged response will likely prove cost-effective because patients achieve many more high-quality years of life after a complete response to a well-tolerated therapy, and they avoid the many medical comorbidities caused by progression of disease. Discontinuation trials after complete responses to immunotherapy will also contribute important information for the design of optimal and cost-effective combination regimens.

RECENT TRIALS OF OTHER COMBINATIONS ACROSS MODALITIES OR PATHWAYS
Rationale

Given the complexity of cell signaling and the multitude of genetic errors characteristic of advanced melanoma tumors, trials are ongoing with various combinations of agents designed to affect multiple targets of growth signaling, combine cytotoxicity with immunotherapy, or otherwise take advantage of synergy between agents with different mechanisms (**Table 2**).

Clinical Trials

Table 2
Other combination trials, 2012 to present

Regimen	Phase	N	ORR	PFS	OS
Preclinical studies revealed that the proteasome inhibitor bortezomib plus cytokine IFN-α synergistically induce apoptosis in human melanoma cells, and combined treatment in a murine model led to improved survival. A phase I study showed[33]:					
IFN α-2B plus bortezomib	I	16	1 PR, 7 SD, 8 PD	2.5 mo	10.3 mo
Preclinical studies showed that bortezomib and sorafenib, a multikinase inhibitor that blocks tumor growth and angiogenesis, modulate expression of BCL-family members and augment cytotoxicity in cell lines. A phase I study showed[34]:					
Bortezomib plus sorafenib	I	11	2 SD, 9 PD	NR	NR
The MET receptor tyrosine kinase is activated in NRAS-mutant melanoma. Oral MET inhibitor tivantinib was studied in combination with sorafenib. Preclinical data indicated synergy between these two agents. A phase I study[35] performed in patients with NRAS-mutant or NRAS-WT melanoma showed:					
Sorafenib plus tivantinib	I	11	1 CR, 3 PR, 3 SD	5.3 mo	NR
NRAS-mutant patients only:		8	1 CR, 1 PR, 2 SD	9.2 mo	NR
A double-blind, randomized, placebo-controlled phase III study showed no improvement in OS with the addition of sorafenib to cytotoxic chemotherapy with carboplatin plus paclitaxel[36]					
Sorafenib plus carboplatin plus paclitaxel vs carboplatin plus paclitaxel	III	823	20 vs 18%, $P = .427$	4.9 vs 4.2 mo	11.3 vs 11.1 mo
A phase II trial in patients with metastatic uveal melanoma was closed early for lack of response[37]					
Sorafenib plus carboplatin plus paclitaxel	II	24	0	4 mo; 6 mo PFS 29%	11 mo
Multikinase inhibitor sorafenib was the foundation of 2 compared regimens: sorafenib plus mTOR inhibitor temsirolimus vs sorafenib plus tipifarnib, an oral farnesyl transferase inhibitor in a randomized phase II trial.[38] Neither combination showed sufficient activity to merit further use					
Sorafenib plus temsirolimus vs sorafenib plus tipifarnib	II	63 vs 39	3 PR vs 1 PR	2.1 vs 1.8 mo	7 vs 7 mo
In preclinical models, bevacizumab, an mAb to VEGF inhibiting angiogenesis and tissue growth, suppressed growth and hepatic establishment of micrometastases, and a potential clinical benefit of the combination of bevacizumab plus alkylating agent dacarbazine. A phase II trial (BEVATEM) showed[39,40]:					
Bevacizumab plus temozolomide	II	35	9/35 SD	3 mo; 6-mo PFS 26%	12 mo

(continued on next page)

Table 2
(continued)

Regimen	Phase	N	ORR	PFS	OS
Temsirolimus is a targeted inhibitor of mTOR kinase activity, blocking progression of the cell cycle past G1 phase. A phase II trial of the combination of temsirolimus and bevacizumab showed[41]:					
Bevacizumab plus temsirolimus	II	16	3 PR in BRAF-WT patients, 9 SD; 1 response duration >3 y	NR	NR
A phase II trial evaluated bevacizumab in combination with oral alkylating agent temozolomide[42]					
Bevacizumab plus temozolomide	II	62	1 CR, 9 PR (16.1%)	4.2 mo	9.6 mo; BRAF-WT 12 mo, BRAF^{V600E} 9.2 mo, $P = .014$
A phase II trial compared bevacizumab as the foundation of 2 regimens: BT vs ABC[43]					
BT vs ABC	II	42 vs 51	1 CR, 9 PR (23.8%) vs 0 CR, 17 PR (33.3%)	3.8 vs 6.7 mo; 6 mo PFS 32.8 vs 56.1%	12.3 mo vs 13.9 mo
Another randomized phase II study evaluated CBP vs CP alone[44]					
CBP vs CP	II	143 vs 71	25.5% vs 16.4%, $P = .1577$	5.6 vs 4.2 mo, $P = .1414$	12.3 vs 8.6 mo, $P = .0366$
Hypomethylating agent decitabine was evaluated in combination with temozolomide, an oral alkylating agent, in a phase I/II trial[45]					
Decitabine plus temozolomide	I/II	35	2 CR, 4 PR, 14 SD	3.4 mo; 6-mo PFS 32%	12.4 mo; 1-y OS 56%
ALT-801 is recombinant human interleukin-2 fused to a single-chain T-cell receptor specific to human p53 peptide antigen presented in the setting of HLA-A2 positivity. This fusion protein showed activity as monotherapy and synergy with cisplatin in melanoma xenograft mouse models. This phase Ib study showed[46]:					
Cisplatin plus ALT-801	Ib	22	NR	NR	6-mo PFS 87%; 12-mo PFS 58%
Angiogenesis inhibitor rh-endostatin in combination with dacarbazine was compared with dacarbazine monotherapy in this randomized, placebo-controlled phase II Chinese trial[47] that showed:					
Dacarbazine plus rh-endostatin vs dacarbazine alone	II	110	NR	5 vs 1.5 mo	16 vs 7 mo; 1-y OS 51 vs 22%
Lenvatinib is an oral, receptor TKI targeting VEGFR1–VEGFR3, FGFR1–FGFR 4, RET, KIT, and PDGFRβ. DTIC upregulates VEGF and has been shown to confer resistance in cell lines. A phase II study was performed to investigate whether combinations of antiangiogenic drugs could potentiate DTIC[48]					
Lenvatinib plus DTIC vs DTIC	II	78	NR	19.1 wk vs 7 wk	NR

(continued on next page)

Table 2
(continued)

Regimen	Phase	N	ORR	PFS	OS
Lenvatinib was given at 24 mg PO daily plus temozolomide 150 mg/m^2 PO on days 1–5 of 28 in this phase Ib trial.[9]					
Lenvatinib plus temozolomide	Ib	32	6 PR	5.4 mo; 6-mo PFS 37%	NR
Plitipepsin is a synthetic form of a peptide isolated from *Aplidium albicans* that triggers apoptosis and blocks VEGF secretion in tumor models. A phase I/II trial of dacarbazine plus plitidepsin vs plitidepsin alone showed[49]:					
Dacarbazine plus plitidepsin vs plitidepsin	I/II	28 vs 16	1 CR, 5 PR, 9 SD vs 0 CR, 0 PR, 2 SD	3.3 vs 1.5 mo	NR
Histone deacetylase inhibitor panobinostat and demethylating agent decitabine were given in combination with temozolomide to overcome development of epigenetically mediated temozolomide resistance in this phase I/II trial.[50] The MTD of this combination has not yet been reached					
Decitabine plus panobinostat plus temozolomide	I/II	17	NR	NR	NR
ERK1/2 is constitutively active in melanoma cells regardless of BRAF mutation status; selumetinib is a highly selective allosteric inhibitor of MEK1/2, suppressing pERK levels in melanoma independently of BRAF and NRAS mutation status. Selumetinib and docetaxel have shown synergy in xenograft models of melanoma. A randomized phase II trial (DOC-MEK)[51] showed:					
Selumetinib plus docetaxel vs docetaxel	II	83	32% vs 14%	6-mo PFS 40% vs 26%	NR
Selumetinib was also tested in combination with cytotoxic alkylating agent dacarbazine vs dacarbazine alone in a phase II double-blind randomized study[52]					
Selumetinib plus dacarbazine vs dacarbazine	II	45 vs 46	1 CR, 17 PR, 13 SD vs 1 CR, 11 PR, 10 SD	5.6 vs 3 mo, $P = .021$	13.9 mo vs 10.5 mo, $P = .39$
YM155 is an inhibitor of survivin, a microtubule-associated protein overexpressed in melanoma and associated with cell viability and regulation of mitosis. An open-label phase II study[53] of YM155 in combination with microtubule-stabilizing chemotherapy agent docetaxel showed:					
Docetaxel plus YM155	II	64	8 PR (12.5%), 33 SD (51.6%)	6-mo PFS 34.8%	1-y OS 50.5%
Everolimus is an oral inhibitor of mTOR, a component of the PI3k/AKT pathway, and has single-agent activity in advanced melanoma. A phase II trial tested everolimus in combination with chemotherapy with DNA cross-linking agent carboplatin and microtubule-stabilizing agent paclitaxel.[54] Because this was not a marked improvement compared with previously published data with carboplatin plus paclitaxel alone, further development was not recommended					
Everolimus plus carboplatin plus paclitaxel	II	70	12 PR, 42 SD	4 mo	10 mo

(continued on next page)

Table 2
(continued)

Regimen	Phase	N	ORR	PFS	OS
Pazopanib is an antiangiogenic inhibitor of VEGFR1, VEGFR2, VEGFR3, PDGFR-β, and c-KIT with activity in melanoma tumor xenografts. A phase II study of pazopanib given in combination with paclitaxel showed[55,56]:					
Pazopanib plus paclitaxel	II	31	32%: 1 CR, 9 PR, 13 SD, 8 PD	NR	NR
PARP inhibitor rucaparib was examined in combination with oral alkylating agent temozolomide in a phase II trial that showed[57]:					
Rucaparib plus temozolomide	II	46	8 PR 17.4%, 8 SD	3.5 mo; 6-mo PFS 36%	9.9 mo
Preclinical data indicated that Src inhibitors sensitize cells to the effects of cytotoxic chemotherapy. Src and c-Kit inhibitor dasatinib was combined with dacarbazine in a phase I trial[58]					
Dasatinib (70 mg PO BID cohort) plus dacarbazine	I	29	4 PR, 17 SD	6-mo PFS 20.7%	12-mo OS 34.5%

Abbreviations: ABC, nab-paclitaxel plus bevacizumab plus carboplatin; BCL, B-cell CLL/lymphoma; BID, twice a day; BT, bevacizumab plus temozolomide; CBP, carboplatin plus bevacizumab plus paclitaxel; CP, carboplatin plus paclitaxel; CR, complete response; ERK1/2, mitogen-activated protein kinase 1/2; FGFR1–4, fibroblast growth factor receptors 1–4; HLA-A2, human leukocyte antigen A2; IFN-α, interferon-alfa; KIT, v-kit Hardy-Zuckerman 4 feline sarcoma viral oncogene homolog; mAb, monoclonal antibody; MET, met proto-oncogene; MTD, maximum tolerated dose; mTOR, mammalian target of rapamycin; N, number; NR, not reported; NRAS, neuroblastoma RAS viral oncogene homolog; ORR, overall response rate; OS, overall survival; PARP, poly ADP ribose polymerase; p53, tumor protein p53; PD, progressive disease; PDGFR-β, platelet-derived growth factor receptor beta polypeptide; pERK, phospho-ERK (phosphorylated ERK); PFS, progression-free survival; PI3k/AKT, phosphatidylinositol-4,5-bisphosphate 3-kinase/v-akt murine thymoma viral oncogene homolog 1; PO, by mouth; PR, partial response; RET, RET proto-oncogene; SD, stable disease; TKI, tyrosine kinase inhibitor; VEGF, vascular endothelial growth factor; VEGFR1–3, vascular endothelial growth factor receptors 1–3; WT, wild-type.

SUMMARY

The current aim of therapy in the treatment of advanced melanoma has shifted from temporary response in a small minority of patients to meaningful durable complete or partial responses in a significant proportion of patients. Although interest in targeted kinase inhibitors continues, these drugs do not lead to durable remissions except in a small number of patients. Immunotherapy has also experienced rapid advances recently but there are still many patients who do not respond. Combination therapy may deliver this goal better than cytotoxic, targeted, or immunotherapy alone.

REFERENCES

1. Sasse AD, Sasse EC, Clark LG, et al. Chemoimmunotherapy versus chemotherapy for metastatic malignant melanoma. Cochrane Database Syst Rev 2007;(1):CD005413.
2. Ives NJ, Stowe RL, Lorigan P, et al. Chemotherapy compared with biochemotherapy for the treatment of metastatic melanoma: a meta-analysis of 18 trials involving 2,621 patients. J Clin Oncol 2007;25(34):5426–34.

3. Flaherty KT, Infante JR, Daud A, et al. Combined BRAF and MEK inhibition in melanoma with BRAF V600 mutations. N Engl J Med 2012;367(18):1694–703.
4. Wolchok JD, Kluger H, Callahan MK, et al. Nivolumab plus ipilimumab in advanced melanoma. N Engl J Med 2013;369(2):122–33.
5. Green DR, Ferguson T, Zitvogel L, et al. Immunogenic and tolerogenic cell death. Nat Rev Immunol 2009;9(5):353–63.
6. Hannani D, Sistigu A, Kepp O, et al. Prerequisites for the antitumor vaccine-like effect of chemotherapy and radiotherapy. Cancer J 2011;17(5):351–8.
7. Kepp O, Galluzzi L, Martins I, et al. Molecular determinants of immunogenic cell death elicited by anticancer chemotherapy. Cancer Metastasis Rev 2011;30(1): 61–9.
8. Nistico P, Capone I, Palermo B, et al. Chemotherapy enhances vaccine-induced antitumor immunity in melanoma patients. Int J Cancer 2009;124(1):130–9.
9. Hong D, Andresen C, Mink J, et al. A phase IB study of lenvatinib (E7080) in combination with temozolomide for treatment of advanced melanoma [abstract 8594]. J Clin Oncol 2012;30(Suppl).
10. Mokyr MB, Kalinichenko T, Gorelik L, et al. Realization of the therapeutic potential of CTLA-4 blockade in low-dose chemotherapy-treated tumor-bearing mice. Cancer Res 1998;58(23):5301–4.
11. DeNardo DG, Brennan DJ, Rexhepaj E, et al. Leukocyte complexity predicts breast cancer survival and functionally regulates response to chemotherapy. Cancer Discov 2011;1(1):54–67.
12. Hersh EM, O'Day SJ, Powderly J, et al. A phase II multicenter study of ipilimumab with or without dacarbazine in chemotherapy-naive patients with advanced melanoma. Invest New Drugs 2011;29(3):489–98.
13. Robert C, Thomas L, Bondarenko I, et al. Ipilimumab plus dacarbazine for previously untreated metastatic melanoma. N Engl J Med 2011;364(26):2517–26.
14. Patel SP, Hwu WJ, Kim KB, et al. Phase II study of the frontline combination of ipilimumab and temozolomide in patients with metastatic melanoma [abstract 8514]. J Clin Oncol 2012;30(Suppl).
15. Wang J, Patel SP, Hwu WJ, et al. Development of brain metastases in patients with metastatic melanoma treated with ipilimumab plus temozolomide [abstract e19014]. J Clin Oncol 2012;30(Suppl).
16. Giacomo AM, Ascierto P, Pilla L, et al. Phase II multicenter trial of ipilimumab combined with fotemustine in patients with metastatic melanoma: the Italian Network for Tumor Biotherapy (NIBIT)-M1 trial [abstract 8513]. J Clin Oncol 2012;30(Suppl).
17. Di Giacomo AM, Ascierto PA, Pilla L, et al. Ipilimumab and fotemustine in patients with advanced melanoma (NIBIT-M1): an open-label, single-arm phase 2 trial. Lancet Oncol 2012;13(9):879–86.
18. Shahabi V, Whitney G, Hamid O, et al. Assessment of association between BRAF-V600E mutation status in melanomas and clinical response to ipilimumab. Cancer Immunol Immunother 2012;61(5):733–7.
19. Lee JT, Li L, Brafford PA, et al. PLX4032, a potent inhibitor of the B-Raf V600E oncogene, selectively inhibits V600E-positive melanomas. Pigment Cell Melanoma Res 2010;23(6):820–7.
20. Boni A, Cogdill AP, Dang P, et al. Selective BRAFV600E inhibition enhances T-cell recognition of melanoma without affecting lymphocyte function. Cancer Res 2010;70(13):5213–9.
21. Frederick DT, Piris A, Cogdill AP, et al. BRAF inhibition is associated with enhanced melanoma antigen expression and a more favorable tumor

microenvironment in patients with metastatic melanoma. Clin Cancer Res 2013; 19(5):1225–31.

22. Wilmott JS, Long GV, Howle JR, et al. Selective BRAF inhibitors induce marked T-cell infiltration into human metastatic melanoma. Clin Cancer Res 2012;18(5): 1386–94.

23. Ji RR, Chasalow SD, Wang L, et al. An immune-active tumor microenvironment favors clinical response to ipilimumab. Cancer Immunol Immunother 2012;61(7): 1019–31.

24. Hooijkaas A, Gadiot J, Morrow M, et al. Selective BRAF inhibition decreases tumor-resident lymphocyte frequencies in a mouse model of human melanoma. Oncoimmunology 2012;1(5):609–17.

25. Flaherty KT, Puzanov I, Kim KB, et al. Inhibition of mutated, activated BRAF in metastatic melanoma. N Engl J Med 2010;363(9):809–19.

26. Nathanson KL, Martin AM, Wubbenhorst B, et al. Tumor genetic analyses of patients with metastatic melanoma treated with the BRAF inhibitor dabrafenib (GSK2118436). Clin Cancer Res 2013;19(17):4868–78.

27. Ribas A, Hodi FS, Callahan M, et al. Hepatotoxicity with combination of vemurafenib and ipilimumab. N Engl J Med 2013;368(14):1365–6.

28. Ascierto PA, Simeone E, Giannarelli D, et al. Sequencing of BRAF inhibitors and ipilimumab in patients with metastatic melanoma: a possible algorithm for clinical use. J Transl Med 2012;10:107.

29. Ascierto P, Simeone E, Chiarion-Sileni V, et al. Sequential treatment with ipilimumab and BRAF inhibitors in patients with metastatic melanoma: data from the Italian cohort of ipilimumab expanded access programme (EAP) [abstract 9035]. J Clin Oncol 2013;31(Suppl).

30. Stuart DD. Intermittent treatment with vemurafenib may prevent lethal drug resistance in melanoma. AACR News 2013. Available at: http://www.aacr.org/ home/public–media/aacr-in-the-news.aspx?d=3083. Accessed December 26, 2013.

31. Romano E, Pradervand S, Paillusson A, et al. Identification of multiple mechanisms of resistance to vemurafenib in a patient with BRAFV600E-mutated cutaneous melanoma successfully rechallenged after progression. Clin Cancer Res 2013;19(20):5749–57.

32. Das Thakur M, Salangsang F, Landman AS, et al. Modelling vemurafenib resistance in melanoma reveals a strategy to forestall drug resistance. Nature 2013; 494(7436):251–5.

33. Markowitz J, Luedke E, Gignol V, et al. Bortezomib and interferon alpha-2b in metastatic melanoma [abstract e20018]. J Clin Oncol 2013;31(Suppl).

34. Sullivan R, Ibrahim N, Lawrence D, et al. A phase I study of the combination of sorafenib (Sor) and bortezomib (Bor) in patients (pts) with metastatic melanoma (MM) [abstract 9076]. J Clin Oncol 2013;31(Suppl).

35. Means-Powell J, Adjei A, Puzanov I, et al. Safety and efficacy of MET inhibitor tivantinib (ARQ 197) combined with sorafenib in patients (pts) with NRAS wild-type or mutant melanoma from a phase I study [abstract 8519]. J Clin Oncol 2012;30(Suppl).

36. Flaherty KT, Lee SJ, Zhao F, et al. Phase III trial of carboplatin and paclitaxel with or without sorafenib in metastatic melanoma. J Clin Oncol 2013;31(3): 373–9.

37. Bhatia S, Moon J, Margolin KA, et al. Phase II trial of sorafenib in combination with carboplatin and paclitaxel in patients with metastatic uveal melanoma: SWOG S0512. PLoS One 2012;7(11):e48787.

38. Margolin KA, Moon J, Flaherty LE, et al. Randomized phase II trial of sorafenib with temsirolimus or tipifarnib in untreated metastatic melanoma (S0438). Clin Cancer Res 2012;18(4):1129–37.

39. Piperno-Neumann S, Servois V, Bidard F, et al. BEVATEM: phase II study of bevacizumab (B) in combination with temozolomide (T) in patients (pts) with first-line metastatic uveal melanoma (MUM): final results [abstract 9057]. J Clin Oncol 2013;31(Suppl).

40. Piperno-Neumann S, Servois V, Bidard F, et al. BEVATEM: phase II single-center study of bevacizumab in combination with temozolomide in patients (pts) with first-line metastatic uveal melanoma (MUM): first-step results [abstract 8546]. J Clin Oncol 2012;30(Suppl).

41. Slingluff C, Petroni G, Molhoek K, et al. Clinical activity and safety of combination therapy with temsirolimus and bevacizumab for advanced melanoma: phase II trial with correlative studies [abstract 8530]. J Clin Oncol 2012;30(Suppl).

42. von Moos R, Seifert B, Simcock M, et al. First-line temozolomide combined with bevacizumab in metastatic melanoma: a multicentre phase II trial (SAKK 50/07). Ann Oncol 2012;23(2):531–6.

43. Kottschade LA, Suman VJ, Perez DG, et al. A randomized phase 2 study of temozolomide and bevacizumab or nab-paclitaxel, carboplatin, and bevacizumab in patients with unresectable stage IV melanoma: a North Central Cancer Treatment Group study, N0775. Cancer 2013;119(3):586–92.

44. Kim KB, Sosman JA, Fruehauf JP, et al. BEAM: a randomized phase II study evaluating the activity of bevacizumab in combination with carboplatin plus paclitaxel in patients with previously untreated advanced melanoma. J Clin Oncol 2012;30(1):34–41.

45. Tawbi HA, Beumer JH, Tarhini AA, et al. Safety and efficacy of decitabine in combination with temozolomide in metastatic melanoma: a phase I/II study and pharmacokinetic analysis. Ann Oncol 2013;24(4):1112–9.

46. Milhem M, Weber JS, Amin A, et al. Clinical experience of a targeted TCR-IL2 fusion protein in combination with cisplatin (CDDP) in patients (pts) with metastatic melanoma [abstract e13088]. J Clin Oncol 2012;30(Suppl).

47. Guo J, Cui CL, Min Tao K, et al. Randomized, double-blind, and multicenter phase II trial of rh-endostatin plus dacarbazine versus dacarbazine alone as first-line therapy for the patients with advanced melanoma [abstract 8554]. J Clin Oncol 2012;30(Suppl).

48. Maio M, Hassel JC, Del Vecchio M, et al. Lenvatinib combined with dacarbazine versus dacarbazine alone as first-line treatment in patients with stage IV melanoma [abstract 9027]. J Clin Oncol 2013;31(Suppl).

49. Plummer R, Lorigan P, Brown E, et al. Phase I-II study of plitidepsin and dacarbazine as first-line therapy for advanced melanoma. Br J Cancer 2013;109(6):1451–9.

50. Xia C, Laux D, Deutsch J, et al. A phase I/II study to evaluate the ability of decitabine and panobinostat to improve temozolomide chemosensitivity in metastatic melanoma [abstract 3056]. J Clin Oncol 2012;30(Suppl).

51. Gupta A, Love S, Schuh A, et al. DOC-MEK: a double-blind randomized phase II trial of docetaxel with or without selumetinib (AZD6244; ARRY-142886) in wt BRAF advanced melanoma [abstract 9068]. J Clin Oncol 2013;31(Suppl).

52. Robert C, Dummer R, Gutzmer R, et al. Selumetinib plus dacarbazine versus placebo plus dacarbazine as first-line treatment for BRAF-mutant metastatic melanoma: a phase 2 double-blind randomised study. Lancet Oncol 2013;14(8):733–40.

53. Steinberg J, Bedikian AY, Ernst D, et al. A phase II, multicenter, open-label study of YM155 plus docetaxel in subjects with stage III (unresectable) or stage IV melanoma [abstract 8587]. J Clin Oncol 2012;30(Suppl).

54. Hauke R, Infante JR, Shih K, et al. Everolimus in combination with paclitaxel and carboplatin in patients with advanced melanoma: a phase II trial of the Sarah Cannon Research Institute (SCRI) [abstract 8556]. J Clin Oncol 2012;(Suppl).

55. Ein-Gal S, Tsang W, Alger B, et al. Updated interim analysis of UCI 09-53: a phase II, single arm study of pazopanib and paclitaxel as first-line treatment for subjects with unresectable advanced melanoma [abstract 9082]. J Clin Oncol 2013;(Suppl).

56. Fruehauf J, Alger B, Parmakhtiar B, et al. A phase II single arm study of pazopanib and paclitaxel as first-line treatment for unresectable stage III and stage IV melanoma: interim analysis [abstract 8524]. J Clin Oncol 2012;30(Suppl).

57. Plummer R, Lorigan P, Steven N, et al. A phase II study of the potent PARP inhibitor, Rucaparib (PF-01367338, AG014699), with temozolomide in patients with metastatic melanoma demonstrating evidence of chemopotentiation. Cancer Chemother Pharmacol 2013;71(5):1191–9.

58. Algazi AP, Weber JS, Andrews SC, et al. Phase I clinical trial of the Src inhibitor dasatinib with dacarbazine in metastatic melanoma. Br J Cancer 2012;106(1):85–91.

Index

Note: Page numbers of article titles are in **boldface** type.

A

Adjuvant therapy, for melanoma, 423–424, **471–489,** 513
    chemotherapy for ocular, 513
    clinical predictors of risk, 471–472
    immunotherapy with interferon, 473–480, 572–575
    indications for, 472–473
    modalities of the near future under trial, 483–484
        immunotherapy with anti-cytotoxic T-lymphocyte antigen 4 antibodies, 483–484
        others, 484
    neoadjuvant, 484–485
    radiation therapy, 480–481
    trials testing other modalities, 481–483
        biochemotherapy, 481
        chemotherapy, 481
        immunotherapy with vaccines, 481, 483
Adoptive T-cell therapies, brief overview of, 549–551
AKT pathway. *See* Phosphoinositol-3-kinase (PI3K) signaling.
Anorectal melanoma. *See* Mucosal melanoma.
Anti-CTLA-4 antibodies, adjuvant immunotherapy for melanoma with, 483–484
    immune checkpoint blockade by, 586–590
Anti-PD-1 antibodies, immune checkpoint blockade by, 590–591
Anti-PD-L1 antibodies, immune checkpoint blockade by, 591–592

B

Biochemotherapy, adjuvant, for melanoma, 481
Biology, of melanoma, **437–453,** 507–509, 540–543
    development of, 438–439
        melanocyte formation, 438
        role of microphthalmia-associated transcription factor, 439
        role of ultraviolet radiation, 438–439
    inflammatory and immune gene signatures in, 540–543
    interaction of immunology and molecular signaling, 446–447
    molecular signaling in, 439–444
        MAPK signaling, 439–440
        oncogene-directed treatments, 444–446
        oncogenic mutations, 441–444
        phosphoinositol-3-kinase signaling, 440–441
    noncutaneous, 507–509
Biomarkers, identification of, in melanoma, 593–594
    immunoprofiling, 593–594

Hematol Oncol Clin N Am 28 (2014) 613–623
http://dx.doi.org/10.1016/S0889-8588(14)00039-2
0889-8588/14/$ – see front matter © 2014 Elsevier Inc. All rights reserved.

hemonc.theclinics.com

Biomarkers (*continued*)
    predictive, 593
    prognostic, 593
Brachytherapy, for locoregional ocular melanoma, 511
BRAF mutation, in melanoma, 441–442
    potential targeted therapy with inhibitors of, 484
    therapies targeting, 493–499
        development of RAF inhibitor resistance, 497–498
        early RAF inhibitor studies, 493–494
        efficacy of selective RAF inhibitors, 494–496
        MEK inhibitor monotherapy and combination therapy, 498–499
        RAF inhibitor toxicity, 497
        RAF inhibitors in patients with brain metastases, 496–497
   resistance mechanisms in targeted therapies for melanoma, **523–536**
      heterogeneity and, 530–531
      other mechanisms mediating BRAF1 resistance, 529–530
      PI3K/AKT pathway in resistance to BRAF and MEK inhibitors, 527–529
      reactivation of MAPK signaling pathway, 524–527
      strategies to overcome BRAF1 resistance, 531–533

C

Cell cycle regulators, mutation of, in melanoma, 443
in BRAF1 resistance, 529–530
Chemotherapy, for melanoma, adjuvant, 481
       for ocular melanoma, 513
     combined with immunotherapy, 602
       with IL-2, 576–577
     for locoregional mucosal melanoma, 511
     for metastatic melanoma, 425–426
CKIT mutation, in melanoma, 442–443
Combinatorial treatment, of melanoma, **601–612**
     immunotherapy plus chemotherapy, 602
     immunotherapy plus targeted therapy, 603
     recent trials of, 604–608
     sequential therapy, 604
Cytokines, in treatment of melanoma, **571–583**
     interferon, 571–575
     interleukin-2, 575–579
     other, 579–560
       GM-CSF, 579
       interleukin-21, 579
   vaccines and, 551–552
Cytotoxic T-lymphocyte antigen 4 (CTLA-4), in adjuvant immunotherapy for
    melanoma, 483–484
inhibitors of, in melanoma therapy, 586–590
     adverse events, 588–589
     evaluating response with, 589–590
     ipilimumab, 587–588
     preclinical studies, 586–587
     trelimumab, 588

D

Diagnosis, of melanoma, 417–418
Drug resistance. *See* Resistance mechanisms.

E

Effector T-cell response, antigen-specific escape from, 549–551
Epidemiology, of noncutaneous melanoma, 507–509
    mucosal, 508
    ocular, 508–509
External-beam radiation therapy, for locoregional ocular melanoma, 512

G

GNAQ/GNA11 mutation, in melanoma, 443
Granulocyte-macrophage colony-stimulating factor (GM-CSF), in immunotherapy
    for melanoma, 579

H

Heterogeneity, and resistance mechanisms in melanoma, 530–531

I

Immune checkpoint blockade, in melanoma therapy, **585–600**
    anti-PD-1 antibodies, 590–591
    anti-PD-L1 antibodies, 590–591
    CTLA-4 inhibitors, 586–590
    identifying a biomarker, 593–594
    in mucosal melanoma, 592
    in uveal melanoma, 592–593
    novel, 594
Immune system, role in melanoma, **537–558**
    background, 537–549
        immunosuppression, tolerance mechanisms, and chronic inflammation induced
            by melanoma, 545–549
        immunosurveillance against primary and relapsing melanoma, 544–545
        inflammation and immunosurveillance, 537–538
        inflammatory and immune gene signatures in melanoma biology, 540–543
        prognostic value of studying immune tumor microenvironment, 538–540
        role in dissemination of melanoma to nodes and distant organs, 543–544
    clinical status of immunotherapy for, 549–554
        cancer vaccines, adoptive T-cell therapies, and antigen-specific escape from
            effector T-cell response, 549–551
        lesional immunotherapy, 552–553
        radiation therapy and, 553–554
        vaccines and cytokines, 551–552
Immunogens, for melanoma, 560–562
Immunology, in melanoma, 422–423
    interaction with molecular signaling, 446–447

Immunoprofiling, to identify biomarkers in melanoma, 593–594
Immunosurveillance, against primary and relapsing melanoma, 544–545
   in melanomagenesis, 537–538
Immunotherapy, in melanoma, 422–423
      as adjuvant therapy, 473–484
         with anti-cytotoxic T-lymphocyte antigen 4 antibodies, 483–484
         with anti-programmed death 1 and L1 agents, 484
         with interferon, 473–480
         with vaccines, 481, 483
      clinical status of, 549–554
         cancer vaccines, adoptive T-cell therapies, and antigen-specific escape from
            effector T-cell response, 549–551
         lesional immunotherapy, 552–553
         radiation therapy and, 553–554
         vaccines and cytokines, 551–552
      combination therapies with, **601–612**
         in sequential therapy, 604
         recent trials of, 604–608
         with chemotherapy, 602
         with targeted therapy, 603
      for advanced ocular and mucosal melanoma, 514–515
      for metastatic melanoma, 426–427
   with melanoma vaccines, 481, 483, 549–551, 551–552, **559–569**
      adjuvant immunotherapy with, 481, 483
      cancer vaccines, overview of, 549–551
      cytokines and, 551–552
      new strategies, 563–566
         NeoVax, 564–566
         WDVAX, 566
      previous approaches in, 560–563
         immunogens, 560–562
         recombinant viral vector-based, 562–563
         whole cell-based, 563
Inflammation, chronic, induced by melanoma, 545–549
   in melanomagenesis, 537–538
   inflammatory gene signatures in biology of melanoma, 540–543
Interferon (IFN), in immunotherapy for melanoma, adjuvant, 473–480, 575
      adjuvant testing, 572–574
      future directions, 575
      initial use in melanoma, 572
      PEG-IFN, 574
      predicting response, 575
      toxicity, 574–575
Interleukin-2 (IL-2), in immunotherapy for melanoma, 575–579
      combined with chemotherapy, 576–577
      combined with other cytokines, 577
      combined with vaccines, 577–578
      initial studies, 576
      other combinations with, 578
      patient selection, 578–579
      toxicity, 578

Interleukin-21 (IL-21), in immunotherapy for melanoma, 579
Ipilimumab, in melanoma therapy, 587–588
    in combination with vemurafenib, 603

K

KIT-mutant melanoma, therapy targeting, 500

L

Lesional immunotherapy, 552–553
Liver-directed therapy, for advanced uveal melanoma, 513–514
Lymph node evaluation, in surgical management of melanoma, 420–421
Lymph node metastases, regional, of melanoma, surgical management of, 461–462
    arguments against routine completion lymphadenectomy, 462
    arguments for routine completion lymphadenectomy, 461–462
    role of postoperative radiation after lymphadenectomy, 462
  role of immune system in dissemination of melanoma, 543–544
Lymphadenectomy, in surgical management of melanoma, 420
  role of postoperative radiation after, 462–463
  routine completion, in regional lymph node metastases of melanoma, 461–462
    arguments against, 462
    arguments in favor of, 461–462

M

MAPK signaling pathway, in melanoma, 439–440
    reactivation of, in resistance to targeted therapy, 524–527
MEDI4736, in melanoma therapy, 591–592
Medical management, of melanoma, historic overview, 421–424
    adjuvant, 423–424
    immunology and immunotherapy, 422–423
    neoadjuvant, 424
MEK inhibitors, in target monotherapy and combination therapy, 498–499
Melanocyte formation, in development of melanoma, 438
Melanoma, 415–612
  adjuvant therapy, **471–489**
    clinical predictors of risk, 471–472
    immunotherapy with interferon, 473–480
    indications for, 472–473
    modalities of the near future under trial, 483–484
      immunotherapy with anti-cytotoxic T-lymphocyte antigen 4 antibodies, 483–484
      others, 484
    neoadjuvant, 484–485
    radiation therapy, 480–481
    trials testing other modalities, 481–483
      biochemotherapy, 481
      chemotherapy, 481
      immunotherapy with vaccines, 481, 483
  biology, **437–453**
    development of, 438–439
      melanocyte formation, 438

Melanoma (*continued*)
        role of microphthalmia-associated transcription factor, 439
        role of ultraviolet radiation, 438–439
    interaction of immunology and molecular signaling, 446–447
    molecular signaling in, 439–444
        MAPK signaling, 439–440
        oncogene-directed treatments, 444–446
        oncogenic mutations, 441–444
        phosphoinositol-3-kinase signaling, 440–441
  combinatorial approaches to treatment, **601–612**
    immunotherapy plus chemotherapy, 602
    immunotherapy plus targeted therapy, 603
    recent trials of, 604–608
    sequential therapy, 604
  cytokines in treatment of, **571–583**
    interferon, 571–575
    interleukin-2, 575–579
    other, 579–560
  historic overview, **415–435**
    diagnosis, 417–418
    future directions, 428–429
    medical management, 421–424
        adjuvant, 423–424
        immunology and immunotherapy, 422–423
        neoadjuvant, 424
    metastatic inoperable (advanced, systemic) disease, 425–428
        chemotherapy, 425–426
        immunotherapy, 426–427
        immunotherapy plus chemotherapy (BCT), 426
        targeted therapy, 427–428
    pathogenesis, 416–417
    prognosis, 418–419
    risk factors, 417
    staging, 418
    surgical treatment, 419–421
        lymph node evaluation, 420–421
        lymphadenectomy, 420
        primary tumor, 419–420
  immune checkpoint blockade, **585–600**
    anti-PD-1 antibodies, 590–592
    CTLA-4 inhibitors, 586–590
    identifying a biomarker, 593–594
    in mucosal melanoma, 592
    in uveal melanoma, 592–593
    novel, 594
  immune system's role in, **537–558**
    background, 537–549
    clinical status of immunotherapy for, 549–554
  noncutaneous, **507–521**
    biology and epidemiology, 507–509
    clinical management, 509–515

advanced, 513–515
locoregional, 509–513
surgical management of, **455–470**
localized disease, 456–461
primary melanoma, 456–458
staging of clinically negative regional lymph nodes, 458–461
metastatic melanoma, 463–466
incidence of resectable cases, 463–464
integration with systemic therapy, 465–466
outcomes with surgery, 464–465
regional lymph node metastases, 461–462
arguments against routine completion lymphadenectomy, 462
arguments for routine completion lymphadenectomy, 461–462
role of postoperative radiation after lymphadenectomy, 462
targeted therapies, **491–505**
BRAF, 493–499
current recommendations, 500
KIT, 500
MAPK pathway in, 492–493
NRAS, 499–500
resistance mechanisms, **523–536**
heterogeneity and, 530–531
other mechanisms mediating BRAF1 resistance, 529–530
PI3K/AKT pathway in resistance to BRAF and MEK inhibitors, 527–529
reactivation of MAPK signaling pathway, 524–527
strategies to overcome BRAF1 resistance, 531–533
vaccines, **559–569**
new strategies, 563–566
NeoVax, 564–566
WDVAX, 566
previous approaches in, 560–563
immunogens, 560–562
recombinant viral vector-based, 562–563
whole cell-based, 563
Melanomagenesis. *See also* Biology *and* Pathogenesis.
inflammation and immunosurveillance in, 537–538
Metastasectomy, for advanced uveal melanoma, 513
Metastatic melanoma, historic overview of inoperable (advanced, systemic) disease,
425–428
chemotherapy, 425–426
immunotherapy, 426–427
immunotherapy plus chemotherapy (BCT), 426
targeted therapy, 427–428
role of immune system in dissemination, 543–544
surgical management of, 463–466
incidence of resectable cases, 463–464
integration with systemic therapy, 465–466
outcomes with surgery, 464–465
Microphthalmia-associated transcription factor (MITF), amplification of, in BRAF1
resistance, 530
role in development of melanoma, 439

Mitogen-activated protein kinase (MAPK) pathway, in cutaneous melanoma, 492–493

Mitotic count, in staging of clinically negative regional lymph nodes in melanoma, 458–461

MK-3475, in melanoma therapy, 591

Molecular signaling, in melanoma, 439–444

     MAPK signaling, 439–440

     oncogene-directed treatments, 444–446

     oncogenic mutations, 441–444

     phosphoinositol-3-kinase signaling, 440–441

MPDL3280A, in melanoma therapy, 591

Mucosal melanoma, **507–521**

   biology and epidemiology, 507–509

   clinical management, 509–515

     advanced, 513–515

     locoregional, 509–513

       adjuvant chemotherapy, 511

       radiotherapy, 510–511

       staging, 509

       surgery, 510

   immune checkpoint blockade in, 592

N

Neoadjuvant therapy, for melanoma, 484–485

Neoadjuvant treatment, for melanoma, 424

NeoVax melanoma vaccine, 564–566

Noncutaneous melanoma. *See* Mucosal melanoma *and* Ocular melanoma.

NRAS mutations, therapy targeting, in cutaneous melanoma, 499–500

NRAS/NF1 mutation, in melanoma, 442

O

Ocular melanoma, **507–521**

   biology and epidemiology, 507–509

   clinical management, 509–515

     advanced, 513–515

       liver-directed therapy, 513–514

       surgery, 513

       systemic therapy, 514–515

     locoregional, 509–513

       adjuvant chemotherapy, 513

       brachytherapy, 511

       other approaches, 512–513

       radiotherapy, 512

       surgery, 512

       surveillance, 513

Oncogene-directed treatments, for melanoma, 444–446

Oncogenic mutations, in melanoma, 441–444

     BRAF, 441–442

     cell cycle regulation, 443

     CKIT, 442–443

     GNAQ/GNA11, 443

NRAS/NF1, 442
PTEN loss, 443–444

P

Pathogenesis, of melanoma, 416–417
Phosphoinositol-3-kinase (PI3K) signaling, in melanoma, 440–441
    in resistance to BRAF and MEK inhibitors, 527–529
Photocoagulation, for ocular melanoma, 512
Photodynamic therapy, for ocular melanoma, 512–513
Predictive markers, for response to therapy with immune checkpoint inhbitors, 593
Prognosis, of melanoma, 418–419
Prognostic markers, for response to therapy with immune checkpoint inhibitors, 593
Prognostic value, of immune tumor microenvironment, 538–540
Programmed death 1 (PD-1), anti-PD-1 antibodies, 590–591
        MK-3475, 591
        nivolumab, 590–591
        preclinical studies, 590
    anti-PD-L1 antibodies, 591–592
        MEDI4736, 591–592
        MPDL3280A, 591
        preclinical studies, 591
    immunotherapy for melanoma with anti-PD 1 and anti-PD L7, 484
PTEN loss, in melanoma, 443–444

R

Radiation therapy, adjuvant, for melanoma, 480–481
    for locoregional mucosal melanoma, 510–511
    for locoregional ocular melanoma, 511–512
        brachytherapy, 511
        external beam, 512
    in immunotherapy designs based on tumor microenvironment, 553–554
    role of postoperative after lymphadenectomy, 462–463
RAF inhibitors, in therapies targeting BRAF in cutaneous melanoma, 483–498
        development of resistance, 497–498
        early studies, 483–494
        efficacy of selective, 494–496
        in BRAF non-V600E mutant melanoma, 496
        in patients with brain metastases, 496–497
        toxicity, 497
Receptor tyrosine kinases, activation of, in BRAF1 resistance, 529
Recombinant viral vector-based vaccines, for melanoma, 562–563
Regional lymph node metastases. *See* Lymph node metastases.
Resistance mechanisms, to targeted therapies for melanoma, **523–536**
        heterogeneity and, 530–531
        other mechanisms mediating BRAF1 resistance, 529–530
        PI3K/AKT pathway in resistance to BRAF and MEK inhibitors, 527–529
        reactivation of MAPK signaling pathway, 524–527
        strategies to overcome BRAF1 resistance, 531–533
Risk factors, for melanoma, 417

S

Sequential therapies, for melanoma, 604
Staging, of clinically negative regional lymph nodes in melanoma, 458–461
    of melanoma, 418
        mucosal, 509
        ocular, 510
Surgical management, of melanoma, **455–470**
        localized disease, 456–461
            mucosal, 510
            ocular, 512
            primary melanoma, 456–458
            regional lymph node metastases, 461–462
            staging of clinically negative regional lymph nodes, 458–461
        metastatic melanoma, 463–466
            incidence of resectable cases, 463–464
            integration with systemic therapy, 465–466
            outcomes with surgery, 464–465
        regional lymph node metastases, arguments against routine completion lymphadenectomy, 462
            arguments for routine completion lymphadenectomy, 461–462
            role of postoperative radiation after lymphadenectomy, 462
Surgical treatment, of melanoma, historic overview, 419–421
            lymph node evaluation, 420–421
            lymphadenectomy, 420
            primary tumor, 419–420
Surveillance, for ocular melanoma, 513
    immunosurveillance against primary and relapsing melanoma, 544–545

T

Targeted therapies, for advanced ocular and mucosal melanoma, 514–515
    for cutaneous melanoma, 427–428, **491–505**
        BRAF, 493–499
        current recommendations, 500
        KIT, 500
        MAPK pathway in, 492–493
        NRAS, 499–500
        resistance mechanisms, **523–536**
    in combination with immunotherapy, 603
        ipilimumab plus vemurafenib, 603
    resistance mechanisms, **523–536**
        heterogeneity and, 530–531
        other mechanisms mediating BRAF1 resistance, 529–530
        PI3K/AKT pathway in resistance to BRAF and MEK inhibitors, 527–529
        reactivation of MAPK signaling pathway, 524–527
        strategies to overcome BRAF1 resistance, 531–533
Transpupillary thermotherapy, for ocular melanoma, 512
Trelimumab, in melanoma therapy, 588
Tumor associated antigens, in melanoma vaccines, 560–562

U

Ulceration, in staging of clinically negative regional lymph nodes in melanoma, 458
Ultraviolet radiation, role in development of melanoma, 438–439
Uveal melanoma. *See also* Ocular melanoma.
   immune checkpoint blockade in, 592–593

V

Vaccines, for melanoma, 481, 483, 549–551, 551–552, **559–569**
      adjuvant immunotherapy with, 481, 483, 577–578
      cancer, overview of, 549–551
      cytokines and, 551–552
      new strategies, 563–566
         NeoVax, 564–566
         WDVAX, 566
      previous approaches in, 560–563
         immunogens, 560–562
         recombinant viral vector-based, 562–563
         whole cell-based, 563
Vemurafenib, in combination melanoma therapy with ipilimumab, 603
Viral vectors, for melanoma vaccines, 562–563
Vulvovaginal melanoma. *See* Mucosal melanoma.

W

WDVAX melanoma vaccine, 566
Whole cell-based vaccines, for melanoma, 563

Printed and bound by CPI Group (UK) Ltd, Croydon, CR0 4YY

07/10/2024

01040499-0002